# Gynecologic Oncology

# Cancer Treatment and Research

WILLIAM L. MCGUIRE, *series editor*

1. R.B. Livingston, ed., Lung Cancer 1. 1981. ISBN 90-247-2394-9.
2. G.B. Humphrey, L.P. Dehner, G.B. Grindey and R.T. Acton, eds., Pediatric Oncology 1. 1981. ISBN 90-247-2408-2.
3. J.J. DeCosse and P. Sherlock, eds., Gastrointestinal Cancer 1. 1981. ISBN 90-247-2461-9.
4. J.M. Bennett, ed., Lymphomas 1, including Hodgkin's Disease. 1981. ISBN 90-247-2479-1.
5. C.D. Bloomfield, ed., Adult Leukemias 1. 1982. ISBN 90-247-2478-3.
6. D.F. Paulson, Genitourinary Cancer 1. 1982. ISBN 90-247-2480-5.
7. F.M. Muggia, ed., Cancer Chemotherapy 1. 1982. ISBN 90-247-2713-8.
8. G.B. Humphrey and G.B. Grindey, eds., Pancreatic Tumours in Children. 1982. ISBN 90-247-2702-2.
9. John J. Costanzi, ed., Malignant Melanoma 1. 1982. ISBN 90-247-2706-5.

# Gynecologic Oncology

*edited by*

C. THOMAS GRIFFITHS, M.D.
Harvard Medical School, Brigham and Women's Hospital, Boston, Massachusetts, USA

ARLAN F. FULLER, Jr., M.D.
Harvard Medical School, Massachusetts General Hospital, Boston, Massachusetts, USA

1983 **MARTINUS NIJHOFF PUBLISHERS**
a member of the KLUWER ACADEMIC PUBLISHERS GROUP
BOSTON / THE HAGUE / DORDRECHT / LANCASTER

**Distributors**

*for the United States and Canada*: Kluwer Boston, Inc., 190 Old Derby Street, Hingham, MA 02043, USA

*for all other countries*: Kluwer Academic Publishers Group, Distribution Center, P.O.Box 322, 3300 AH Dordrecht, The Netherlands

**Library of Congress Cataloging in Publication Data**

Main entry under title:

Gynecologic oncology.

(Cancer treatment and research ; v. 10)
1. Reproductive organs, Female--Cancer.
I. Griffiths, C. Thomas.  II. Fuller, Arlan F.
III. Series.  [DNLM: 1. Genital neoplasms,
Female.  W1 CA693 v. 10 / WP 145 G99651]
RC280.G5G886   1983      616.99'465      82-14491

ISBN 0-89838-555-5 (this volume)

**Copyright**

© 1983 by Martinus Nijhoff Publishers, Boston.

All rights reserved. No part of this publication may be reproduced, stored in a retrieval system, or transmitted in any form or by any means, mechanical, photocopying, recording, or otherwise, without the prior written permission of the publishers,
Martinus Nijhoff Publishers, 190 Old Derby Street, Hingham, MA 02043, USA.

PRINTED IN THE NETHERLANDS

# Contents

Foreword to the Series . . . . . . . . . . . . . . . . . . . . . vii
Preface . . . . . . . . . . . . . . . . . . . . . . . . . . . . . . ix
List of Contributors . . . . . . . . . . . . . . . . . . . . . . . xiii

1. Evidence for a Viral Etiology of Squamous Cell Carcinoma of the Cervix . . . . . . . . . . . . . . . . . . . . . . . . . . . . 1
   LAURE AURELIAN
2. Tumor Markers in Gynecologic Malignancies . . . . . . . . . 63
   JOHN R. VAN NAGELL
3. Hormonal Receptors in Endometrial and Ovarian Neoplasia . 81
   GEORGE S. RICHARDSON and DAVID T. MACLAUGHLIN
4. Germ Cell Tumors of the Ovary: Pathology, Behavior and Treatment . . . . . . . . . . . . . . . . . . . . . . . . . . . . . . 103
   ROBERT J. KURMAN and EDMUND S. PETRILLI
5. Treatment of Advanced Trophoblastic Disease . . . . . . . . 155
   RICHARD H. J. BEGENT and KENNETH D. BAGSHAWE
6. The Immunobiology of Ovarian Carcinoma . . . . . . . . . . 187
   ROBERT C. BAST Jr. and ROBERT C. KNAPP
7. Lymph Node Metastases from Gynecologic Cancer – Biological Concepts and Therapeutic Implications . . . . . . . . . . . 227
   ARLAN F. FULLER Jr.
8. Radiation Therapy of Ovarian Carcinoma . . . . . . . . . . 263
   ALON J. DEMBO and RAYMOND S. BUSH

9. Heavy Particle Radiation Therapy in Gynecological Malignancies . . . . . . . . . . . . . . . . . . . . . . . . . 299
ROBERT D. HILGERS, STEVEN E. BUSH and FRANCISCO AMPUERO

10. Growth of Gynecologic Neoplasms in Tissue Culture and as Heterografts . . . . . . . . . . . . . . . . . . . . . 313
CHARLES E. WELANDER and JOHN L. LEWIS Jr.

11. Clinical Trials in Gynecologic Oncology: Cooperative Group Research . . . . . . . . . . . . . . . . . . . . . . . 343
GEORGE C. LEWIS Jr., JOHN BLESSING and JOHN R. KELLNER

Subject Index . . . . . . . . . . . . . . . . . . . . . 385

# Foreword to the Series

Where do you begin to look for a recent, authoritative article on the diagnosis or management of a particular malignancy? The few general oncology textbooks are generally out of date. Single papers in specialized journals are informative but seldom comprehensive; these are more often preliminary reports on a very limited number of patients. Certain general journals frequently publish good indepth reviews of cancer topics, and published symposium lectures are often the best overviews available. Unfortunately, these reviews and supplements appear sporadically, and the reader can never be sure when a topic of special interest will be covered.

Cancer Treatment and Research is a series of authoritative volumes which aim to meet this need. It is an attempt to establish a critical mass of oncology literature covering virtually all oncology topics, revised frequently to keep the coverage up to date, easily available on a single library shelf or by a single personal subscription.

We have approached the problem in the following fashion. First, by dividing the oncology literature into specific subdivisions such as lung cancer, genitourinary cancer, pediatric oncology, etc. Second, by asking eminent authorities in each of these areas to edit a volume on the specific topic on an annual or biannual basis. Each topic and tumor type is covered in a volume appearing frequently and predictably, discussing current diagnosis, staging, markers, all forms of treatment modalities, basic biology, and more.

In Cancer Treatment and Research, we have an outstanding group of editors, each having made a major commitment to bring to this new series the very best literature in his or her field. Martinus Nijhoff Publishers has made an equally major commitment to the rapid publication of high quality books, and world-wide distribution.

Where can you go to find quickly a recent authoritative article on any major oncology problem? We hope that Cancer Treatment and Research provides an answer.

WILLIAM L. MCGUIRE
Series Editor

# Preface

At the turn of the century gynecology had achieved independence from surgery in most medical schools; although gynecologists were surgeons, their interests were turning toward nonsurgical aspects of their specialty. In 1900, merely two years after the Curies' discovery, radium was first used as a treatment for carcinoma of the cervix. In that day cervical cancer claimed more women's lives than any other malignancy and was described by William P. Graves, the second professor of gynecology at Harvard as follows: 'Cancer of the cervix may rightly be termed of all tumors one of the most deadly and most ghastly. It kills by slow torture, causing in later stages months of agonizing pain and producing a discharge of such a foul and nauseating character as to repel proper medical assistance. Nurses declined to care for these cases, while many public hospitals closed their wards to them as patients.' In late twentieth century parlance the dramatic results of radium therapy would indeed have been called a 'breakthrough', and radium techniques, later combined with external irradiation, were developed by gynecologists, no longer just surgeons. Pathology was the basic science of gynecology and gynecologists with a special interest in pathology served as pathologist to the departments of gynecology. As late as 1970 six months of the three-year residency program in obstetrics and gynecology at Harvard were devoted to formal training in pathology. After the observation in the early 1950s that nitrogen mustard could induce regression of ovarian cancers, clinical trials with this agent and its congeners were carried out by gynecologists. In 1961 Howard W. Jones, Jr. of Johns Hopkins Medical School admonished gynecologists to become further involved in cancer chemotherapeutic research and then added a prophetic warning that 'a new specialty might arise which would include gynecological cancer in its ken.'

As we entered the last quarter of the twentieth century gynecologic oncology became formally recognized as a subspecialty of obstetrics and gynecology. At the same time, it became apparent that the era of multimodality expertise had waned; a gynecologic oncologist would function primarily as a surgeon but also as a consultant by virtue of erudition in the natural history of a particular class of diseases. The establishment and rapid growth of the specialties of radiation oncology and medical oncology had so expanded the therapeutic potential in gynecologic cancer that no one person or specialty could be qualified to undertake the broad range of complex therapies. In addition, a small but active group of pathologists had attained special knowledge through fellowship training in the field of gynecologic pathology.

Only 202 gynecologists in the United States have been certified for special competence in gynecologic oncology. In order to maintain their identity, much less their visibility, gynecologic oncologists cannot function merely as surgical technicians. Expansion of their knowledge to include the latest developments in all phases of cancer research and treatment which pertain to the female genitalia has become even more important at a time when keeping abreast has become all the more difficult.

With these thoughts in mind we designed this first volume in the series on gynecologic malignancies for the gynecologic oncologist in particular. We selected subjects for the chapters based upon our perception of need for scholarly reviews of certain complex, rapidly moving areas. Our goal has been to synthesize all currently available information in selected areas in a manner that will enable the clinician to reconcile his clinical observations with related scientific observations.

In a traditional sense we began with carcinoma of the cervix and some exciting new information brilliantly espoused by Aurelian that increases the probability of a viral etiology. We then turned to radiation therapy with chapters on irradiation for ovarian cancer by Dembo and Bush and on heavy particle therapy for gynecologic malignancy by Hilgers and associates. The former authors, having induced the revival of interest in radiotherapy for ovarian cancer whereas the latter authors introduce an altogether new biophysical approach to the deliverance of lethal radiation to the cancer cell.

Recent advances in pathological research and their clinical application are demonstrated in the chapter on germ cell tumors of the ovary by Kurman and Petrilli. Utilizing immunoperoxidase histochemical techniques Robert Kurman in collaboration with Henry J. Norris at the Armed Forces Institute of Pathology established embryonal carcinoma of the ovary as a distinct entity and clearly defined the influence on prognosis of the histologic counterparts of mixed germ cell tumors of the ovary. Some newer biologic concepts of lymph node metastasis in gynecologic cancer, particularly as a manifestation of systemic disease, are presented by one of us (AFF Jr.).

The victories of cancer chemotherapy are exemplified by accomplishments in the management of choriocarcinoma. Innovations in the treatment of advanced trophoblastic disease and its complications have come from the Charing Cross Hospital in London and Richard H.J. Begent and Kenneth D. Bagshawe of that institution have presented their approach to these diseases. Clinical trials by cooperative groups have become the means whereby the efficacy of rational chemotherapeutic regimens are evaluated. The scientific approach to group trials as well as the bureaucratic mechanisms involved in their conduct are described best by those qualified, George C. Lewis, Jr. and his associates at the Gynecologic Oncology Group headquarters.

We have selected three areas of basis preclinical research in which clinical application has begun to emerge. The identification of estrogen and progesterone receptor proteins in the cytosol of endometrial carcinomas has been with us for some time and that of ovarian neoplasms only recently. Relevance of this knowledge to treatment has been slowed by the infrequency of recurrent endometrial cancer wherein receptor status and endocrine responsiveness can be correlated. George. S. Richardson and David T. MacLaughlin, have been active investigators in this field for more than a decade and have contributed a succinct 'state of the art' review. Cell cultures of gynecologic cancers have a long history dating from the successful passage of HeLa cells into immortality by George Gey in the late 1940s. Although cell cultures in soft agar for clonogenic assays of chemotherapeutic sensitivity have dominated the scene in recent years, other *in vivo* and *in vitro* techniques need review. We have chosen two modern experts in gynecologic cancer cell culture, Charles E. Welander and John L. Lewis Jr. of Sloan-Kettering Memorial Hospital to review this field. Finally, clinical applicability of long-term studies of the immunobiology of ovarian carcinoma has now arrived. Clinical trials of immunodiagnostic techniques are underway and immunotherapy is now moving from nonspecific to specific immunostimulants. Robert C. Bast and Robert C. Knapp who have developed a monoclonal antibody to a purified ovarian cancer antigen have contributed a chapter on the immunobiology of ovarian carcinoma.

The usefulness of tumor markers in monitoring therapy is well brought out in the chapters on germ cell tumors of the ovary, trophoblastic disease, and immunobiology, but we felt that for completeness a summary on tumor markers in gynecologic cancer in general was needed. John R. van Nagell has contributed more than any other to the application of a broad range of oncofetal antigens and other biochemical markers to gynecologic cancer in general. Van Nagell's summary of this subject overlaps somewhat with the aforementioned chapters but we believe that the information presented is more complementary than repetitive. Accordingly these areas are cross-referenced in the text.

The selection of authors for this volume was easy. We simply asked those investigators whom we felt were best qualified to address the subject. Despite admitted bias in the selection of topics, we certainly hope that oncologists other than those of the gynecologic genre will find this volume useful. If by good fortune more than a few of the topics we have selected satisfies a broader readership our purpose shall be more than fulfilled.

C. Thomas GRIFFITHS, M.D.<br>
Arlan F. FULLER Jr., M.D.

# List of Contributors

AMPUERO, Francisco, M.D., Cancer Research and Treatment Center, University of New Mexico School of Medicine, Albuquerque, NM 87131, USA.

AURELIAN, Laure, Ph.D., Division of Comparative Medicine, Department of Biochemistry and Biophysics, The Johns Hopkins Medical Institutions, Baltimore, MD 21205, USA.

BAGSHAWE, Kenneth D., M.D., F.R.C.P., F.R.C.O.G., Department of Medical Oncology, Charing Cross Hospital, Fulham Palace Road, London, W6 8RF, England.

BAST, Robert C., Jr., M.D., Sidney Farber Cancer Institute, 44 Binney Street, Boston, MA 02115, USA.

BEGENT, Richard H. J., M.D., M.R.C.P., Department of Medical Oncology, Charing Cross Hospital, Fulham Palace Road, London, W6 8RF, England.

BLESSING, John, Ph. D., Gynecologic Oncology Group, Roswell Park Memorial Institute, Kress Building, 666 Elm Street, Buffalo, NY 14263, USA.

BUSH, Raymond S., M.D., F.R.C.P.(C), Ontario Cancer Institute, 500 Sherbourne Street, Toronto, M4X 1K9, Canada.

BUSH, Steven E., M.D., Cancer Research and Treatment Center, University of New Mexico School of Medicine, Albuquerque, NM 87131, USA.

DEMBO, Alon J., M.B., F.R.C.P.(C), Radiation Oncology Department, Princess Margaret Hospital, The Ontario Cancer Institute, 500 Sherbourne Street, Toronto, M4X 1K9, Canada.

FULLER, Arlan F., Jr., M.D., Massachusetts General Hospital, Vincent 1, Fruit Street, Boston, MA 02114, USA.

GRIFFITHS, C. Thomas, M.D., Gynecologic Oncology, Brigham and Women's Hospital, 75 Francis Street, Boston, MA 02115, USA.

HILGERS, Robert D., M.D., Cancer Research and Treatment Center, University of New Mexico School of Medicine, Albuquerque, NM 87131, USA.

KELLNER, John R., B.S., Gynecologic Oncology Group Headquarters, 1234 Market Street, Suite 430, Philadelphia, PA 19107, USA.

KNAPP, Robert C., M.D., Brigham and Women's Hospital, 75 Francis Street, Boston, MA 02115, USA.

KURMAN, Robert J., M.D., Departments of Obstetrics and Gynecology and Pathology, Georgetown University School of Medicine, 3800 Reservoir Road, N.W., Washington, DC 20007, USA.

LEWIS, George C., Jr., M.D., Department of Obstetrics and Gynecology, Jefferson Medical College, 1025 Walnut Street, Philadelphia, PA 19107, USA.

LEWIS, John L., Jr., M.D., Memorial Sloan-Kettering Cancer Center, 1275 York Avenue, New York, NY 10021, USA.

MACLAUGHLIN, David T., Ph.D., Massachusetts General Hospital, Vincent 1, Fruit Street, Boston, MA 02114, USA.

VAN NAGELL, John R., Jr., M.D., Division of Gynecologic Oncology, University of Kentucky Medical Center, 800 Rose Street, Lexington, KY 40536, USA.

PETRILLI, Edmund S., M.D., Department of Obstetrics and Gynecology, Georgetown University School of Medicine, 3800 Reservoir Road, N.W., Washington, DC 20007, USA.

RICHARDSON, George S., M.D., Massachusetts General Hospital, Vincent 1, Fruit Street, Boston, MA 02114, USA.

WELANDER, Charles E., M.D., Bowman Gray School of Medicine, Wake Forest University, Winston-Salem, NC 27103, USA.

# 1. Evidence for a Viral Etiology of Squamous Cell Carcinoma of the Cervix

LAURE AURELIAN

## 1. CAUSE AND EFFECT: A PERSPECTIVE

For nearly 100 years, Koch postulates have served as a reference point in evaluating the causal relationship of an agent to the disease with which it is associated. The concepts that served as the basis of Koch postulates, their historic evolution, and their limitations in reference to the study of chronic disease etiology have recently been reviewed by Evans [1]. Briefly, there are three postulates: (1) the agent occurs in every case of the specific disease under scrutiny and within circumstances that account for pathological changes in the clinical course, (2) the agent never occurs in any other disease as a fortuitous parasite, and (3) after isolation and growth in pure culture, the agent can induce the disease in humans [6]. While many diseases fulfill these criteria, a number of infectious agents (viz. leprosy, cholera, typhoid, diphtheria) do not meet them all, thereby casting doubt on their causal relationship to the disease.

Two major problems are the inability to produce the disease anew in an experimental host, and the identification of persistence of the organism in asymptomatic infections. These are particularly significant in the case of viral diseases. As early as 1937, in his presidential address before the American Society for Immunology, Rivers [3] pointed out that blind adherence to Koch's postulates might sometimes act as a hindrance rather than an aid, particularly when applied to viruses because the disease may not be caused by the action of a single agent, and the infectious agent may not be grown in a pure state on defined medium. In establishing his criteria for viral causality of disease, Rivers pointed out that the presence of a virus need not be identified in every case of disease; asymptomatic carriers exist and it is not essential to grow the virus *in vitro*. In establishing proof of causation, Rivers suggested that the specific virus must be associated with the disease with a

*Griffiths, C. T. and Fuller, A. F. (eds.), Gynecologic Oncology.*
© *1983, Martinus Nijhoff Publishers, Boston. ISBN 0-89838-555-5.*
**Printed in The Netherlands.**

certain degree of regularity and it should not occur in the sick individual as an incidental finding. The latter is to be determined by seroconversion, a concept of utmost significance, as it enables the differentiation of the patient from the asymptomatic carrier: 'If a virus is the actual cause of a disease, immune substances are virtually absent from the patient's serum at the onset of illness and make their appearance during the period of recovery' [3]. As technology improved and virus isolation became a 'commonplace occurrence' [4] the wide dissemination, high prevalence, numerous immunologic types, and frequent isolation of viruses from persons who are healthy or have only mild illnesses led Huebner [4] to the conclusion that epidemiologic criteria of causation must be added to the original Koch and Rivers postulates in order to develop a reasonable method for establishing causality.

At present, as the causative agents of many clinical entities have been established, it is still evident that there are a number of common illnesses for which no etiologic agent could be identified, while other illnesses with identical clinical presentations are produced by different agents. Fulfillment of a set of special criteria has enabled the establishment of a causal relationship between a virus and a given syndrome. These include the original Koch postulates, primarily concerned with the nature of the agent (virologic criteria), consideration of the circumstances under which infection occurred (epidemiologic criteria) and finally recognition of the role played by the host in determining whether infection results in clinical disease (immunologic/seroepidemiologic/host-determined criteria).

Consideration of these historical developments is particularly important to an understanding of the role of viruses in the causation of human cancer because of complications generated by the nature of the host, the absence of totally valid animal models and the contradictions introduced by the infectious identity of the putative agent, and the chronic nature of the disease. Difficulties in establishing a cause and effect relationship arise from: (1) the long incubation period between exposure to the suspected agent and cancer development, (2) the relatively low incidence of most cancers *versus* the ubiquity of the viruses suspected of being oncogenic in humans, (3) the possibility that cancer may result as a consequence of reactivated virus, rather than as a direct consequence of primary infection, (4) the probable role of environmental and/or genetic co-factors, (5) the difficulty in reproducing the disease in animal models, and (6) the impossibility of human experimentation. The historical perspective is important because it underscores the fact that insurmountable as these complications appear at first glance, they are not significantly different from those that were originally faced by the students of the microbial (particularly viral) causality of infectious disease. Accordingly, the student of tumor virology will find it relatively easy to investigate his problem in the context of the conditions and elements of causality already established for viral diseases.

Evans [1] has recently synthesized the epidemiologic, immunologic/seroepidemiologic and virologic criteria of disease causation in a unified concept applied to the role of viruses in human cancer. This concept is based on the assumption, derived from experimental study [5], that virus-induced carcinogenesis depends on the persistence and expression of transforming viral gene(s) (Section 3.1). Evans' assumption stresses the need to establish the specificity of a particular effect, and points out the concept of multiple causation in chronic diseases including cancer. Table 1 summarizes the presently available data on HSV-2 and cervix cancer (*the herpesvirus hypothesis*) within the context of the criteria put forth by this unified concept of cau-

*Table 1.* Koch postulate revisited: 'the herpesvirus hypothesis'[a].

1. *Neoplastic transformation:* induced by HSV-2 or specific HSV-2 DNA sequences. Viral genetic information is maintained and expressed (ICP 10).
2. *Reproduction of disease:* cervically infected Cebus monkeys develop dysplasia; mice develop dysplasia and cancer[b].
3. *Presence* of virus and viral DNA in cervical tumor.
4. *Expression:* viral mRNA and antigens/proteins (ICP 10, ICP 12, ICP 14, ICSP 11/12, VP 143) expressed in cervical tumor cells.
5. *Cancer-associated* immune response has characteristics indicative of continuous virus expression.
   a. Antibody to ICP 10/AG-4 is IgM. It reflects tumor progression.
   b. CMI response directed against AG-e (ICP 12 and ICP 14) reflects lymphoid effector function that is driven by continuous antigen expression.
6. *Frequency:* exposure to HSV-2 (virus-specific antibody and CMI responses) more common in cancer cases than in controls matched for other disease associated variables. Calculated relative risk: 2.03–17.45.
7. *Immunologic specificity:* humoral and CMI response is HSV-2 specific. Similar response is not seen with other viruses (CMV, HSV-1) nor in other cancers (breast, vulva, ovary, vagina).
8. *Incidence:* women with HSV-2 infections at higher risk of developing cervix cancer than uninfected ones as shown in prospective studies.
9. *Temporally:* HSV-2 infection precedes by a mean of 6 years the development of the earliest precancerous lesion(dysplasia).
10. *A spectrum:* dysplasia and carcinoma *in situ* follow exposure to HSV-2 and precede cancer. Prevalence of virus-specific antibody is identical in all three.
11. *Elimination or modification of HSV-2 should reduce incidence of cervical cancer:* unstudied.
12. *Biologic and epidemiologic sense:* human virus; persists in infected host without causing cell death (latencey) and is sexually transmitted, as is cervix cancer. Association is not a co-variable of promiscuity.
13. *Co-factors:* poorly studied. Potential candidates are: estrogenic hormones, sperm DNA and/or proteins, immunologic factors, other viruses.

---

[a] Adapted from Evans AS: Yale J Biol Med 49: 175, 1976.
[b] Wente *et al.*, Gyn Onc 12: 590, 1981

sality. In the following sections, we will critically consider this evidence and demonstrate the strength of this association, pointing out areas in which further research is necessary.

## 2. HERPES SIMPLEX VIRUS

Humans are the natural host for 5 immunologically distinct herpesviruses: (1) herpes simplex virus type 1 (HSV-1) which primarily infects the oropharyngeal pathway, (2) herpes simplex virus type 2 (HSV-2) primarily infecting the genital tract, (3) varicella zoster virus, (4) cytomegalovirus and

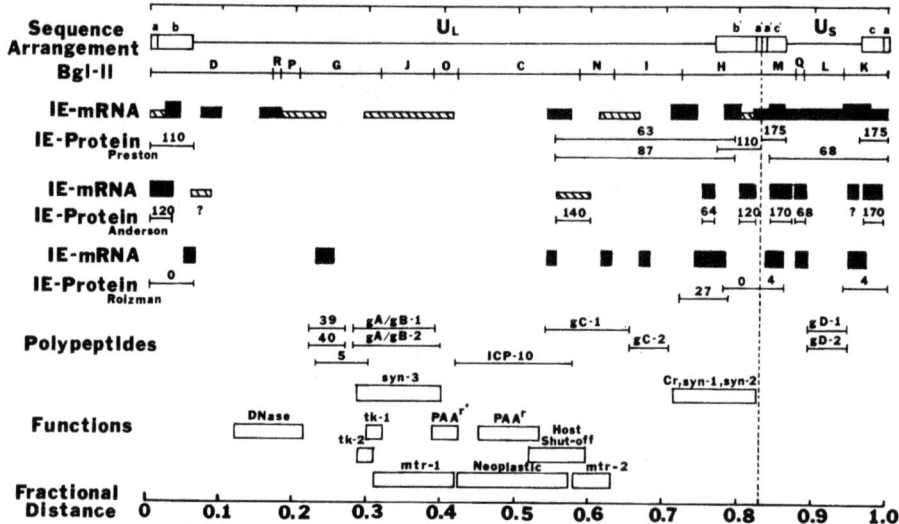

*Figure 1.* Location of templates specifying HSV immediate early messenger RNA (mRNA), proteins and functions in the prototype sequence arrangement of viral DNA. Bgl II restriction endonuclease map of HSV-2 DNA (Bgl II) is shown in order to locate transforming functions mtr-1 (HSV-1 morphologic transformation), mtr-2 (HSV-2 morphologic transformation) and neoplastic (HSV-2 neoplastic transformation). Three studies describing HSV-1 'immediate early' mRNA species (major ( ■ ), minor ( ▨ )) and related proteins (identified by molecular weight $\times 10^{-3}$) are listed according to authors [63, 183, 184]. HSV-2 immediate early mRNA has not been studied. Proteins reported by Anderson *et al.* [183] were translated in vitro. Listed proteins include: (i) HSV-1 and HSV-2 glycoproteins (respectively identified), (ii) major capsid protein (5), virion protein possibly involved in DNA packaging (39), virion protein that may have protein kinase activity (40), regulatory protein VP 175 (4), and two other 'immediate early' proteins (0,27) (Roizman's nomenclature [149] is used), and (iii) ICP 10 the viral protein immunologically identical to AG-4 (our nomenclature is used [14]). Listed functions are thymidine kinase (tk), DNAse, DNA polymerase (PAA$^r$ [185] and PAA$^r$ ($\times$36)) syncytia formation (Cr. syn.), host shut-off genes, morphologic transformation mtr-1 (HSV-1) and mtr-2 (HSV-2), and neoplastic transformation (neoplastic).

(5) Epstein-Barr virus (EBV), shown to cause infectious mononucleosis. Historically, most of the evidence points towards the early recognition of HSV-1; the word 'herpes' has appeared in the medical literature for at least 2500 years. However, our modern view of herpes can be traced to Willan, who, in 1914, restricted the term to conditions characterized by localized groups of vesicles and a short self-limited disease with mild constitutional symptoms [6]. Bateman [7] described two varieties of herpes, '*herpes labialis*' and '*herpes praeputialis*' and in 1735, the French physician, Jean Astruc, first described the genital condition in a classical fashion and defined it as being sexually transmitted [8].

The herpesviruses are large (150–200 nm) enveloped DNA viruses with icosahedral symmetry. The envelope, a triple-layered-membraneous structure, is acquired by budding of the capsids through an infected cell membrane. Viral DNA is a linear and double-stranded helix possessing a high guanine and cytosine base composition (67 and 69 moles, respectively, for HSV-1 and HSV-2) and a relatively high ($97 \times 10^6$ daltons for HSV) [9] molecular weight. HSV-DNA contains two large sets of reiterated sequences at the termini, and in inverted form internally [10]. These sequences effectively subdivide the viral DNA into two components of which the largest (left) is designated L, and the smallest (right) is designated S (Figure 1). The L and S components structurally resemble prokaryotic DNA sequences capable of excision and insertion into the same or different DNAs. The viral DNA sequence (located within the inverted repeats) bears some homology to eukaryotic cell (DNA) (Hayward, personal communication). Conceivably, both the inverted positions of the L and S segments of viral DNA relative to each other, and the capacity of the virus to cause nonproductive infection (Section 2.1) may hinge on the ability of the L and S components to insert and excise into either host or viral DNA.

Antigenic and biologic markers capable of differentiating between HSV-1 and HSV-2 were described and are summarized in Table 2. Nevertheless, the viruses are closely related antigenically and their DNAs share 47–50% of their nucleotide sequences under relatively stringent hybridization conditions [11]. Analyses of restriction endonuclease digests of HSV-DNA have revealed that epidemiologically unrelated isolates of the same serotype are not identical. The major differences seen were occasional deletions and the presence or absence of restriction endonuclease cleavage sites [12]. Consistent with these differences in viral DNA within (intratypic) and between (intertypic) serotypes, very few of the HSV-1 proteins have electrophoretically identical counterparts in HSV-2. Specific variations in the electrophoretic mobilities of proteins from various isolates of the same serotype have also been described [13, 14]. Antigenically distinct or related HSV-1 and HSV-2 proteins have been identified [15, 18], as have proteins that possess

*Table 2.* Properties of HSV serotypes.

| Property | HSV-1 | HSV-2 |
| --- | --- | --- |
| *Site of infection* | Primarily nongenital | Primarily genital[a] |
| *Transmission* | Primarily nonsexual | Primarily sexual |
| *Source of virus* | Excretors (saliva)[b] | Execretors (genital secretions)[b] |
| *Biochemical properties* | | |
| % G+C content of viral DNA | 67 | 69 |
| Homology of viral DNA | Approximately 50% | |
| Viral proteins by electrophoretic mobility | Some differences | |
| *Antigenic properties* | Mostly cross-reactive with intratypic variation | |
| *Biologic properties* | | |
| Pock size CAM[c] | Small | Large |
| Plaque size CE cells[c] | None or small | Yes or large |
| CPE in other cells | Tight adhesion of rounded cells | Loose aggregation, propensity for syncitia formation |
| *Growth cycle* | Some differences | Dependent on cell type |
| Titers in RK[c] | $6 \times 10^7$ | $8 \times 10^5$ |
| Particle to PFU ratio in RK cells | 36 | 2000 |
| % enveloped virus in RK cells | 38 | 6.8 |
| Microtubules | No | Yes |
| *Sensitivity to inactivation* | | |
| Temperature (37 °C) log/loss/hr | 0.07 | 0.27 |
| IUdR | Less resistant | More resistant |
| Interferon | More resistant | Less resistant |
| *Neurotropism* | More | Less |
| *Virulence* ($PFU/LD_{50}$) | 4.0 | 0.5[d] |

[a] HSV-1 infection of genitalia appears to differ in various population groups.
[b] The existence of asymptomatic carriers is becoming increasingly evident.
[c] CAM: Charioallantoic membrane of fertilized eggs; CE: chick embryo cells; RK: rabbit kidney cells.
[d] Done in mice. Large variation in various isolates.

both serotype-specific and cross-reactive antigenic determinants [19]. These findings compounded by the fact that various serologic assays identify different antigenic determinants, underscore the difficulties related to the typing of human HSV-specific antibody, a problem of major significance to the student of *'the herpesvirus hypothesis'* of cervical cancer (Section 6).

## 2.1. HSV infections in vivo: herpetic disease

Two questions merit consideration: (1) is infection with HSV-1 restricted to the face? (2) Do herpetic infections display site (viz. cervix *versus* vulva) localization?

Recent studies indicate that the localization of HSV-2 infection to the genitalia and of HSV-1 to the face is by no means absolute. In Atlanta, 5–10% of genital infections yielded HSV-1 [21] and similar isolation rates were reported in Houston, where nine of 67 (13%) genital isolates were typed as HSV-1 [22]. Smith *et al.* [23] reported that of 65 genital isolates in England, 11 had antigenic and biologic properties commensurate with HSV-1 and one half of the isolates obtained from female genitalia in Japan were HSV-1 [24].

In females, HSV-2 most commonly infects the cervix; HSV-1 is only rarely isolated above the vaginal introitus [21], suggesting that HSV-2 is commonly transmitted during coitus, and that HSV-1 infection of the genitalia may result from either self-inoculation or oral genital contact. More difficult to interpret is the observation that HSV-1 infection of the genitalia is more prevalent in females than in males as suggested by the data of Josey *et al.* [21]. Moreover, Kawana and his colleagues [24] reported that as many as 50% of the female genital isolates were HSV-1, whereas all the male genital isolates were HSV-2. One possible interpretation of these sex differences in the rate of HSV-1 infections of the male and female genital organs is that HSV-1 cannot routinely infect the male genitalia. Since genital cells are under strict hormonal control and viruses are well known to be affected by hormones [25], this is not an unreasonable interpretation.

A significant aspect of the HSV infection of the multicellular host is the observation that the virus can persist indefinitely in its natural host in an asymptomatic state, causing periodic recurrent lesions in the presence of high levels of circulating antibody (*latency*). Recurrences are induced by exposure to a variety of stress conditions including fever, menstruation, and emotional stress. Two basic questions pertain to this phenomenon: (1) what is the nature of the interaction between the virus and the cell in which it persists in the interim between recurrent lesions, and (2) what is the mechanism that might render an individual susceptible to recurrent disease and allow him to terminate the recurrence once it has been initiated?

Two hypotheses have been advanced by Roizman [26] to explain the mechanism of virus persistence in the absence of clinical disease. The first one, designated the 'dynamic state', suggests that persistence results from continuous multiplication of the virus in confined pockets of chronically infected tissue. It predicts the successful isolation of infectious virus in the interim between recrudescences. According to the alternative hypothesis, designated the 'static state', the viral genome is maintained in a nonreplicating state and resumes a productive infection when the cells are induced as a consequence of provocation by stress. Although a rigorous differentiation between these two hypotheses is difficult, there is merit in discussing their independent requirements and predictions. Since cell death, defined as the inhibition of host macromolecular functions, occurs relatively early in the reproductive cycle of the virus, the static state hypothesis predicts that 'immediate' transcription of viral DNA does not occur in the cells that harbor the virus in the interim between recurrences. Thus, the static state may be the result of (a) the absence of the specific polymerase capable of transcribing viral DNA early in infection, (b) inactivity of the transcriptase possibly because the cells are nonreplicating, and (c) insertion of the L and S components of viral DNA into cellular DNA, thus falling under cellular regulatory control. However, experimental evidence appears to support the 'dynamic state' hypothesis. Thus, virus was recovered both from neuronal and non-neuronal tissue of asymptomatic hosts using the co-cultivation procedure [27, 29] and from homogenates of dorsal root ganglia of asymptomatic animals, provided highly sensitive indicator cells were used [30]. Furthermore, examination of serial sections of freshly excised ganglia from quiescent hosts revealed the presence of complete HSV virions [31] and virus-specific RNA [32] in rare, histologically abberant, neurons. Finally, virus was isolated from various sites and body fluids of asymptomatic humans with or without a history of recurrent disease [28, 33–37]. Nevertheless, these data are not incompatible with virus persistence in adjacent cells of the same tissue, or in cells from other tissues, in a static nonreplicating state.

Central to the 'dynamic state' hypothesis is the notion of a homeostatic relationship between the virus and the host during quiescence. This interpretation argues that in the interim between recurrences, the rate of virus replication and its spread to adjacent tissues is, by definition, limited to the extent compatible with a clinically asymptomatic state. Changes in the relative permissiveness of host cells, in the virulence or antigenicity of the virus, or in the host immune response, could result in a temporary disequilibrium favoring virus replication and recurrent disease. Recent studies from other laboratories and our own [27, 38] suggest that virus-specific cell-mediated immunity (CMI) plays a pivotal role in the maintenance of this homeostatic relationship. This control probably occurs at the level of the conversion of immune memory to active CMI effector responses capable of eliminating infected cells and stopping viral spread. If prompt and efficient, this response would check viral spread early, conceivably resulting in little or no symptomatology. In contrast, a lag in the generation of an anamnestic response would temporarily favor the replication of the virus resulting in clinically apparent recurrent disease due to viral cytopathic effect or im-

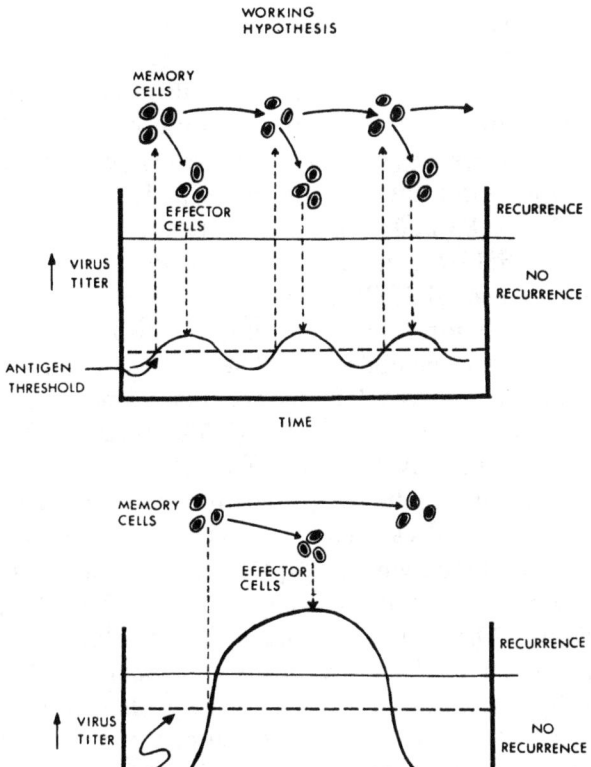

*Figure 2.* Schematic representation of the hypothetical mechanism of recurrent HSV lesions visualizes recurrent symptomatic disease as resulting from virus replication above a certain threshold. (A) The efficient conversion of virus specific immune memory (memory cells) into effector cell functions, expressed as a function of time and antigen dose (antigen threshold) maintains the virus titers at levels below those required for the induction of symptomatic (recurrence) disease. (B) The inefficient conversion of immune memory into effector cell functions requires longer time of exposure to antigen and higher antigen doses and results in the increase in virus titers above the cut-off point for symptomatic recurrent lesions.

mune destruction of infected tissue (Figure 2). The impairment in the generation of an anamnestic effector function could conceivably result from decreased numbers of appropriate lymphoid cells, ineffective interaction of immune and accessory cells, or the intervention of active suppression [27].

## 2.2. HSV-2 infections: epidemiologic considerations

HSV-2 prevalence rates in asymptomatic individuals sexually active with multiple partners (prostitutes, sexually transmitted disease clinic patients) are higher than those observed in randomly selected healthy subjects and indicate a sexual pattern of transmission of the virus. Moreover, comparison of the rates of virus isolation from asymptomatic, randomly selected individuals of both sexes suggests that males may preferentially shed virus while in an asymptomatic state. Centifanto et al. [37] reported the isolation of HSV-2 from 27 of 183 males (14.8%) seen during 5 months in a university urology clinic. Subjects, ranging in age from 15 to 85 years, had no previous history of genital HSV infection and were symptom-free at the time of specimen collection. The distribution of virus-positive cultures varied with the site of specimen collection. The highest isolation rates [(9 of 31 (20%)] were obtained from vas deferens specimens and prostatic fluids [3 of 13 (23.1%)]. This compares to 11 of 144 (7.6%) from urethral swabs. Similar results were obtained by Deardourff et al. [39], who isolated HSV-2 from 15% of 273 asymptomatic males (positive cultures were most frequent in prostatic fluid (29%) and vas deferens (26%) specimens), and by Jeansson and Molin [40], and Goodwin et al. [41], who reported the isolation of HSV-2 from urethral swabs of 3.1% of 130 and 2 of 12 asymptomatic males, respectively. The failure of other investigators [42, 43] to isolate virus from vas deferens and urethral samples probably reflects the relative insensitivity of their isolation procedures since virus was isolated from only 40% of active HSV-2 lesions (in at least one of these studies) compared to rates as high as 80-100% in other laboratories [42].

In most asymptomatic female populations studied to date, the rates of virus isolation or herpetic cytopathology associated with virus replication, are significantly lower than those reported in asymptomatic males. Routine examination of the cervical smears of asymptomatic women screened for cervical cancer revealed cells diagnostic of gential herpetic lesions at prevalence rates ranging between 0.03 to 1.5% in different population groups [44, 45]. Similarly, Jeansson and Molin [46] reported and isolation rate of 0.50% among 200 healthy asymptomatic women. Kleger et al.al. [47] isolated HSV-2 from only 2 of 1899 (0.1%) women seen in a cervical cytology clinic, and the highest isolation rates reported in asymptomatic females were 6.4-10% [48]. The relatively high rates of virus isolation from asymptomatic males as compared to asymptomatic females does not appear to be due to technical differences since, in the same laboratory, only one of 1,300 (0.03%) cultures of cervical and vaginal smears from 32 healthy asymptomatic females, was found to be HSV-2 positive [49] as compared to an overall isolation rate, by the same laboratory, of 14.8% from asymptomatic males [37]. In this context, it may be interesting that Duenas and colleagues [48] found that the rate of HSV-2 isolation from asymptomatic prostitutes decreased with age (<19 years = 12%; 20-29 years = 6%; >30 years = 2.8%) possibly representing a virus/host cell interaction that becomes increasingly nonpermissive due to estrogenic control of the virus replicative cycle. This interpretation is particularly significant to the student of HSV-2 and cervical cancer since: (1) the latter occurs at an older age (Section 8), (2) it is associated with nonpermissive HSV-2 infection (Section 4.3), and (3) an HSV-2 associated cancer has not yet been identified in males, possibly due to the persistence of the virus as a permissive rather than nonpermissive infection.

*2.3. HSV-2: a sexually transmitted disease*

Direct evidence concerning the sexual transmissability of genital herpes infections is derived from a number of observational studies of the sexual contacts of infected consorts. In many of these studies recently reviewed by Kessler [50] and by Aurelian and Strand [51], herpetic infections were diagnosed clinically in the contacts, and, sometimes, in their consorts, but serological measurements or virus isolation were not undertaken. In other investigations, laboratory tests were performed on the contacts, the consorts or both: measurement of HSV-2 antibodies, virus isolation or cytological diagnosis through visualization of characteristic multinucleated giant cells in exfoliate smears, were variously employed. Special attention was usually given to the temporal relationships between the reported coital experiences and the subsequent manifestations of genital disease in contacts and consorts. That genital herpes is a sexually transmitted disease (STD) is also suggested by clinical studies of prostitutes, and patients seen in venereal disease clinics who had an increased prevalence of clinically manifest disease and of serologically and virologically confirmed infections when compared with control populations (Section 2.2). Possibly the best clinical evidence of the sexual transmission of HSV-2 to date, is found in the investigations of Nahmias and Rawls and their respective colleagues [51, 52]. Eight female contacts of seven male patients with virologically confirmed HSV-2 penile infections were examined within one week of the initial detection of the herpetic lesions in their consorts; seven of eight contacts gave evidence of a current genital HSV-2 infection of either the vulva or the cervix, and virus was isolated from each of them [51]. Rawls and his co-workers examined 30 female contacts of 30 males with clinical genital herpes infections; HSV-2 was successfully isolated from the penile lesions of 53 percent of the male patients and from the genital secretions of 33 percent of their female contacts [52]. This prevalence of HSV-2 isolates was markedly greater than the prevalence of HSV-2 infections in a control group of women from the same clinic.

## 3. THE HERPESVIRUS HYPOTHESIS: ONCOGENIC POTENTIAL OF HSV-2

### 3.1. Neoplastic transformation

In principle, cancer could be viewed as a population of cells that have escaped regulatory controls, and thereby achieved immortality. Therefore, the *in vitro* transformation of cultured mammalian cells is a system particularly amenable to the study of the basic processes of viral oncogenesis. In the case of the herpesviruses, the invariable consequence of productive infection of permissive cells is cell death. Consequently, early studies of viral transformation were performed with virus whose lytic functions were inactivated. Selection of transformants was based on morphologic and growth alterations including, in some cases, neoplastic potential, or the transfer of the virus-encoded thymidine kinase (tk) gene to mouse cells previously lacking this function [53].

From the standpoint of the '*herpesvirus hypothesis*' of cervical cancer, two problems merit further scrutiny. Is the maintenance of a neoplastically transformed phenotype a function of the persistence or expression of specific viral gene(s), and by analogy to the progression from precursor cervical lesions to frank carcinoma (Section 3.2), is neoplastic potential *in vitro* acquired by a cell's progression through qualitatively different stages of autonomy?

3.1.1. *Transforming HSV-DNA sequences.* Several recent reports have attempted to localize the viral genes responsible for transformation (Figure 1). Camacho and Spear [54] reported that nucleotide sequences contained in a fragment of HSV-1 DNA that spans map coordinates 20–45, were sufficient to cause morphologic but not tumorigenic transformation of hamster embryo cells. Originally carrying viral glycoproteins, the cells were found to be free of viral DNA sequences at later passages [55]. Similarly, Reyes *et al.* [56] reported that transfection with a HSV-1 DNA fragment spanning map units 31–41 (mtr-1) (Figure 1) resulted in morphologic transformation of mouse cells as defined by focus formation. However, the focus-inducing function of HSV-2 DNA was localized in another DNA fragment (mtr-2) spanning map coordinates 58–63. Cells morphologically transformed by these DNA sequences were not tumorigenic. On the other hand, studies from other laboratories (Walboomers, personal communication) and our work [57] demonstrated that HSV-2 DNA sequences capable of inducing the neoplastic transformation of hamster embryo fibroblasts were localized in a fragment ('neoplastic') spanning map coordinates 43–58. Cells transformed by this fragment expressed viral antigens (including ICP 10, Section 4.1; 5.1) for at least 60 passages [57].

Another approach [58] towards the localization of the viral transforming

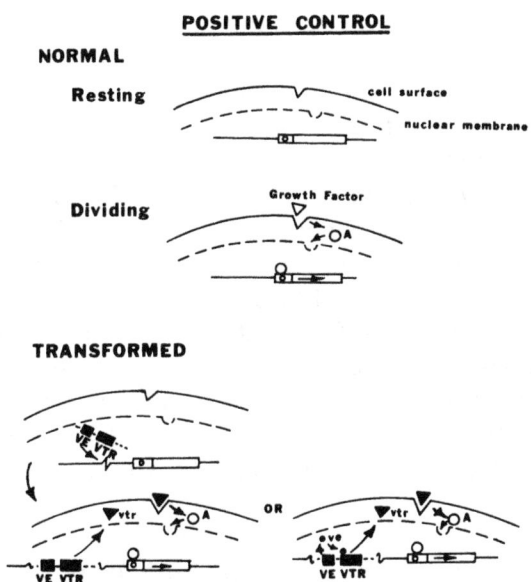

*Figure 3.* Schematic representation of the hypothetical mechanism of virus-induced transformation, according to the positive control of DNA synthesis/cell division. A regulatory host-encoded cytoplasmic factor (A), posited as the activator of DNA synthesis/cell division, is induced by the interaction of growth factors with the cell surface. It acts directly on the operator (O) of the gene regulating DNA synthesis or by interaction with the nuclear membrane. Transformation is visualized as resulting from an imbalance in growth regulation. It is postulated that a virus gene (VTR) codes for a transforming protein (vtr) that: (i) mimicks the action of the growth factors thus inducing activator (A) molecules, or (ii) mimicks the action of the activator itself (not shown). Another viral gene (VE) that is not absolutely necessary for transformation and may or may not be retained in transformed cells, significantly enhances transformation frequency by producing an 'enhancer' protein (ve). This protein acts by stabilizing the VTR gene in the host cells (integration) or by turning on the 'maintained' VTR gene. According to the negative control interpretation of DNA synthesis (not shown), a repressor (R) of DNA synthesis acts by binding the DNA thus preventing its replication (resting cells). Protein 'vtr' is posited as blocking (R) by binding it or its DNA attachment site. (62).

sequences is based on a hypothetical mechanism of transformation discussed in Section 3.1.4. and schematically diagrammed in Figure 3. Maintenance of a transformed or neoplastic phenotype depends on the persistence and expression of specific transforming viral gene(s) (designated VTR). Only cells that retain VTR have the selective advantage required for the establishment of stable neoplastically transformed cell lines. Accordingly, Galloway and her colleagues attempted to identify viral DNA sequences that were common to a cell line transformed by UV-inactivated HSV-2, its clones and subclones, and two lines established from tumors induced by one of the subclones. To this end, restriction endonuclease fragments of HSV-2

DNA spanning almost the entire genome, were made highly radioactive *in vitro* and a small amount was hybridized with large quantities of unlabeled DNA isolated from both the transformed cells and the tumor cell line. Whereas the original transformed line retained an extensive set of viral DNA sequences, a greatly decreased number of sequences was observed in the subclones and particularly in the tumor lines. Significantly, the only two blocks of viral DNA sequences common to all the cells, including the two tumor lines, were those homologous to the Bgl II G fragment (map units 21–31) (Figure 1) and to the Xba I D fragment (map units 45–72). However, since sequences homologous to fragments that overlap the right-hand end of the Xba I D fragment (spanning map units 58–72) were not present in some of the lines, we conclude that the only sequences common to all the lines were those spanning positions 45–48 and overlapping virtually the entire fragment (designated *neoplastic*) that possesses neoplastic potential (Figure 1).

*3.1.2. Expression of viral genes in transformed cells.* Traditional carcinogenesis is a multi-step process that includes an 'initiation' followed by a 'promotion' phase [59]. Although promotion is not well defined in viral carcinogenesis, transforming functions of DNA tumor viruses have been shown to reside in two distinct complementation groups, respectively responsible for initiating and maintaining a transformed phenotype. Viruses having a defect in the capacity for maintenance can cause morphologic transformation (apparently a criterion of initiation) but most of the transformed cells fail to establish neoplastically transformed lines. Results of HSV-2 induced transformation are compatible with the lack of expression of viral functions related to the 'promotion'/'maintenance' phase by the vast majority of morphologically transformed cells which, therefore, fail to develop into stable lines. Indeed, approximately 96% of morphologically altered foci do not grow into stable lines [60, 61] and viral DNA sequences that induced morphologic transformation differ from those that induce neoplastic transformation (Section 3.1.1). However, in some cells, maintenance functions appear to be expressed and neoplastic lines can be established, albeit at a significantly (>30) fold lower frequency [61]. Furthermore, viral functions expressed between 0–4 hours post infection enhance the frequency of both morphologic and neoplastic transformation [61]. As such, presently available data on HSV-2 induced transformation functionally define 'enhancer' gene(s) and putative 'maintenance' VTR gene(s) [5, 62]. The exact identity of the enhancer gene(s) and their relationship to putative 'initiator' functions is unclear. Viral functions known to be expressed by 4 hours p.i. include (1) induction of chromosomal lesions, (2) inhibition of $\alpha$-amanitin sensitive RNA polymerase [63] (the host polymerase most probably involved in the immediate early transcription of viral DNA) [64], (3) increased thymidine metabolism such as transport and phosphorylation [65], and (4) stimulation of cellular DNA synthesis [65]. This is particularly significant since all these viral functions could support any one of the hypothetical interpretations of the mechanism of action of enhancer functions: (1) regulation of the expression of the 'promotion/maintenance' gene(s), (2) integration of the 'promotion/maintenance' gene(s) into the host genome, or (3) interaction with host cellular functions in order to trigger morphologic transformation, rendering the cells more susceptible to permanent neoplastic transformation when they are exposed to the viral 'promotion/maintenance' gene(s) (VTR).

The 'maintenance' (VTR) gene(s) are particularly significant to the '*herpesvirus hypothesis*' of cervical cancer since identification of such gene(s) could reasonably be expected in cervical tumor cells. Recent data indicate that neoplastically transformed lines contain viral DNA [61, 66] express virus-specific mRNA [61] and viral antigens or proteins [61]. One of the latter is designated ICP 10. It is a 160,000 dalton 'immediate early', DNA-

Table 3. Expression of viral antigen(s) and tumorigenic potential of HSV-2 transformed lines

| Cells[a] | % complement fixed with IgG from | | | Tumorigenicity[b] |
|---|---|---|---|---|
| | HSV-2 | Anti-AG-e | Anti-ICP 10 | |
| SHE | 0 | 0 | 0 | − |
| HBU-2 | 0 | 0 | 0 | − |
| HBU-0 | 0 | 0 | 3.5 | − |
| HBU-1 | 63.0 | 83.7 | 20.2 | + |
| HBU-2A | 0 | 10.2 | 0 | − |
| HBU-2B | 25.7 | 0 | 0 | − |
| HBU-2C | 25 | 10 | 6.7 | − |
| HBU-2D | 5.7 | 0 | 23 | + |
| HBU-4 | 22.9 | 55 | 0 | − |
| HBU-4B | 67.9 | ND | 12.8 | + |
| HBU-4C | 76.9 | ND | 16.3 | + |
| HBU-4A | 90.2 | ND | 23.1 | + |
| HBU-4D | 0 | 0 | 15.4 | + |
| HBU-6A | 88.9 | ND | 43 | + |
| HBU-8A | 91.1 | ND | 77.2 | + |

[a] Extracts of HSV-2 transformed (HBU series) (ptp 25–62) and normal hamster cells (SHE) assayed against IgG from antisera to total viral antigens (HSV-2), AG-e and ICP 10 (1/4 dilution). Reaction considered positive if > 10% complement is fixed.
[b] Newborn hamsters (5–12 animals/line) were injected subcutaneously with $2 \times 10^6$ cells. A negative line is one that does not cause tumors in any animal.

binding protein [147, 148] found in all the transformed lines studied in our laboratory including those established with the specific 'neoplastic' HSV-2 DNA fragment (Figure 1; Section 3.1.1). It is a reasonable candidate for the viral gene product (vtr) involved in the 'promotion/maintenance' phase of transformation (Figure 3), since its expression correlates well (99% confidence level; $p \leq 0.01$, according to Kendall's coefficient of rank correlation) with anchorage independent growth, and with tumorigenicity (Table 3). The expression of a 160,000 dalton protein was also correlated with the acquisition of tumorigenic potential in a line of HSV-2 transformed rat cells following exposure to the tumor promoting agent 12-0-tetradecanoyl-phorbol-13-acetate (TPA) (Kucera, personal communication).

Another viral antigen (AG-e) consisting of the 'immediate early' protein ICP 12 (MW: 140,000) and late structural protein ICP 14 (MW: 130,000) [86] is also expressed in some of the transformed cells. However, its expression does not appear to correlate with tumorigenic potential (Table 3). In this context, it is particularly significant that the viral DNA sequences (mtr-2) that induce morphologic, but not tumorigenic transformation overlap with viral DNA sequences that code for an 'immediate early' (IE) protein of 140,000 dalton (Figure 1) [67] possibly similar to our ICP 12. Other viral proteins identified in neoplastically transformed cells include VP 143 [68] a protein that might be similar to our ICP 12 and three proteins that co-migrate on SDS-acrylamide gel electrophoresis with ICP 7/8: an 'immediate early', 175,000 dalton protein that may represent the regulatory protein VP 175, ICP 22, a DNA-binding protein and ICP 35 a protein that may represent the viral thymidine kinase [149].

*3.1.3. Progression/selection.* HSV-2 transformed hamster embryo fibroblasts display a progressive acquisition of phenotypic alterations associated with the neoplastic state. Thus, morphologic alterations and growth in low concentrations of serum are first detected at post-treatment passage (ptp) 4-8. Cells enter crisis at ptp 8-10 and recover at ptp 12-24. Anchorage independence is first detected at ptp 24-37 and increases with cell passage. The appearance of anchorage independence is virtually simultaneous (ptp 24-54) with the acquisition of tumorigenic potential for newborn hamsters and unlike growth in low serum concentrations, anchorage independence correlates well with tumorigenicity [62]. Viral antigen expression precedes anchorage independence by 13-14 passages and persists thereafter [62]. This temporal acquisition of the transformed phenotype appears to be due to a progressive passage of the cells through qualitatively different stages, since clones isolated at early (ptp 8) or intermediate (ptp 25) passage did not express anchorage independence until they reached ptp 35-55. However, it should be pointed out that not all cells within a population reached an identical stage at the same time. Thus, clones isolated at a passage (ptp 35), when the parental line already expressed a low (5%) cloning efficiency in 0.3% agarose, grew well in semi-solid medium within 3 or 20 independent passages [62].

The concept that the acquisition of a neoplastic potential results from the progressive passage of the cells through qualitatively different stages has been disputed by Kucera et al. [69]. These investigators found that foci of HSV-2 transformed rat cells at early passage, produce small numbers of colonies in soft agar. Lines established from these colonies were tumorigenic, eliminating the requirement for long (up to 2 years) *in vivo* latent periods described for low passage rat transformants [70]. These contradictory conclusions may reflect different mechanisms of virus-induced transformation operative under various selection pressures (i.e. continuous passage vs growth in semi-solid medium) brought to bear on the HSV-2 infected cells in the transformation assay.

*3.1.4. Mechanism of transformation: a hypothesis.* The concepts considered above are similar to those developed for other tumor viruses. Thus, cells transformed by the DNA tumor virus SV 40 express two virus-specific tumor antigens; T antigen (94,000 daltons) predominantly nuclear, and t antigen (20,000 daltons) predominantly cytoplasmic, as well as cell-encoded tumor antigen NVT (50,000–56,000 daltons) [71]. In SV 40 cells that are transformed but not productively infected, a stable association is observed between T and NVT [72]. This association is believed to be responsible for the induction of DNA synthesis in arrested cells [73]. Synthesis of T antigen, in turn, appears to be regulated by another viral gene product normally expressed early in infection [76]. The role of t antigen in SV 40 transformation is to destabilize the actin cables that are involved in cellular adhesion, mobility, morphology, and in the organization of the cell surface [75]: and that correlate with a reduced serum requirement for growth. Taken *in toto,* the data suggest that transformation by SV 40 probably involves the coordinated effect of the two viral antigens: t antigen disrupts the normal organization of cellular structure and control thus permitting stable integration of the transforming gene(s) and T antigen (interacting with NVT) regulates DNA synthesis and ultimately accounts for the tumorigenic characteristics of the cells.

Based on these interpretations, it seems reasonable to conclude that in virus-induced transformation, the development and maintenance of a transformed phenotype usually depends on the persistence and expression of a specific viral transforming gene designated VTR. This gene codes for a protein (vtr) that is capable of interacting with the host cell in such a fashion as to irreversibly commit the cell to continuous DNA synthesis and cell divi-

*Table 4.* ICP 10: a hypothetical HSV-2 vtr[a].

1. HSV-2 specific viral protein. MW: 160,000 daltons.
2. Phosphorylated, DNA binding.
3. Synthesis begins at 3 hours p.i. Phosphorylated by 4 hrs p.i.
4. 'Immediate early' – made in presence of cycloheximide (8 hrs) and actinomycin D (4 hrs).
5. Antigenic in phosphorylated state. Non-phosphorylated, immunologically related, 160,000 daltons protein present in HSV-2 virions.
6. Genetically linked to viral DNA polymerase.
7. Expressed in HSV-2 transformed cells including those transformed by viral DNA sequences that map at 43–58 units on viral genome.
8. Expression in transformed cells, correlates well with anchorage independent growth and tumorigenicity.
9. Expressed in cervical tumor cells (biopsied and exfoliated).
10. Immunologically identical to AG-4; it reflects the progression of the cervical tumor.

[a] Postulated vtr (viral transforming protein) is encoded by transforming viral DNA sequences (VTR) that persist in transformed/tumor cells and are involved in the promotion/maintenance of a transformed/tumorigenic phenotype (Figure 3).

sion. Another viral gene designated VE codes for viral functions (ve) that enhance the frequency of transformation by creating conditions conducive to the maintenance (integration) or expression of the VTR gene (Figure 3). Analogous to the T antigen of the DNA tumor viruses, a good candidate for the postulated vtr protein of HSV-2 is ICP 10, a serotype specific, 'immediate early' DNA-binding protein, the properties of which are summarized in Table 4. Significantly, ICP 10 is expressed in cells transformed by the viral DNA sequences that induce neoplastic transformation and span map coordinates 43–58 on the viral genome (Figure 1). Its expression correlates well with anchorage independence and tumorigenicity. Recently, we have shown that ICP 10 is genetically linked to the viral DNA polymerase [148] (Figure 1), thereby giving rise to various speculations as to its possible involvement in the stimulation of host cell DNA synthesis. Expression in the transformed cells of other viral proteins such as ICP 12 or ICP 14 does not correlate with tumorigenicity (Section 3.1.2) thus suggesting that these may not represent the putative vtr. However, such proteins may play a role in the 'initiation' process or may represent the putative 've' protein(s). Alternative hypotheses for the mechanism of HSV-induced transformation that do not require the maintenance and expression of viral genes have been discussed by Aurelian *et al.* [62].

How does our hypothesis contend with the observation that tumorigenicity is acquired as a progressive passage through qualitatively different stages? The expression of a transformed phenotype such as reduced serum requirement (altered membrane receptors for growth factors), loss of contact inhibition (membrane mediated cell-to-cell communication), anchorage independent growth (membrane attachment to surface), and tumorigenicity (alteration of cell surface so as to become unresponsive to growth controls and insensitive to the immune system) can be considered to be different stages in the alteration of cell membranes. Given that all these membrane effects are interrelated, it may be postulated that the progressive acquisition of morphologic alterations, growth in low serum concentrations, anchorage independence and tumorigenicity, represent the progressive loss of response to a cell-encoded repressor molecule that regulates cell division or the progressive accumulation of a cell-encoded activator molecule that induces cell division. According to this interpretation, the initial transforming event would produce an imbalance in the rate of production of the regulatory molecules per cell cycle, but subsequent cell divisions would be required before the full effect of this imbalance could be observed. Assuming that a finite number of regulatory molecules is essential in order to regulate cellular DNA synthesis, and that those functions associated with neoplastic transformation, such as morphologic alteration, growth in low serum concentration, and anchorage independence, are controlled by contiguously regulated cellular genes, it follows that quantitative defects in regulatory molecules would fail to regulate the expression of these genes in a cascading, interlocking order. Alternatively, it may be argued that at consecutive stages in its life cycle, the cell may differentiate or retrodifferentiate. The cumulative effect of these changes in differentiation will determine the cell's ultimate fate: immortality (neoplastic transformation) or senescence (normal life and death) [62].

## 3.2. Animal model of HSV-2 induced anaplasia

A unique characteristic of squamous cervical cancer is the recognition of the precursor lesions, dysplasia and CIS. Briefly, experimental studies have demonstrated that once the epithelial abnormalities, defined as atypia or dysplasia, are present, carcinoma of the cervix will develop without further application of the carcinogen [76]. Koss and co-workers [77], showed that 10 out of 25 untreated dysplasias progressed to either CIS or invasive cancer. Stern and Neely [78] demonstrated that the rate of progression to CIS was 106/1000 in patients with dysplasia compared to a control population rate of 5.1/1000. The rate of progression to invasive carcinoma was 11/1000 in patients with dysplasia as compared to a rate of 1.5/1000 for controls. Follow-up studies reviewed by Koss [76] revealed that only 23–40% of the mild to moderate dysplasias regressed or improved, when 5–20% progressed. In 107 patients with severe dysplasia, 40% of the lesions culminated in CIS and, in 2 patients, early invasive epidermoid carcinoma of the cervix developed. Evidence from these and other studies [79] led to the concept of the progression of at least a proportion of pre-neoplastic lesions to frank invasive disease. Since the necessary co-factors (Section 10) may not be reproducible, the most reasonable animal model of HSV-2 carcinogenesis is one that evidences progression through precursor lesions. In one study [80] (in previously immunized mice inoculated with live HSV-2), lesions histologically commensurate with dysplasia (5.2%) and invasive cancer (10.5%) were observed and compared to a 3.2% incidence of pre-cancerous lesions in uninfected animals. Unimmunized mice were also inoculated intravaginally with live HSV-2 but a high mortality resulted such that only 5% of the animals survived more than 1 year. Only 2 of 50 surviving mice thus inoculated developed cervical dysplasia or CIS [80]. In another murine study, cytopathologic evidence of pre-invasive lesions similar to those in humans was detected in 50% of animals inoculated with inactivated HSV-2. In 35% of these animals, the changes progressed to invasive cancer [81]. In hamsters inoculated with live HSV-2, the high mortality rate masked any potential oncogenic activity [81], however, rabbits inoculated *in situ* with a nucleic acid extract of HSV-2 infected cells developed uterine leiomyosarcomas [82]. Extracts of uninfected cells did not produce the disease. Finally, 35% of Cebus monkeys vaginally infected with HSV-2 developed severe dysplasia 5–6 years later [83]. This observation is particularly significant since the mean age for the development of dysplasia is 5 years older than the mean age of infection with HSV-2 (Section 8), and since approximately 20% of human dysplasias persist or progress to CIS or invasive cancer [76]. There is no compelling reason to assume that the virus interaction with Cebus and human cervical cells is identical, and that cervical dysplasia in the Cebus monkey will progress to invasive cancer. Moreover, all required co-carcinogens may not be available and operative in the Cebus: Nevertheless it may be argued that the monkey is the best and most promising model for human disease. However, it should be remembered that this assumption implies that the first cases of cervical carcinoma in the HSV-2 infected Cebus monkeys should be observed in the years 1997–1999, i.e., 23–25 years post infection with HSV-2 (Section 8), if the animal's life span permits it.

## 4. HSV GENETIC INFORMATION IN CERVICAL TUMOR CELLS

The following predictions pertaining to cervical tumor cells are a natural extension of the transformation data presented in Section 3.1: (1) tumor cells should maintain at least those viral DNA sequences involved in neoplastic transformation (designated VTR in Figure 3), (2) they should express viral mRNA and viral proteins. Among these, ICP 10, AG-e (ICP 12 and/or ICP 14) and VP 143, are reasonable candidates since they are found in the transformed cells, (3) the expression of at least one of these proteins (vtr) should reflect the growth of the cervical tumor. ICP 10 is a good candidate since it correlates with the tumorigenic potential of the HSV-2 transformed cells (4). Continuous expression of the persistent VTR gene should give rise in the cancer patient to antigen-driven humoral and cellular immune responses (such as 19S immunoglobulin, or effector-type CMI responses) that are specific to the putative vtr protein (possibly ICP 10). These immune responses are not expected in vtr negative normal controls even if these subjects were previously exposed to HSV-2 and retained a virus-specific immune memory. Furthermore, removal of the tumor burden should eliminate the source of the vtr protein that drives the immune response, with patients converting to a vtr negative immune status. Tumor recurrence, on the other hand, would be associated with the re-expression of the vtr protein resulting the reappearance of the specific antigen-driven immunity.

*Table 5.* HSV-2 proteins in cervical tumor and dysplastic cells.

| Reference | Anti-serum[b] to | % positive subjects[a] | | |
|---|---|---|---|---|
| | | Normal | Dysplasia | Cancer |
| Aurelian et al. [154, 150] | HSV-2 | 0 | 82.2–72 | 91.6 |
| Aurelian et al. [150] | AG-e | 0 | 61.5 | 72.7 |
| Pacsa et al. [155] | HSV-2 | 9.4 | 61 | 94 |
| Adelusi et al. [156] | HSV-2 | 0 | ND | 100 |
| Minhui et al. [157] | HSV-2 | 9 | ND | 100 |
| Smith et al. [87] | AG-e | 0 | 72.6 | 91.4 |
| Smith et al. [87] | ICP 12 | 0 | 61.5 | 100 |
| Smith et al. [87] | ICP 14 | 0 | 53.8 | 75 |
| Athanasiu et al. [158] | HSV-2 | 0 | ND | 33.3 |
| Dreesman et al. [88][c] | ICSP 11/12 | 0 | 10.6 | 40 |
| Dreesman et al. [88] | ICSP 34/35 | 0 | 10.6 | 40 |
| Klacsmann et al. (in prep.)[d] | ICP 10 | 0 | 90 | 100 (80) |

[a] Exfoliated cervical cells collected by the irrigation procedure were stained by the immunofluorescent assay in all cases except those reported by Athanasiu et al. [158], and Dreesman et al. [8], who used frozen sections of cervical biopsies. Results are expressed as the percent of patients with staining cells.
[b] Antisera against total viral antigens (HSV-2), antigen AG-e, (consisting of proteins ICP 12 and ICP 14) and proteins ICP 12, ICP 14, ICP 10, ICSP 11/12 (Mw = 140,000) and ICSP 34/35 (MW = 54,000).
[c] Immunoperoxidase staining.
[d] Frozen sections of cervical biopsies from cancer patients and normal control women were stained with immunoperoxidase. Staining was observed in 8 of 10 (80%) cervical cancer biopsies but not in normal tissue. Exfoliated cervical cells, collected by the irrigation procedure, were stained in immunofluorescence. Staining was observed in anaplastic cells from 90% of patients with dysplasia and all those with invasive cancer (Figure 4).

## 4.1. Viral proteins

The viral proteins enumerated in Table 5 have been identified in cervical tumors using various serologic assays. One of these, designated ICP 10/AG-4, is the viral protein whose expression correlates with anchorage independent growth and tumorigenicity in HSV-2 transformed cells (Section 3.1.2). This protein was identified in 5 of 6 cervical tumors but not in normal cervical tissue or in a biopsy from an adenocarcinoma of the cervix by complement fixation [85]. Eight of ten tumors were stained positively by the immunoperoxidase procedure with antiserum to ICP 10 [141]. Exfoliated anaplastic cells from 58% of patients with cervical dysplasia and 100% of those cells from patients with invasive cancer stained with anti-ICP 10 serum in indirect immunofluorescence (Figure 4) thus indicating the ability of ICP 10 to reflect tumor growth. The staining of the cervical tumor cells localized in both the nucleus and the cytoplasm and was virus and tumor-specific. Pre-immune serum and serum adsorbed with extracts of

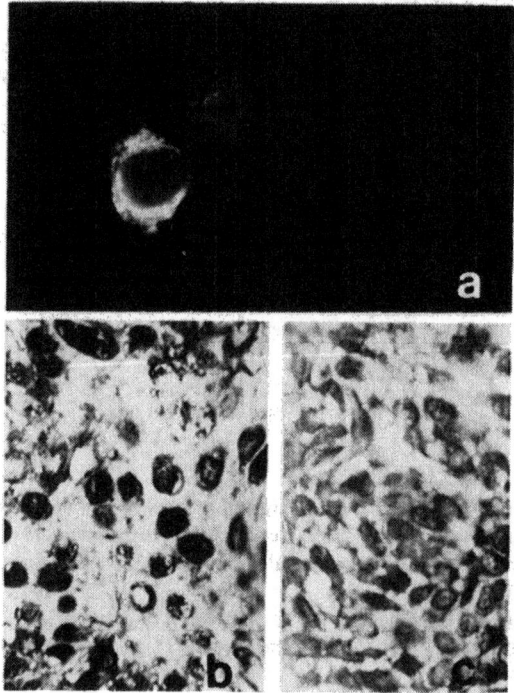

*Figure 4.* (b) Frozen section of cervical biopsy from a patient with invasive cancer stained in immunoperoxidase with antiserum to ICP 10. Staining localized in the nucleus and cytoplasm ($\times 320$). (c) Serial section as in (a) stained with pre-immune rabbit serum ($\times 320$). (a) Exfoliated cervical atypical cells from patient with mild dysplasia stained in indirect immunofluorescence with antiserum to ICP 10 ($\times 600$).

ICP 10-positive, HSV-2 infected cells did not stain cervical tumor cells or normal cervical tissue.

Another viral antigen expressed by cervical tumor cells is AG-e (Table 5), an antigen that consists of viral proteins ICP 12 and ICP 14 [86]. Antiserum prepared against purified AG-e stains exfoliated cells from patients with cervical cancer or dysplasia in indirect immunofluorescence. The staining is virus-specific and is not observed in normal cervical cells from the same individuals or from normal control women (Figure 4). Unlike the situation in normal cervical cells or cultured cells permissively infected with HSV-2, in which AG-e staining is both cytoplasmic and nuclear, the staining in the anaplastic cells is cytoplasmic. The antigenicity or immunogenicity of the AG-e antigen does not depend on the structural interaction of the ICP 12 and ICP 14 proteins, since antisera against these two proteins will independently stain the exfoliated anaplastic cells from 66.6% (ICP 12) and 61% (ICP 14) of all the patients with dysplasia and cancer studied in this series. Approximately one half of these patients expres both ICP 12 and ICP 14 [87] (Section 11).

VP 143 is a third protein described in HSV-2 transformed cells and also in cultured cervical carcinoma by indirect immunofluorescent staining with specific antiserum [89]. VP 143 has a molecular weight (MW) similar to that of both ICP 12 and ICSP 11/12. The latter is a protein recently described by Dreesman et al. [88], in cervical carcinoma and dysplastic cells from 38% of patients based on immunoperoxidase staining with specific antiserum. In all cases, normal cells were negative. It is not clear whether these 3 proteins are identical. However, they have similar MW's and at least ICSP 11/12 and ICP 12 bind DNA.

Other viral proteins were described in cervical tumor cells but not in transformed cells. These include: (1) ICSP 34/35, a 54,000 dalton DNA-binding protein identified by immunoperoxidase staining in 38% of cervical biopsies from patients with dysplasia and invasive cancer [88], (2) HSV-TAA recently shown to be a 70,000 dalton glycoprotein [90] probably induced, but not encoded by HSV-1 and HSV-2, and (3) an antigen described by Gall and Haines [91] as a line of identity in immunodiffusion between extracts of HSV-2 infected cells and cervical cancer tissue. This antigen has not been further identified.

Two comments seem pertinent from the standpoint of the predictions made by the '*herpesvirus hypothesis*' of cervical cancer. First, comparison between the number of patients that have exfoliated anaplastic cells staining with antisera to total viral antigens and the number of patients with anaplastic cells that recognize antisera to AG-e (ICP 12/ICP 14) or ICP 10 reveals that a higher proportion of patients with cervical dysplasia react with antisera to total virus antigens than with antisera to any one of the purified viral proteins. Exfoliated atypical cells from patients with cancer reacted with all antisera almost equally well, suggesting that progression from the precursor to the neoplastic lesion involves a loss in the expression of viral genetic information, possibly due to a decrease in the complexity of persistent viral DNA sequences. Such a loss has been described in transformation (Section 3.1.1). The second comment that is pertinent with respect to these findings is the identity of the viral proteins presently identified in the cervical tumor. ICP 10 is expressed in neoplastically transformed cells and its expression correlates with tumorigenicity (Section 3.1.2). Consequently, ICP 10 may reflect growth of the cervical tumor. Consistent with this expectation, anti-ICP 10 serum stains cells from 45.5% of patients with mild dysplasia compared with 70% of patients with moderate dysplasia and 100% of patients with lesions ranging from marked dysplasia to invasive cancer. On the other hand, AG-e (ICP 12/ICP 14) is also expressed in the HSV-2 transformed cells but its expression does not correlate with tumorigenicity (Section 3.1.2). Consistent with this finding, anti-AG-e serum stains cells from only 50-57.7% of patients with all stages of dysplasia (mild, moderate, marked) and from 87.5% of those with invasive cancer. In this context, it should be remembered that of the two proteins in AG-e, ICP12 (possibly similar to VP 143 and ICSP 11/12) might be the protein encoded by viral DNA sequences spanning map units 55-61 on the viral genome (Figure 1). These DNA sequences overlap those of mtr-2 responsible for morphologic transformation, suggesting that the 140,000 dalton protein that they encode might be involved in 'initiation' processes (Section 3.1.2). The other protein in AG-e, ICP 14, is viral glycoprotein C (18) that has been mapped between map units 65-72 on the HSV-2 genome (Figure 1). The possibility that the adjacent location of the DNA sequences coding for these viral proteins is not fortuitous but rather results from the direct or indirect involvement in the carcinogenic process of the entire set of sequences spanning map units 43-72, must be given serious consideration.

*4.2. Viral messenger RNA*

Using the *in situ* hybridization procedure, McDougall *et al.* [92], have recently described the presence of viral messenger RNA (mRNA) in frozen sections of cervical tumor biopsies. Lesions, diagnosed as mild to severe dysplasia, CIS and invasive cancer, were studied. The viral DNA probe was extracted from HSV-2 infected cells, labeled *in vitro* with $_3$H-nucleotides and shown to be virus-specific by its inability to hybridize with sequences of normal human cell DNA. That the reaction was specific was evidenced by the absence of hybridization with DNA from SV-40, bacteriophage lambda, and adenovirus type 2 and by 90% reduction in autoradiographic grains after treatment with ribonuclease. Viral mRNA was demonstrated in 60% of intraepithelial lesions (dysplasia or CIS) as compared to 5% of non-neoplastic epithelial tissues. These investigators failed to detect viral mRNA in 5 invasive cervical tumors. However, this is probably due to technical difficulties, since data generated in other laboratories; ( [93] Wilkie, personal communication) suggest that virus-specific mRNA is, indeed, expressed in biopsies from CIS and invasive cervical tumors.

*4.3. Viral DNA*

The presence of viral DNA in the cervical tumor cells has been more difficult to establish. The rate of re-association between radiolabeled HSV-2 DNA probe and DNA from cervical cancer cells, was measured by Frenkel et al. [94], who demonstrated the presence in the cervical tumor cells of a segment representing 39% of the HSV-2 genome at a concentration of 3.4 copies per cell. The kinetics of hybridization of the viral DNA sequences in sheared DNA, suggested that these sequences were covalently linked to host DNA regions in the proximity of the reiterated regions. On the other hand, biopsies from cervical cancer cases were negative when examined by hybridization procedures capable of detecting only 0.25 to 1 virus genome equivalent/cell [95].

Many reviewers have focused on the negative DNA hybridization data, although as previously discussed [96], these are not technically comparable to Frenkel's original studies. In principle, the assay for viral DNA sequences in transformed or tumor cells is based on the fact that renaturation of labeled viral DNA probe is accelerated in the presence of excess unlabeled DNA containing sequences that are homologous to the probe. The detection of the viral DNA sequences hinges on the magnitude of the difference between the self-renaturation of the probe, and the renaturation observed in presence of transformed cell DNA. Analysis of the factors that affect the magnitude of this difference [96] has revealed that a maximal difference will be observed in the test only if the homologous sequences in the transformed cell DNA are in vast excess over those in the probe DNA. Consequently, the amount of tumor DNA in the assay mixture, and the specific number of tumor cells in the tissue being investigated, will determine the positive or negative outcome of the hybridization studies.

Since sequences corresponding to maximum 10% of the viral genome suffice to cause neoplastic transformation (Section 3.1.1), and since most specimens available for study weigh less than 2.5 gm and consist of connective tissue with approximately 20% tumor cells, it can be easily estimated that the experimental conditions necessary for the detection of viral DNA in the tumor mass are not met. Frenkel's successful report involved a 70-gram tumor mass consisting of 50% tumor cells. Since suitable tissue for such experimentation is generally not available, current studies in many laboratories are designed to circumvent these difficulties by cloning specific restriction endonuclease-generated fragments of HSV-2 DNA, and using these as probes in hybridization assays. It therefore seems premature to draw final conclusions on the presence of the viral DNA in cervical tumors. It should be stressed, however, that the presence of viral proteins and mRNA in the tumor cells constitutes strong evidence in support of the maintenance of viral DNA in the tumor cells. Furthermore, the presence of viral DNA in the cervical cancer cells considered independently of all the rest of the evidence for the association of HSV-2 with cervical cancer, does not in itself prove that the virus plays a role in the etiology of cervical cancer.

*4.4. Infectious virus*

Originally, HSV-2 was isolated from cells in cultures derived from a precursor cervical lesion (severe dysplasia) and maintained at high pH [97]. Despite dramatic pronouncements to the contrary, the isolate did not result from chance contamination since it was obtained from parallel cultures of the same line and differed from laboratory strains with respect to both biologic properties including the formation of aberrant lamellar structures [98] and the restriction endonuclease cleavage pattern of its DNA [57]. More recently, HSV-2 has been repetitively isolated from biopsy material obtained from one patient with Stage I cervical carcinoma and from cervical discharge and blood clots obtained from three other patients with cervical cancer [99]. In another study, HSV-2 was also isolated from a patient with invasive cervical carcinoma by the co-cultivation procedure [100]. Virus could not be isolated from homogenates of the same cervical tumor tissue, consistent with the significantly lower sensitivity of this procedure. Possibly some of the cells in the cervical tumor mass are latently infected and thereby maintain the entire viral genome (Section 2.1) whereas other cells may maintain only viral transforming DNA sequences and are thereby neoplastically transformed (Section 3.1.1). Indeed, cytopathologic changes commensurate with a productive HSV infection were seen in patients with dysplasia, CIS and invasive cancer [101]. In at least one case, the changes were localized to the paracervical neurons within the cervical tumor mass [102]. Underscoring the role of the host cell in the regulation of the persistence and expression of viral DNA sequences, however, virus was also isolated from a cell line established from the 18th *in vivo* passage of tumors induced in hamsters by a HSV-2 transformed hamster cell line following exposure to 40 µg/mg of 5-iododeoxyuridine for 3 days. This isolation did not result from extraneous contamination since virus could not be isolated from parallel cultures treated with arginine or Ara-c [103]. Infectious virus was also retrieved from a line established from a rat tumor induced by HSV-2 transformed rat cells (J.C.M. MacNab, personal communication).

5. CERVICAL CANCER ASSOCIATED IMMUNE RESPONSE INDICATIVE OF CONTINUOUS VIRUS EXPRESSION

*5.1. ICP 10/AG-4: antigen-driven humoral response reflects the progression of the cervical tumor*

The transformation data (Section 3.1.2) predict that ICP 10, the viral protein that correlates with tumorgenicity (Table 3) might be a good candidate for the putative 'vtr' protein (Table 4) in cervical cancer patients. According to this prediction, ICP 10 should induce an antigen-driven immune response that reflects the progression of the tumor in patients with cervical cancer. Fulfilling this prediction, 44 to 85% of patients with cervical cancer have demonstrable levels of IgM antibody (antigen-driven humoral response) to ICP 10/AG-4. A similar response to ICP 10/AG-4 is virtually

*Table 6.* Summary of findings on prevalence of antibody to early viral antigens among cervical cancer patients and controls.

| Location | Antigen | Percent with antibodies | | References |
|---|---|---|---|---|
| | | Cancer | Controls | |
| Maryland | AG-e | 85 | 12 | Aurelian et al., 1973 [85] |
| Texas | VP 134 | 93 | 40[a] | Anzai et al., 1975 [108] |
| Pennsylvania | AG-4 | 78 | 29 | Notter and Docherty, 1976 [164] |
| North Carolina | AG-4 | 55 | 0 | Heise and Kucera, 1976 [163] |
| Japan | AG-4 | 75 | 14[b] | Kawana et al., 1976 [161] |
| Japan | AG-4 | 52 | 17[c] | Kawana et al., 19678 [162] |
| Japan | ICSP 8/15 | 71.4 | 16 | Ito et al., 1978 [112] |
| Texas | AG-4 | Reactivity only with CaCx sera | | Melnick, 1978 [159] |
| North Carolina | AG-4 | 44 | ND[d] | Heise et al., 1979 [105] |
| Maryland | AG-4 | 72.5 | 14[e] | Aurelian et al., 1980 [104] |
| Australia | AG-4 | 75 | 10–20[f] | Arsenakis et al., 1980 [160] |

[a] Breast cancer patients: 30%.
[b] Proportion among HSV-2 positive patients.
[c] Proportion among HSV-2 positive and HSV-2 negative patients.
[d] Prevalence increases to 77% post therapy, primarily by radiation.
[e] Cancers at other sites: 7.7%. Patients with latent HSV-2 lesions: 14.3%. Patients with primary HSV-2 lesions: reflects tumor progression.
[f] Dysplasia: 40%; CIS: 60%; Primary HSV-2: 58%; Primary HSV-1: 10%; Cancer at other sites: 20%.

absent in normal individuals or in patients with cancer at other sites (Table 6). However, since ICP 10 is a virus coded protein, patients with primary HSV-2 infections develop a specific antibody response that precedes the development of neutralizing, primarily IgG, antibody to HSV-2 and disappears one to seven months after infection [104]. Consistent with the strict regulation of anamnestic responses which are antigen-driven, subjects whose immune systems are not continuously exposed to the antigen are virtually AG-4 seronegative. This group would include those with a history of recurrent HSV-2 disease, or HSV-2 seropositive control women without cancer.

In a recent study [104] sera obtained under code from 1325 individuals were assayed blindly for AG-4 antibodies. Furthermore, a proportion, (209 subjects) with cervical neoplasia were followed prospectively for 6 years with blood samples drawn at intervals of 6–12 months. The results obtained from those patients studied at only one time interval prior to therapy may be summarized as follows:

(1) The prevalence of AG-4 antibody is significantly higher in patients with cervical cancer (72.4%) ($x^2 = 160.7$; $p \ll 0.001$), CIS (63%) ($x^2 = 99.5$; $p \ll 0.001$) and dysplasia (49.6%) ($x^2 = 69.7$; $p \ll 0.001$) than in control women without cancer (11.7%); the response is specific for cervical cancer.

(2) Antibody to AG-4 reflects the progression of the neoplastic lesion. Thus, 92% of patients successfully treated by surgical procedures are virtually AG-4 negative whereas 96% of those with recurrent disease are AG-4 seropositive. On the other hand, some of the patients treated by radiation convert to AG-4 positivity after treatment, presumably due to antigen release from lysed tumor cells or release of antibody previously bound by the tumor cells. Furthermore, only 32.1% of patients diagnosed as mild dysplasia are AG-4 seropositive as compared to 52.2%, 56.5%, 61.3% and 85.7% of those with moderate dysplasia, marked dysplasia, CIS and Stage I invasive cancer, respectively (Table 7) (linear correlation coefficient $r = 0.64$). The frequency of AG-4 seropositivity, however, is significantly lower in patients with more advanced stages of invasive disease. This finding is consistent with the conclusion by Heise *et al.* that the lack of an AG-4 response is correlated with an increased risk of an unfavorable clinical outcome [105] and may reflect the immunodeficiency of patients with advanced cancer. Indeed, patients with advanced or recurrent cervical carcinoma display decreased delayed hypersensitivity responses, depressed erythrocyte rosette formation, a decreased number of total lymphocytes [106] and nonspecific lymphocytotoxic antibody [107]. The virus-specific antibody, primarily IgG, reflects a state of immune memory and is not affected by this immunological defect related to tumor burden.

(3) The loss in AG-4 reactivity at 4 to 24 weeks after surgery was similar

Table 7. AG-4 antibodies in patients with various stages of cervical anaplasia[a].

|  | No. assayed | AG-4 positive | |
| --- | --- | --- | --- |
|  |  | No. | % |
| Dysplasia |  |  |  |
| mild | 28 | 9 | 32.1 |
| moderate | 46 | 24 | 52.2 |
| marked | 62 | 35 | 56.5 |
| CIS | 75 | 46 | 61.3 |
| Invasive[b] |  |  |  |
| I | 35 | 30 | 85.7 |
| II | 17 | 9 | 59.2 |
| III | 24 | 6 | 20.8 |
| Total | 76 | 44 | 57.9 |
| Controls[c] | 264 | 31 | 11.7 |
| Cancer at other sites[d] | 78 | 6 | 7.7 |

[a] Sera collected once, at diagnosis and prior to treatment.
[b] Stage I: invasive cancer confined to the cervix.
Stage II: invasive cancer involving parametria (but not extending to the pelvic wall) or involving the upper two-thirds of the vagina.
Stage III: invasive cancer extending all the way out to the pelvic side wall or involving the lower third of the vagina.
[c] Frequency of AG-4 seropositivity is significantly higher ($p \ll 0.001$) in patients with dysplasia, CIS, and invasive cancer.
[d] Includes lung, stomach, pancreas, breast, ovary, endometrium, vulva, vagina, adenocarcinoma of the cervix, colon, kidney, prostate, bladder, nasopharynx, oropharynx. Positives are: endometrium (2), colon (1), nasopharynx (1), adenocarcinoma of the cervix (1), and oropharynx (1).

to that observed following primary HSV-2 infection and reflected the normal catabolic rate of the immunoglobulin following the removal of the source of antigen driving its synthesis.

Of the 209 patients with cervical dysplasia, CIS or invasive cancer studied prospectively, 152 were first assayed for AG-4 antibody prior to treatment, whereas the other 57 patients were entered into the study at least one year after they had been treated for cervical neoplasia. Eighty-seven of the 152 patients entered into the study prior to therapy converted from a state of AG-4 seropositivity prior to treatment to one of seronegativity thereafter. None developed recurrent disease during the follow-up interval. Twelve patients that were AG-4 seropositive at entry remained positive after treatment; seven of these (58.3%) had persistent neoplasm and 3 expired. Twenty patients were AG-4 seronegative at entry into the study and converted to positivity during the follow-up interval. Nine of these 20 patients converted to AG-4 seropositivity in conjunction with recurrence of cervical neoplasia.

Similar observations were made with respect to the 57 patients entered into the study after previous treatment for cervical neoplasia. In this series, 38 patients were entered as AG-4 seronegative. The largest proportion (26) remained seronegative throughout follow-up, consistent with the interpretation that seronegativity follows successful surgical treatment. Twelve converted to AG-4 seropositivity during the follow-up. Nine of the 12 developed recurrent disease and 4 expired. Nineteen patients were entered into the study as AG-4 seropositive. Eleven of these 19 patients (57.9%) had recurrent disease at which time they were positive for AG-4 antibody (Figure 5).

There are two salient features of this follow-up study. First, the majority of patients entered into the study prior to therapy were successfully treated and converted from a state of AG-4 seropositivity to one of seronegativity. Recurrent disease was not observed in any one of these 87 patients during the 6-year study interval. On the other hand, patients that remained AG-4 seropositive or converted to AG-4 seropositivity following treatment displayed some level or recurrent disease during the follow-up period. The second finding of this series that merits special attention is that nine patients entered into the study while free of neoplastic disease had herpetic

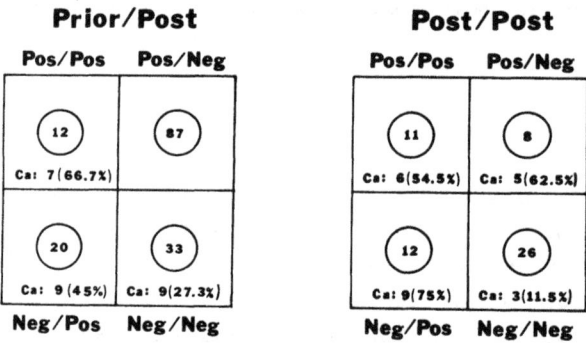

*Figure 5.* AG-4 seropositivity in patients with various degrees of cervical anaplasia studied prior to therapy and followed at 6-month intervals for 6 years (prior/post) or entered into the study at various intervals after treatment for cervical anaplasia and followed in a similar fashion (post/post). Pos/Neg: positive for AG-4 antibody at entry into the study converted to AG-4 seronegativity during follow-up. Pos/Pos: positive for AG-4 antibody at entry into the study remained AG-4 positive throughout study interval. Neg/Pos: negative for AG-4 antibody at study onset, converted to AG-4 seropositivity during follow-up. Neg/Neg: AG-4 seronegative at study onset and throughout follow-up. Ca: Recurrent disease defined as at least one abnormal Papanicolaou smear during follow-up.

cervicitis alone. During the study interval these patients developed cervical neoplasia preceded or accompanied by conversion to AG-4 seropositivity. One of them (No. 229) converted to AG-4 seropositivity 10-12 months after the diagnosis of cervical HSV-2. At that time, she was still considered cytologically and clinically normal. Seventeen months after her HSV-2 diagnosis, the patient remained AG-4 seropositive and a cytologic diagnosis of dysplasia was made. Two months thereafter, she was treated surgically for Stage I invasive cancer. By that time, the AG-4 antibody titer had increased significantly. In the two other patients (Nos. 646 and 613) entered into the study at the time of HSV-2 diagnosis, CIS and marked dysplasia were diagnosed within 5 and 6 months respectively (Figure 6).

The temporal relationship between the development of AG-4 antibody and clinical status was studied in patients with recurrent neoplasia. The data are summarized in Figure 7 for 5 patients in this category. Patient 369 was AG-4 seropositive at the time of hysterectomy for microinvasive cervical cancer. AG-4 antibody titers declined after operation and the patient was considered negative for tumor on both clinical and cytological grounds.

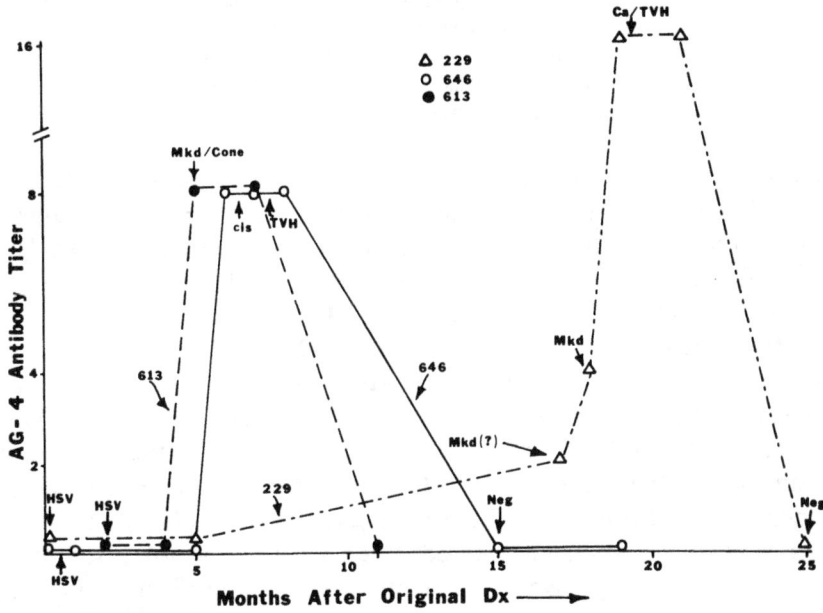

*Figure 6.* Temporal relationship of HSV infection and cervical anaplasia as reflected by the development of the AG-4 antibody. Patients (No. 229, 646, and 613), entered into the study at the time of diagnosis of recurrent HSV infection were AG-4 seronegative. AG-4 seropositivity preceded (No. 229) or coincided (Nos. 613 and 646) with the development of marked dysplasia (mkd), CIS or Stage I invasive cancer (Ca). It was lost following tumor removal whether by hysterectomy (TVH) or conization (Cone).

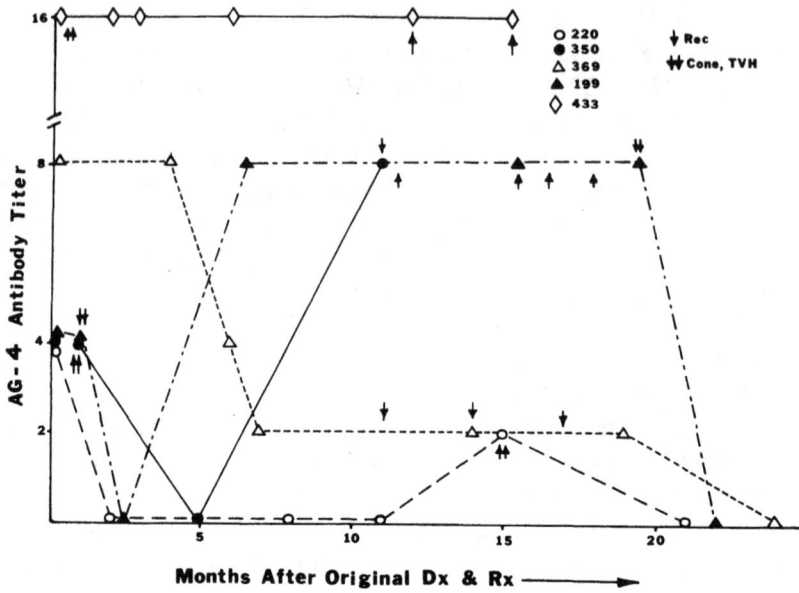

*Figure 7.* AG-4 antibody during follow-up of patients treated for cervical anaplasia. Patients entered into the study at time of diagnosis and surgical treatment, or 2–8 weaks prior to surgical treatment (↓↓), were AG-4 seropositive. Treatment resulted in antibody loss in all but one patient (No. 433). Recurrent disease (↓) was preceded (Nos. 369, 199, 433) or coincided (Nos. 220, 350) with a return in AG-4 seropositivity.

Approximately 7 months after surgery, when AG-4 antibody titers had reached relatively low levels, the humoral immune response plateaued and the patient remained AG-4 seropositive for approximately 1 year. During this interval her cytologic smears were consistently abnormal, at least moderate dysplasia. Significantly, five months later, the patient returned to the clinic with negative cytology and AG-4 antibody and both assays remained negative throughout the rest of the study period. Patient 199 was AG-4 seropositive at the time of histologic diagnosis for CIS. Therapeutic conization was followed by the disappearance of the AG-4 antibody. Six months after conization, the patient was AG-4 seropositive while clinically and cytologically free of tumor. Shortly thereafter, however, her cytologic examinations consistently revealed marked dysplasia while AG-4 antibody titers remained relatively high. She was again treated by conization (9 months after the original cone) and again converted to an AG-4 seronegative state. Since that time, she has been free of tumor on both clinical and cytological grounds and has remained AG-4 seronegative. Patient 433 was entered into the study at the time of diagnosis of Stage IIB cervical cancer with a high titer of AG-4 antibody. She was treated one month later by radical Wertheim hysterectomy and remained AG-4 seropositive despite negative clinical and cytological findings. One year after entry into the study, however, recurrent disease was diagnosed and she later expired with metastatic lesions.

## 5.2. Antibody to VP134 in patients with cervical cancers

A second cervical cancer-associated viral antigen is VP 134, an 'early' HSV-1 protein; its HSV-2 analog has a molecular weight of 143,000 daltons. VP 134 has been described in HSV-2 transformed cells and in cell lines established from cervical tumor biopsies [89]. IgG antibodies to VP 134 were identified in sera from cervical cancer patients but not in sera from patients with breast cancer or from normal women [108]. It is not clear whether these antibodies vary with the course of the disease.

## 5.3. AG-e: antigen-driven CMI response in patients with cervical neoplasia

AG-e (consisting of proteins ICP 12, ICP 14) is expressed in HSV-2 transformed cells (Section 3.1.2) and cervical tumor cells (Section 4.1); it induces a specific antigen-driven immune response in patients with cervical cancer. Thus [109], lymphocytes from 75% of patients with cervical dysplasia, CIS

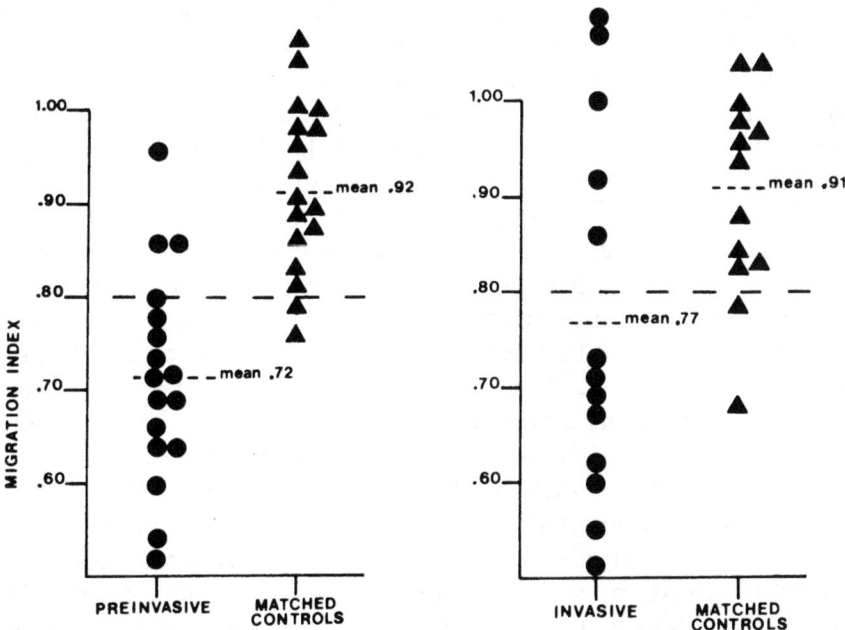

*Figure 8.* AG-e mediated leukocyte migration inhibition (LIF) in patients with dysplasia and CIS (preinvasive) or invasive cancer and their matched controls. Migration indices lower than 0.8 represent a positive response.

or invasive cancer, respond to AG-e in leukocyte migration inhibition (LIF), an antigen-driven effector cell CMI assay. This can be compared with responses of lymphocytes from 13% of matched control women without cancer ($p<0.01$) and from 16% of patients with other neoplasma (Figure 8). Patients with cervical cancer, as well as normal control women without cancer also have positive titers for IgG antibody to ICP 12 and ICP 14 by immunoprecipitation and SDS-acrylamide gel electrophoresis [18]. IgG antibody reflects a state of immune memory and does not vary with clinical status, in contrast to IgM, which may reflect an antigen-driven humoral response. It should be pointed out that Rivera *et al.* [110] have recently confirmed the ability of lymphoid cells from cervical cancer patients, but not controls, to specifically respond in LIF assay against HSV-2 antigens; the identity of these antigen(s) is still unclear.

## 5.4. *Immune response to miscellaneous viral antigens in patients with cervical neoplasia*

Numerous other studies have demonstrated that immune responses to as yet unidentified HSV-2 antigens play a role in the natural history of cervical cancer. Thus, reminiscent of the AG-4 responses, virus-specific non-IgG antibody (predominantly IgM) to an unidentified HSV-2 antigen, has been described in 8% of women with normal cervical smears compared to 20%, 41% and 74% of women with dysplasia, CIS, and invasive cancer, respectively. Most of these women lost their IgM antibodies following irradiation or hysterectomy, while this treatment did not modify the proportion of women with IgG antibodies to the virus [111]. It would be particularly important to identify the antigen that induces this response and compare it to AG-4.

In another study [112], sera from 71.5% of cervical cancer patients but only 16% of sera from patients with other malignancies, were shown to precipitate two 'early' viral proteins designated ICSP 8 (MW: 172,000) and ICSP 15 (MW: 128,000) by SDS-acrylamide gel electrophoresis of the precipitates. On the other hand, sera from HSV convalescent patients precipitated eight viral proteins among which one, ICSP 11, (MW: 151,000) was most prominent. Comparisons of ICSP 8 to our ICP 10/AG-4, and of our ICP 12 to ICSP 11 is warranted, particularly in view of the $\pm 10\%$ difference in molecular weights reported by various laboratories. Serum antibodies to 'immediate early' antigens were also described in patients with cervical cancer but not in control women, using the anti-complement immunofluorescence assay with cells infected in presence of cycloheximide or hydroxyurea [113].

Women with progressive cervical lesions display decreasing levels of neutralizing antibody to HSV-2, and lack activity to presently uncharacterized antigen(s) on the surface of the HSV-2 infected cells [114]. More recently, it has also been reported that virus-specific ADCC activity is lower in cervical cancer patients with advanced disease than in disease-free patients [115]. An increased frequency (27.8%) of serum IgA antibodies to HSV-2, and significantly higher serum IgA levels (308.5+4 WHO units/ml) were observed in patients with cervical cancer as compared to normal women (3.6%; 189±73.2 WHO units/ml [116]. More recently, Gilman et al. [117] assayed sera from 105 patients with cervical cancer and from 231 matched controls in immunoprecipitation/SDS acrylamide gel electrophoresis against extracts of HSV-2 infected cells. Comparison of the precipitates obtained from those sera that were HSV-2 positive in neutralization revealed that only one protein (MW: 38,000) was preferentially precipitated by sera from cancer patients matched to the controls for sexually related variables. Finally, complement fixing antibodies to HSV-TAA (Section 4.1) were detected in the sera from a higher proportion of patients with cervical carcinoma than from controls. Consistent with the conclusion that this is a virus-induced cell-coded protein, a similarly high frequency of HSV-TAA antibody was also observed in sera from patients with cancer of the head and neck. HSV-TAA was also shown to induce a delayed hypersensitivity skin reaction in patients with cervical cancer but not breast cancer and a significant ($p<0.005$) inhibition of the migration of leukocytes from patients with cervical cancer but not from controls [118].

## 6. FREQUENCY OF EXPOSURE TO HSV-2 AND SPECIFICITY OF THE ASSOCIATION TO CERVICAL CANCER

Case control epidemiologic studies designed to identify antibody to HSV-2 as an indication of previous infection with the virus, provided the bulk of the early evidence associating HSV-2 with cervix cancer. A higher prevalence of antibodies to HSV-2 was found among women with cervical cancer than among control women; with very few exceptions, the differences were statistically significant. These differences were apparent regardless of the population studied, the epidemiologic study design, or the method used for antibody assay. Whether the results were expressed as the percent of women positive for antibody to HSV-2 or as the mean titers of HSV-2 antibody, these differences persisted (Table 8). Although these studies were extensively reviewed [119, 120], it seems worthwhile to critically consider the data within the context of the unified concept of causality (Table 1).

As discussed in Section 2.1, studies designed to identify antibodies to HSV-2 must circumvent the close antigenic similarity between HSV-2 and HSV-1. In all the studies summarized in Table 8, the assays involved quan-

*Table 8.* Summary of findings on prevalence of HSV-2 antibody among cervical cancer patients and controls.

| Location | Serologic[a] method | Antibodies to HSV-2 | | | | Reference |
|---|---|---|---|---|---|---|
| | | Cases | | Controls | | |
| | | % | Titer | % | Titer | |
| Mayland | KN | 100 | | 67 | | Aurelian et al., 1970 [165] |
| Texas | KN | 71.1 | | 21.6 | | Rawls et al., 1969 [166] |
| Texas | MN  black | 80 | | 52 | | Adam et al., 1972 [167] |
| | white | 54 | | 23 | | |
| West Virginia | MN | 51.9 | | 23.3 | | Rawls et al., 1973 [119] |
| Georgia | MN | 82.7 | | 34.6 | | Nahmias et al., 1970 [51] |
| Massachusetts | MN | 42 | | 17.7 | | Catalano and Johnson, 1971 [127] |
| Illinois | KN | 48 | | 18 | | Plummer and Masterson, 1971 [168] |
| Cali, Columbia[b] | IF | 90 | | 68 | | Munoz et al., 1975 [169] |
| England[c] | KN | — | 0.96 | — | 0.41 | Skinner et al., 1971 [170] |
| Denmark | KN | 85.2 | | 47 | | Vestergaard et al., 1972 [171] |
| Belgium | KN | 83.3 | | 32.6 | | Sprecher-Goldberger, 1976 [172] |
| Sweden | MHA | 81 | | 17 | | Christensen and Epsmark, 1976 [173] |
| Yugoslavia | MN | 40 | | 25 | | Kessler et al., 1974 [174] |
| Hungary | NEUT | 50 | | 9 | | Pacsa et al., 1975 [175] |
| Czechoslovakia | NEUT | 50 | | 21 | | Janda et al., 1973 [176] |
| Israel | NEUT | 15 | | 7 | | Menczer et al., 1975 [177] |
| Uganda | MN | 81 | | 71 | | Adam et al., 1974 [137] |
| Nigeria | IF | 71 | | 11 | | Adelusi et al., 1975 [178] |
| South Africa | KN | 87 | | 64 | | Freedman et al., 1974 [135] |
| Taiwan[d] | MN | 61 | | 0 | | Kao et al. 1974 [179] |
| Japan[e] | KN | 75 | 1.41 | 71 | 0.61 | Kawana et al., 1974 [180] |
| West Indies | CF | 91 | | 77 | | Ory et al., 1974 [181] |
| England | CF | 80 | | 12 | | Skinner et al., 1977 [122] |
| India | IHA | 64.5 | 2.64 | 36.2 | 1.89 | Seyth et al., 1978 [182] |

[a] Neutralization kinetics (KN), microneutralization (MN), indirect immunofluorescence (IF), neutralization in culture tubes (NEUT), mixed hamadsorption (MHA), complement fixation (CF), indirect hemagglutination (IHA).
[b] Percent with antibody titers ≥ 1/160.
[c] Antibody titers expressed as mean constant of neutralization K.
[d] Percent with antibody titers ≥ 1/32.
[e] Titers expressed as constant of neutralization were calculated by Rawls and Adam [166].

titation of antibody activity to both viruses and comparison of the relative activities against HSV-1 and HSV-2. The specific serologic assay and the criteria used for establishing HSV-2 seropositivity differed, however, thus explaining the variation observed among the results of different studies. Indeed, in a direct comparison between a specific modification of the kinetics of neutralization assay and the microneutralization assay, only 41 of 108 sera testing positively in the former assay were positive in the latter assay. Eighteen of 22 sera (81.8%) testing negative in neutralization kinetics, however, were also negative in microneutralization [121], suggesting that the former assay is more sensitive in differentiating between antibody to HSV-1 and antibody to HSV-2. Consistent with this finding, analysis of the data in the literature indicates that in only one study in which the kinetics of neutralization was used, did less than 72% of the cancer cases have antibody to HSV-2. In 7 studies the mean of positive results using the kinetics of neutralization was 79.6%. Thirteen studies utilized other neutralization tests; and in only three was the percentage of cancer cases with HSV-2 antibodies greater than 70%, with the mean for these studies being 50.8% [119].

In order to overcome these difficulties, Skinner and co-workers [122] prepared type-specific antigen by adsorption of general antigen with heterologous immune sera until all type-common immunoprecipitating or complement fixing material was eliminated. This type-specific antigen was used in complement fixation with sera from cases of cervical cancer and controls. The prevalence of type-2 specific antibody in patients with invasive cervical carcinoma was 80%, significantly higher ($p<0.001$) than the 12% found in controls. Case control differences for patients with CIS and dysplasia were less striking but still statistically significant. As could be expected from the usual chronology of HSV-1 and HSV-2 antibody acquisition, it was uncommon to find HSV-2 specific antibodies in absence of co-existing type-1 specific antibodies. However, HSV-1 specific antibody in the absence of HSV-2 specific antibody, was identified more frequently in the control group than in the carcinoma group.

A significantly higher rate of exposure to HSV-2 in cervical cancer patients than in controls was also demonstrated in CMI assays (such as lymphocyte blastogenesis) reflecting the development of immune memory. Here again, criteria for HSV-2 specific response had to be developed. One such criterion was expressed as the ratio of $^3$H-thymidine label incorporated in presence of HSV-2 to that incorporated in presence of HSV-1 antigen [123]. Using this procedure, Smith and co-workers [124] reported that the blastogenic response (HSV-2/HSV-1 = $104\pm44$) was virtually identical in cancer cases and in patients with an established history of recurrent HSV-2 disease ($132\pm36$), whereas it was significantly lower in matched controls ($67\pm41$) and in patients with an established history of HSV-1 ($38\pm13$)

lesions. HSV seronegative individuals who were never exposed to either HSV serotype were also unresponsive in lymphocyte blastogenesis. Similar conclusions were reached by Thiry et al. [111], using an extract of HSV-2 transformed hamster cells as an antigen. She found positive results using the lymphoproliferation assay in 40% of patients with cervical carcinoma compared to 2% of normal women. The frequency of the response was intermediate in cases of dysplasia and CIS. Significant differences ($p<0.0001$) were also found between normal subjects and patients with cervical dysplasia or carcinoma, when lymphocytes were stimulated by HSV-2, but not by HSV-1 virions.

In conclusion, although presently available data probably underestimate the level of HSV-2 seropositivity and virus-specific immune memory (reflected as CMI responsiveness) in various population groups, these epidemiologic studies have demonstrated a significantly higher rate of exposure to HSV-2 in patients with cervical cancer than in control women. The neoplasm was not associated with a humoral or cellular response to other viruses including HSV-1, cytomegalovirus and adenovirus [125, 129]. Furthermore, there was no association between the antibody to HSV-2 and cancers at other sites [51, 85, 104, 108, 109, 119, 120].

## 7. CERVICAL CANCER: INCIDENCE IN HSV-2 INFECTED WOMEN

The '*herpesvirus hypothesis*' predicts that women with HSV-2 infections are at higher risk of developing cervical cancer than are noninfected ones. Supporting this prediction, an increased risk of subsequent cervical neoplasia was reported in patients with cytologically detected HSV-2 when compared to women without evidence of HSV-2 infection: Naib et al. [126] calculated that the rate of cervical neoplasia in patients with genital herpes detected cytologically was 15-fold higher than that found in control women, and at least 6-fold higher than that found in a general hospital population. Catalano and Johnson [127] demonstrated that the risk of cervical cancer was increased in HSV-2 infected patients; they found that 5 of 14 women who developed CIS had HSV-2 antibodies, compared to 2 of 20 women in their control group. In a larger scale prospective epidemiological study (Section 8), the rate of cervical dysplasia was found to be 8-fold greater in patients with evidence of prior HSV-2 infection than in a control group without HSV-2 disease [128]. These values are in agreement with the relative risk values calculated from retrospective epidemiologic studies by Thomas and Rawls [129], ranging between 2.03–17.45 for invasive cancer; 1.94–7.91 for CIS and 0.7–7.58 for dysplasia.

8. TEMPORAL ASSOCIATION

Data generated in retrospective and prospective studies support the prediction that infection with HSV-2 precedes the development of the earliest detectable precancerous lesions. Using sensitive serologic assays, a significantly higher prevalence of antibodies to HSV-2 was demonstrated in patients with CIS or dysplasia than in matched controls (Section 6; Table 8). Thomas and Rawls [129] found that the relative risk of CIS in those patients with evidence of prior HSV-2 infections was inversely related to probable age at risk of first exposure to HSV-2, suggesting that virus infection at an early age precedes the onset of the cervical neoplasia. Rare studies, in which statistically significant differences between women with pre-invasive cervical lesions and controls were not observed with respect to the occurrence of HSV-2 antibodies, used relatively insensitive assays [119, 120]. A prospective study of 56,418 hospitalized women [130] established that the peak age for detection of cervical HSV-2 infections was 10 to 11 years earlier than the peak age at diagnosis of 235 cases of CIS and was 28 years earlier than the peak age at diagnosis of 220 cases of invasive carcinoma [130]. The average age reported for patients with a cervical lesion was: herpetic infection – 20 years; dysplasia – 25 years; CIS – 31 years; invasive cancer – 48 years. Similarly, in a prospective follow-up study of 872 women with herpetic infection and 562 HSV seronegative controls, Nahmias et al. [128] found that the rate of cervical dysplasia was 2-fold higher and that of CIS was 8-fold higher, in the herpes patients than in the control group. Consistent with the conclusion that HSV-2 infection precedes the development of cervical neoplasia, Pacsa et al. [131] found HSV-2 antigens in cervical cells from 36 to 530 (6.8%) normal women. In our own longitudinal ICP 10/AG-4 study (Section 5.1), we identified 4 women in whom cervical infection with HSV-2, diagnosed by cytopathology, seroconversion, and virus isolation, preceded the development of the cervical neoplasia by six months to three years [129].

9. BIOLOGIC AND EPIDEMIOLOGIC SENSE: HSV-2 AND THE NATURAL HISTORY OF CERVICAL CANCER

HSV-2 biologically and epidemiologically fits the carcinogenic model in a convincing fashion. An obligatory, intracellular parasite (an intuitively appealing requirement for carcinogenic potential), the virus causes latent infections characterized by virus persistence in the infected host (Section 2.1). Since cancer is a means of cellular immortality, the propensity of the virus to persist in its natural host without causing cell killing is an important prerequisite for carcinogenicity.

## 9.1. Cervical cancer: a sexually transmitted disease

Since the original observations of Rigoni-Stern over a century ago [132], it has been repeatedly demonstrated that factors associated with coitus and marriage play a role in the etiology of cervical cancer [121]. Mean age at first coitus is lower and the proportion initiating coitus at an early age is higher among cervical cancer cases than among controls. Similarly, cervical cancer patients have had more coital partners on the average, than other women. Finally, the proportion of cervical cancer claiming virginity is essentially nil, in contrast to control populations. Rotkin [133] focused attention upon coital onset in mid-adolescence as a possible initiating factor in cervical carcinogenesis, posing a hypothesis involving: 'the female at risk as the host, the male coital partner as the donor, and the intervening vector as his contribution.' Data from six studies on contraceptive practices in women with cervical cancer provide indirect support of this hypothesis by demonstrating that the use of barrier methods of contraception, such as the condom, is less common among cervical cancer patients than among controls [121]. However, direct evidence for the male role in the transmission of cervical cancer was provided by Kessler [50], who sought to answer the basic question: 'Is the risk of developing cervical cancer increased among wives of men who at some other time in their lives were married to other women who developed cervical cancer?' At the time of publication, 4178 probands with cervical cancer had been identified. A total of 726 husbands of these probands had been studied and 625 second wives traced. Among these, 14 second wives with cervical cancer were detected compared to a total of 4 cancers among the control wives matched for demographic and marital characteristics. The difference is highly significant and it confirms the suggestion that cervical cancer behaves as an infectious disease, in regard to transmission.

## 9.2. Promiscuity and the association of HSV-2 with cervical cancer

The evidence that patients with cervical cancer have higher prevalence of antibody to HSV-2 than controls, suggest the independent association of cervical cancer and HSV-2 with promiscuity, the *promiscuity hypothesis* [134]. According to this hypothesis, HSV-2 is not etiologically related to cervical cancer but rather represents another marker of promiscuity. Presently available data do not support this hypothesis. Cancer cases and controls did not differ with respect to other sexually transmitted diseases such as syphilis and trichomoniasis, although the frequency of HSV-2 antibodies was significantly higher in cancer cases than in controls [134]. Similar results were obtained by Freedman *et al.* [135] and Schneweis *et al.* [136]. Using another approach to study the interrelationship of sexual behavior, HSV-2 and cervix cancer, Adam *et al.* [137] have determined the influence of age at first coitus, age at first pregnancy, age at first marriage, number of marriages, and number of sexual partners on the distribution of antibodies to HSV-2 among cancer cases and controls. An excess of antibody to HSV-2 among women with cervical cancer was found when one or all of these factors were included in the statistical analysis; the greatest relative risk (4-fold) was associated with antibodies to HSV-2.

In a recent study [129], sera from 75 women with CIS, 84 women with squamous dysplasia, and 132 controls, were analyzed for HSV-2 antibodies by the chromium release complement-dependent cytotoxicity assay. CIS and severe dysplasia were more frequently associated with HSV-2 both in terms of the increased frequency of positivity and the high titers of antibody. Consistent with the belief that the association between HSV-2 and cervical neoplasia is not the result of two co-variables of promiscuity, previous exposure to the virus remained a relative risk of about 2 after adjustment for 12 potentially confounding variables in a multiple linear regression equation. After multiple regression adjustments, the presence of HSV-2 antibodies was the only variable that was independently related to CIS ($p<0.05$). The authors interpreted these observations as supportive of a causal relationship between HSV-2 and CIS, and indicative of the involvement of HSV-2 in the genesis of those dysplastic lesions that appear to be CIS precursors [76-78].

*9.3. The male role*

Kessler's studies on the high risk male (Section 9.1) have confirmed the hypothesis that the male plays a distinct role in the etiology of cervical cancer. Assuming that the male is a reservoir of HSV-2 infections, and that the vas deferens is a primary site for successful virus isolation (Section 2.3), it follows that HSV-2 should be isolated from sperm or seminal fluid from sexual partners of cervical cancer patients at a rate significantly higher than that in sexual partners of normal control women. Furthermore, female partners of vasectomy patients should be at a lower risk of developing cervical cancer. However, it should be pointed out that the latter prediction is not restricted to HSV-2. It also applies to an alternative theory consistent with the male role in cervical carcinogenesis that posits the spermatozoan as the most likely cervical carcinogen [138].

Kunkel *et al.* [139] found a significantly higher prevalence of antibody to HSV-2 in husbands of cervical cancer than control subjects, and the risk of cervical cancer has recently been shown to be significantly lower (4.9-fold) in women whose husbands had had vasectomies [140]. Furthermore, in a preliminary study designed to verify the premise that HSV-2 could be isolated with higher frequency from coital partners of cervical cancer patients than controls, single ejaculates obtained from coital partners of 2 patients with cervical cancer and 8 randomly selected controls without cancer, were assayed for infectious virus and viral antigens. HSV-2 and viral antigen were detected in the spermatozoa from the coital partners of the cervical carcinoma partners but not in those of the coital partners of the control women [141]. Although final conclusions must await the results of further studies, the data are consistent with an asymptomatic carrier state in coital partners of patients with cervical cancer in whom infectious HSV-2 appears to persist in the spermatozoa, possibly as a chronic low grade infection (Section 2.1). From the standpoint of the *'herpesvirus hypothesis'*, virus replication in the spermatozoa is not essential, since the transmission by direct contact with infected tissue or seminal fluid is efficient. The finding of virus in spermatozoa or seminal fluid, however, is consistent with the relatively high rate of virus isolation from vas deferens specimens obtained from asymptomatic males and the reduced risk of cervical cancer in women whose husbands have had vasectomies [140]. This finding also supports the alternative hypothesis that the spermatozoan is the cervical carcinogen [138].

## 10. CO-FACTORS

In the previous sections we have considered the *'herpesvirus hypothesis'* to the exclusion of possible co-factors. Little, if any, information is presently available on co-carcinogens. These could act at both the *'initiation'* and *'promotion/maintenance'* phase of the tumorigenic process. Endocrine factors, spermatozoan DNA or basic proteins, immunologic imbalance, genetic and/or physiologic defects or infection with other viruses qualify as potential co-factors and have been discussed in detail by Aurelian [141]. In this context, a virus that has recently received particular attention as a possible cervical co-carcinogen is the papillomavirus. Indeed, Syrijanen [142] reported the co-existence of condylomatous lesions with cervical dysplasia. The general consensus, however, is that condylomatous lesions are only misdiagnosed as dysplasia. In a recent study using the immunoperoxidase staining with a broadly cross-reactive antiserum of the group, human papillomavirus antigen was detected in the nuclei of 21 of 34 (60%) condylomata while all other lesions including dysplasia, CIS or carcinoma were negative [143]. Similar results were reported by Woodruff *et al.* [144], who found papillomavirus antigen in 3 of 3 biopsies from women diagnosed as condyloma/atypia as compared to 3 of 8 women diagnosed as dysplasia and 2 of 4 normal women. Although the relative risk of mild dysplasia was found to be increased with a positive history of cytomegalovirus, adenovirus, trichomonas vaginalis, mycoplasma pneumoniae or HSV-2, the risk of

CIS was increased only in the presence of previous infection with HSV-2 [129]. The data suggest that, consistent with its frequent reversibility, mild dysplasia is a nonspecific response of the cervical epithelium to various chronic inflammatory stimuli apparently including papillomavirus; the significant data factor for CIS is a history of HSV-2 infection. Significantly, in a 3-year study, the rate of progression of CIS and invasive cancer was found to be identical in women with lesions diagnosed as both dysplasia and condyloma, as compared to women diagnosed as having dysplasia alone [145]. This finding suggests that condyloma does not increase the risk or accelerate the progression to CIS or invasive cancer.

## 11. 'THE HERPESVIRUS HYPOTHESIS' AND THE CLINICIAN

To the clinician, the *herpesvirus hypothesis* holds the promise of unique markers for cancer screening, diagnosis and treatment evaluation. The ultimate aim of automation of cervical cytology is the development of cancer screening procedures that are reliable, efficient, reproducible, and of low cost. As medical instrumentation becomes increasingly sophisticated, devices capable of better fulfilling these needs will be developed. However, the major problem for cervical cancer screening is the relative infrequency of atypical cells in abnormal specimens, which leads to false-negative results. Progress in the field indicates that this problem could be best resolved by the development of highly specific and sensitive markers of premalignant cellular changes. Such markers should be associated with the premalignant lesion with sufficient frequency to be reliable, and should have a clearly understood biological basis. The *herpesvirus hypothesis* provides the solution to this dilemma by demonstrating that viral antigens are expressed in neoplastic cervical cells but not in normals. In a recent study with the broader specificity serum (anti-AG-e), exfoliated cervical cells from 18 patients with dysplasia, CIS or invasive cancer, were stained in triplicate with antisera to antigen AG-e and its two constituent proteins ICP 12 and ICP 14 (Section 4.1). The respective pre-immune sera were used as controls. Staining, primarily cytoplasmic, was observed with all immune sera but not with pre-immune controls but only in the neoplastic cells. The patterns of reactivity with the three antisera differed. Some patients preferentially recognized one or the other of the anti-ICP sera. All but two patients had atypical cells, however, that reacted with the broader specificity serum (anti-AG-e) [87]. Consistent with this finding, our recent data indicate that the antiserum prepared against total viral antigens identifies the highest proportion of patients with earliest premalignant changes (Table 9). This represents the most promising marker for screening and potential automation. The

*Table 9.* Immunofluorescent staining of anaplastic cervical cells from patients with various cytopathologic diagnoses.

| Cytopathologic diagnosis | No. | % Patients staining[a] with | |
|---|---|---|---|
| | | Anti-HSV-2 | Anti-AG-e |
| Squamous metaplasia | 12 | 25.0 | 4.0 |
| *Dysplasia* | | | |
|   mild | 44 | 61.3 | 56.8 |
|   moderate, moderate-marked | 26 | 76.9 | 57.7 |
|   marked | 14 | 85.7 | 50.0 |
| Cancer | 23 | 95.8 | 87.5 |
| Normal | 190 | 0.1 | 0 |
| Chlamydia/condyloma | 8 | 0 | 0 |
| HSV cervicitis | 6 | 100 | 100 |

[a] Pre-immune sera are nonreactive. Staining is restricted to anaplastic cells. Normal and inflammatory cells do not stain.

reactivity with all the HSV antisera is virus-specific. Therefore, pre-immune sera do not stain atypical cells; the reactivity is abrogated by adsorption with extracts of HSV-2 infected but not mock-infected cells, and staining with the HSV antisera is observed in HSV-2 infected cervical cells. That the cells staining for HSV antigens are indeed atypical was demonstrated by marking the fluorescence positive cells, restaining with Papanicolaou stain, relocating them with a microslide Field Finder and classifying them by an independent cytopathologist. The results of these studies demonstrated that in 88% of the patients, the majority (90.6%) of the fluorescent cells were neoplastic (Figure 9). In 1.5% of the patients, the fluorescent cells were inflammatory and in rare cases (10–20%), some of the fluorescent positive cells (20.6%) were classified as metaplastic [86, 150].

The potential use of the HSV antigens in cancer screening was further explored in two independent efforts. In one of these, a blind study was designed to determine the ability of the immunofluorescent staining to accurately predict the results of cytologic or histologic diagnoses. A high degree of correlation was observed. Fifteen of 16 fluorescent antibody (FA) positive patients (93.8%) were diagnosed as having at least dysplasia and conversely only 1 of the 17 patients (5.9%) diagnosed by cytologic criteria as having dysplasia, was FA negative. Of the 10 patients with FA negative cells, eight were considered normal, inflammatory, benign disease or condylomatous and only one was atypical. Correlation was impossible in one case due to technical difficulties. Correlation with routine diagnostic cytopathology was

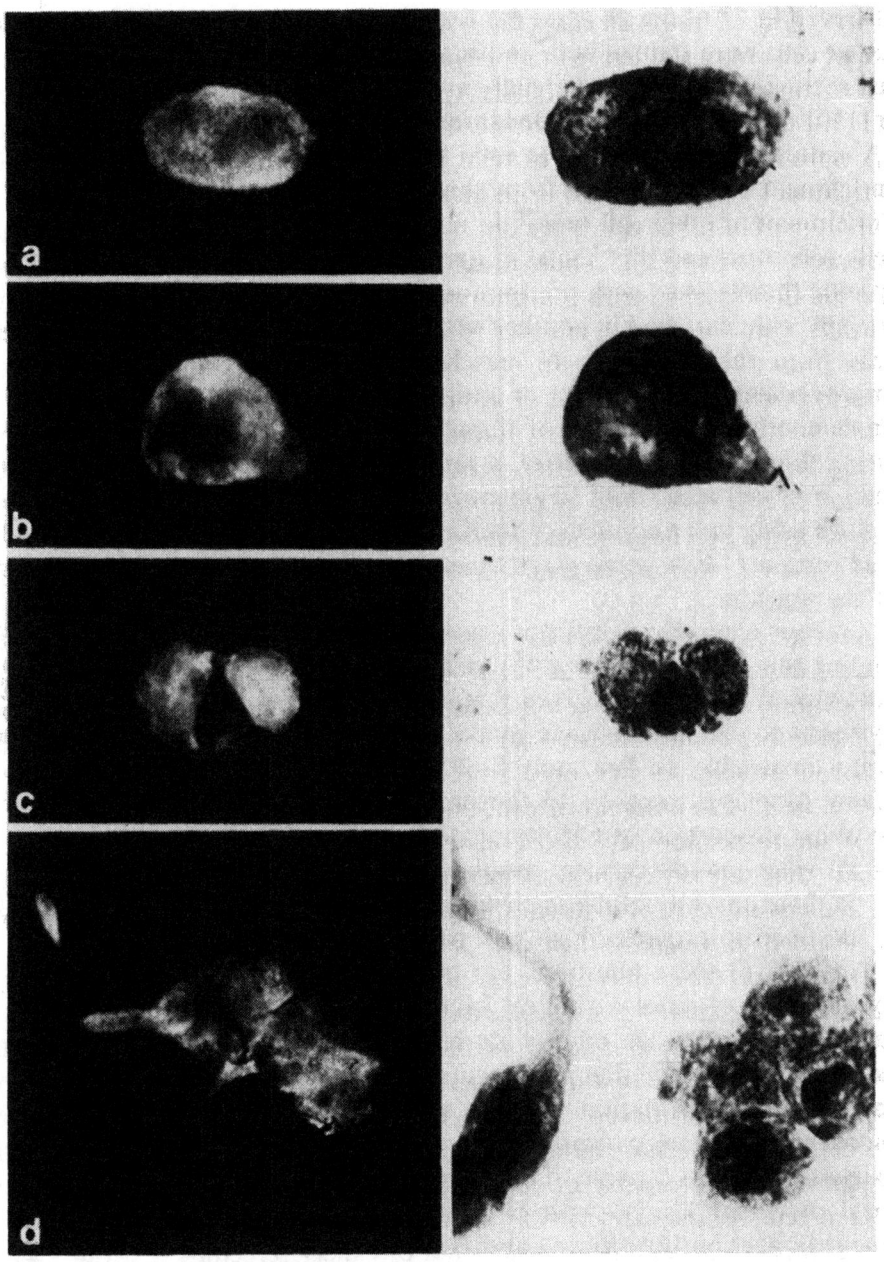

*Figure 9.* Cell by cell analysis of cells stained by indirect immunofluorescence with antiserum to AG-e (left) and restained by the Papanicolaou technique (right). (a) Cell from patient with mild dysplasia ($\times 800$). (b) Cell from patient with moderate dysplasia ($\times 800$). (c) Cells from patient with CIS ($\times 480$). (d) Cells from patient diagnosed as invasive cancer ($\times 800$).

observed in 22 of the 26 cases (84.6%) studied in this series [87]. In another series, cells were stained with antisera to total viral antigens and analyzed by cell sorting with the commercially available fluorescence activated cell sorter [150] (FACS II, Becton, Dickinson). Although the data are preliminary, FA staining with antiserum to total HSV-2 antigens resulted in the specific enrichment of atypical cells from abnormal specimens in a selected window. Enrichment of other cell types did not occur and the enrichment in atypical cells was virus-specific. Thus, in one patient who displayed low-level nonspecific fluorescence with pre-immune serum atypical cells staining nonspecifically were enriched in another window while specifically staining atypical cells from this patient were enriched in the correct window. A further improvement in enrichment of antigen-positive cells could be achieved by implementing a parameter of fluorescence per unit area on the machine. Using fluorescence and scatter, a ratio of fluorescence over some approximation of cell area could be obtained for each cell. Such studies, as well as studies using two fluorescence markers (viz. viral antigens and total nucleic acid content [146]), could greatly increase the resolving and screening power of the machine.

Another clinically significant aspect of the '*herpesvirus hypothesis*' is the finding that AG-4 seropositivity reflects the growth of the cervical tumor. Although it is generally agreed that cervical neoplasia runs the gamut from dysplasia to CIS and invasive cancer, progression from one level to the next is not invariable. In fact, only 5–20% of mild dysplasias and 40% of the severe dysplasias progress to cancer [76–78]. Several questions remain:
— What proportion of CIS lesions eventually become invasive?
— At what rate do cervical dysplasias progress to CIS or invasive?
— Is there any way of distinguishing between premalignant lesions that are destined to progress (high risk patient) and those which are not?

Answers to these questions are not readily available. The diagnosis of dysplasia necessitates a surgical excision which may remove the lesion in question or otherwise modify its biologic behavior. It seems reasonable, however, to conclude that if a precursor lesion is indeed destined to undergo malignant transformation whereas another is not, the two types may be biochemically, immunologically or otherwise distinguishable. In theory, the existence of a test capable of differentiating between these two types of cervical precursor lesions with or without invasive potential could have a major impact on the efficacy and yield of cancer screening programs when combined with exfoliative cytology. For example, if a patient's initial smear is classified as inconclusive, atypical or suggestive of neoplasia, the physician may not be certain as to his course of action. He may wish to observe the patient for a period of time, obtain repeat cytologic smears, and re-examine her later. However, should the woman be unreliable, transient or potentially noncompliant, he may feel constrained to take a biopsy or perform conization earlier than is his usual practice. Improvement in the diagnostic precision of the initial cytologic smear could, when applied to precancerous lesions, prevent unnecessary procedures and lead to more rational clinical management. These issues become particularly relevant in our present-day cost-efficient and consumer-oriented society, in which the cost of the cytologic procedure compared with its effectiveness (cost/benefit ratio) and the possible increase in morbidity associated with mass screening are loudly-voiced criticisms.

The potential use of AG-4 serology as an adjunct to exfoliative cytology was examined for 15 patients whose cytologic reports were inconsistent. In all but one case (Table 10), AG-4 serology correlated well with the absence of neoplasia in subsequent hysterectomy specimens. This could be due to the fact that the surgical excision of the biopsy itself was curative; alternatively, it could reflect the AG-4 negative status of atypical lesions that are not premalignant. Presently available data do not differentiate between these

Table 10. Correlation between AG-4 seropositivity and pathologic diagnosis.

| Patient No. | Initial Cytology/Bx. | AG-4[a] | Subsequent Cone (TVH, TAH) |
|---|---|---|---|
| 413 | Dysplasia (mo.) | – | CC, SM |
| 450 | Dysplasia (mkd.) | – | Atypia of atrophy |
| 473 | Dysplasia (mkd.) | – | Condyloma |
| 521 | Dysplasia (mo.) | | CC, SM |
| 541 | Dysplasia (mkd.) | – | CC, SM |
| 576 | Dysplasia | | CC, SM |
| 578 | Dysplasia (mkd.) | | CC, SM |
| 592 | CIS | – | Atypia of viral origin |
| 597 | Dysplasia | – | CC |
| 106A | SM | 4 | CIS |
| 679 | Inconclusive | 8 | CC, SM |
| 724 | Dysplasia (mo.) | – | CC, SM |
| 752 | Dysplasia (mo.) | – | CC, SM |
| 559 | Dysplasia (mo.) | – | CC, SM |
| 732 | Dysplasia (mo.) | – | CC, SM |

TVH = total vaginal hysterectomy.
TAH = total abdominal hysterectomy.
CC = chronic cervicitis.
SM = squamous metaplasia.
CIS = carcinoma *in situ*.

[a] Antibody titer expressed as the reciprocal of the highest serum dilution that fixes ≥10% complement.

two interpretations for most of the patients studied in this series. The exception are patients No. 450, 473, and 592, whose AG-4 seronegativity was associated with an unrelated diagnosis, and patient No. 106A, whose AG-4 seropositivity proved to be an early warning of neoplastic disease in a patient diagnosed with squamous metaplasia (Table 10).

Table 11. Correlation between AG-4 seropositivity and clinical status post treatment for cervical anaplasia.

| Patient No. | | Initial Diagnosis[a] | AG-4[b] | Subsequent Diagnosis[c] |
|---|---|---|---|---|
| 194 (post rad.) | | Dysplasia (mild) | 16 | Metastatic Ca. |
| 221 (post cone) | | Inconclusive | 2 | Mod. dysplasia |
| 350 (post cone) | 5/76 | Dysplasia (mild) | 4 | CIS |
| | 6/76 | Negative | 4 | |
| | 10/77 | Inconclusive | 4 | |
| | | 3/78 Recurrent (?) | 8 | Dysplasia (mild) |
| 215 (post rad.) | 5/76 | Negative | 4 | |
| | 7/76 | Negative | 4 | |
| | | 1/77 Expired | | Metastatic disease |
| 340 (post rad.) | 5/76 | Negative | 0 | |
| | 9/76 | Negative | 2 | |
| | | 5/77 Recurrent (?) | 2 | Vulvar CIS |
| 490 (post TVH) | 8/76 | Negative | 4 | |
| | 9/76 | Negative | 8 | |
| | 4/77 | Negative | 4 | |
| | | 3/78 Recurrent (?) | 4 | Dysplasia |
| 449 (post rad.) | 7/76 | Negative | 4 | |
| | | 7/76 Recurrent (?) | 8 | |
| | | 9/76 Recurrent | 16 | Liver metastases |
| | | 12/76 Expired | | |
| 219 (post rad.) | 5/76 | Negative | 0 | |
| | 2/77 | Negative | 2 | |
| | 1/78 | Negative | 4 | ? |
| | 9/79 | Negative | 16 | |

[a] Clinical, cytology and/or histology.
[b] Titer expressed as reciprocal of highest serum dilution that fixes ≥10% complement.
[c] Clinical, histology, exploratory.
Post rad. = 1–5 years after treatment by radiation for invasive carcinoma.
Post cone = 1 year after treatment by conization.
Post TVH = 1 year after treatment by total vaginal hysterectomy.
ND = Not done.

If AG-4 serology proves to be a diagnostic adjunct to exfoliative cytology, women showing suggestive exfoliate findings without AG-4 antibodies could be reassured and seen less frequently. This physician could direct more of his time and attention to those patients who are at considerably greater risk of developing cervical cancer. The advantage of such an approach in terms of lowering the cost while still retaining all the benefits of the screening program and reducing unnecessary morbidity associated with screening is obvious.

AG-4 testing has another potential clinical benefit serving as a simple method for monitoring the therapeutic procedure for patients with dysplasia, CIS and early invasive cancer. This conclusion is exemplified by the data summarized in Table 11 for a number of patients followed prospectively. Thus, patient 215 was considered clinically negative for 12 months while AG-4 seropositive, but she died with metastatic disease. Patient 340 was considered negative for 8 months while AG-4 seropositive. When the possibility was finally considered that she might have recurrent disease, vulvar CIS was found. Patient 449 was first considered negative and then a recurrence was identified within the same month. She was consistently AG-4 seropositive and expired with disseminated metastatic disease. Since patients with recurrent cervical neoplasia appear to become AG-4 seropositive prior to the development of a large tumor mass, periodic serologic testing of cervical cancer patients should provide their physicians with an early warning of clinical recurrence or metastases that could lead to more effective control and increased survival. It should be pointed out, however, that there is also a small proportion (9.6%) of patients, e.g. No. 219, for whom there is no correlation between AG-4 seropositivity and clinical status. At present, we cannot determine whether such patients may still develop neoplastic disease, or whether this represents a false-positive response. In this context, it may be particularly significant that the level of AG-4 seropositivity in the control groups ranges between 7.7% (cancer at other sites) and 11.7% (normal controls) (Table 7).

AG-4 seropositivity may also fail as a prognostic tool in the largest proportion of patients with advanced tumors since the majority of these are AG-4 negative at the outset (Table 7). At this stage of disease, however, the clinician rarely needs evidence of persistent disease in managing his patient.

## 12. CONCLUSIONS AND PERSPECTIVES

Thirteen criteria have been enumerated whose fulfillment should convince us that a virus is causally related to a particular malignancy [1]. With respect to the association of HSV-2 with cervical cancer, the evidence pertaining to these criteria is summarized in Table 1. Although this evidence has been previously reviewed, final conclusions have differed. Three basic points of view have emerged. One of these, based on the misrepresentation of the data, argues that the association of HSV-2 with cervical cancer is, at best, fortuitous. Reviewers subscribing to this point of view argue that seroepidemiologic data are inconsistent and even contradictory, that early antigens are of doubtful specificity, and that consistent antibody patterns were not demonstrated in cancer and control subjects using these antigens in double blind studies. They state that the virus isolated from cervical cancer cells is a laboratory contaminant and that transformation is not caused by HSV-2, but rather by activated retrovirus [151]. In reality, none of these comments are valid. The evidence presented in detail in this chapter, demonstrates that the seroepidemiologic data associate HSV-2 with cervical cancer in an impressively consistent fashion in various geographic areas (Table 8). The early antigens have been purified and their protein identity and their viral specificity is well established as are their properties and involvement in the virus replicative cycles (Tables 4, 5). Double blind studies performed with these antigens have consistently associated their presence with cervical cancer (Table 6). The virus isolated from cervical cancer cells is not a laboratory contaminant since it differs from established HSV-2 strains both in biologic properties [98] and in restriction endonuclease cleavage patterns of its DNA [57]. In all but two cases (Section 2.1.2), HSV-2 transformed cells were shown to express HSV-2 antigens at late passages. Finally, HSV-1 DNA sequences (map positions 29–32; 87–97) that induce mouse retrovirus [156] differ from those (map positions 30–45) that cause morphologic transformation [54]. HSV-2 DNA sequences capable of activating retrovirus are unknown.

Among those reviewers who argue that the association of HSV-2 with cervical cancer is fortuitous, some, nevertheless, believe that another herpesvirus, EBV, is causally related to human tumors. Therefore, it may be profitable to compare the two systems. Unlike EBV, the association of HSV-2 with cervical carcinoma does not suffer from the limitations of a peculiar geographic and racial distribution, and prospective studies consistently indicate that women with cervical HSV-2 infections are at a significantly higher risk of developing cervical cancer (Section 6, 7). On the other hand, in the one prospective survey on EBV and Burkitt lymphoma (BL), only 14 tumor cases were identified. Antibodies against virus capsid antigen (VCA) were equally distributed among cancer cases and controls. Titers, prior to BL development, were virtually identical in the two groups. Antibody titers against the early antigen (EA) increased in 8 of the 14 BL patients but only after development of the tumor, suggesting that at least this antigen is unrelated to tumor growth [153]. Viral antigens were readily identified in both Burkitt and cervical tumors. Despite recent progress in this area, however, the protein identity of most of the EBV antigens is still largely unknown while that of the HSV-2 antigens in the cervical tumors is well established (Section 3.1.2). The critics of the *'herpesvirus hypothesis'* correctly point out that while HSV-2 DNA has been difficult to identify in cervical tumors, EBV DNA has been readily demonstrated in cell lines from Burkitt tumors, although only 6 of the 14 BL tumors in the prospective study were positive for viral DNA [153]. The oncogenic potential of both viruses has been established in both animal models and in *in vitro* transformation. While the specific HSV-2 DNA sequences capable of causing neoplastic transformation of cultured mammalian cells have been identified (Section 3.1.1), those of EBV have not. The obvious conclusion of this comparison is that each system has its respective strengths and weakenesses, underscoring the fallacy of accepting only one of the two systems as causally related.

The second point of view that has emerged from the review of the evidence associating HSV-2 with cervical cancer is based on an approach that places different emphasis on the various criteria of causality. Thus, some reviewers might consider the epidemiologic evidence associating HSV-2 with cervix cancer as highly significant, while others consider it tantalizing but inconclusive. The latter argue that detection of viral DNA in the cervical tumor cells is the only evidence that will fulfill a causal relationship between HSV-2 and cervical cancer. Although demonstration of viral DNA in cervical tumor cells is of utmost significance, fulfillment of this criterion will not add substantive evidence in support of a causative link between HSV-2 and cervical cancer. Presence of HSV-2 DNA in the tumor cells could be due to infection of cervical cells by the virus, after neoplastic transformation, or it could be the result of the common co-existence of two sexually transmitted diseases (HSV-2 and cervix cancer) in the promiscuous woman. In fact, it can be reasonably argued that the presence of viral messenger RNA and proteins in the cervical tumor cells, and the correlation of at least one of these proteins (ICP 10) with both tumorigenic potential in transformed cells (Section 3.1.2) and active cervical tumor growth (Section 5.1), are a much more significant criterion of causality. They confirm the presence of viral DNA in the cervical tumor cells and indicate that this DNA plays an active role in the neoplastic process. For those who, nevertheless, persist in advocating the supremacy of one criterion of causality over the others, further studies designed to validate their favorite criterion and resolve any contradictions that it may present, seem warranted. We have discussed at least some of the contradictions, technical difficulties, and criticisms pertaining to each criterion. Some of the solutions are obvious, some will remain the challenge of those interested in that particular problem.

The last point of view that has emerged from the analysis of the evidence associating HSV-2 and cervical cancer is advocated by the writer. It argues that, like our precedessors in the infectious diseases, we do not have all the facts. Indeed, even the criteria for causality may have to be modified as new knowledge is gained and as our horizons broaden. However, short of preventing cervical tumor by vaccination, or inducing tumor regression by anti-viral therapy, all the criteria in the unified concept of causality [1] have been studied and have been fulfilled within the limits of time and technology. Little additional observational data on these specific criteria could be acquired that would add fundamentally to our appreciation of the etiologic role of the virus in cervix cancer. Each criterion standing alone does not provide convincing evidence that HSV-2 plays a causal role in cervical cancer. In its consistency, however, the cumulative evidence is most compelling. Critical acceptance of the available evidence and a willingness to continue the search for a better understanding of the regulatory interplay between viruses and host, particularly, the human host, will make the real difference between light and darkness, knowledge and ignorance, and, ultimately, life and death.

## GLOSSARY

*Permissive vs nonpermissive infection.* Permissive infection is characterized by virus replication and the generation of viral progeny. In the case of the herpesviruses it results in cell death. Nonpermissive infection is characterized by the failure of the virus to replicate in the cell that it has infected. The outcome of such an infection may be the maintenance of the viral genetic information and continuous cellular replication.

The terminology implies that the restriction occurs at the level of the host cell that is incapable of supporting virus growth.

*Productive infection.* Another term for permissive infection.

*Transfection.* Infection with viral nucleic acid rather than virus particles.

*Transformation.* Acquisition by cells cultured *in vitro* of properties that are correlated with neoplastic potential. These include morphologic changes, fibrinolytic activity, growth in medium containing low (1–2%) serum concentrations, and anchorage independent growth (i.e. growth in medium containing agar or agarose). However, it must be stressed that neoplastic potential does not always follow the acquisition of the above properties. The term neoplastic transformation defines a cell line that, besides the *in vitro* properties listed above, is also capable of causing tumors when inoculated into normal syngeneic animals. The terms oncogenic or tumorigenic transformation are synonymous.

*Hybridization.* A procedure designed to identify the presence in cells of specific (viz. viral) nucleic acid or sequences thereof. It uses a radioactively labeled DNA probe rendered single stranded and measures its rate of reassociation in the presence and absence of unlabeled DNA extracted from the cells under investigation. If nucleic acid sequences homologous to the probe are present in the cells, the rate of reassociation of the labeled DNA strands is accelerated. *In situ* hybridization is a modification of this procedure in which the entire cell is exposed to the labeled DNA probe and the outcome is quantitated by autoradiographic procedures in which silver grains are counted on the exposed cells.

*Map coordinates (or units)* define the location of the specific DNA sequences on the viral genome.

*Restriction endonuclease.* Enzymes that recognize specific cleavage sites on the DNA molecule. They are used in the definition of genetic maps, preparation of specific DNA fragments and determination of genetic variability.

*Post treatment passage.* Defines the specific passage of the cells following exposure to a chemical or viral carcinogen. *In vitro,* primary cells have a finite life and, therefore, they can only sustain a limited number of passages. On the other hand, transformed cells are immortal (established lines) and can be transferred indefinitely.

*Crisis.* Cells exposed *in vitro* to chemical or viral carcinogens go through a period of poor growth, termed crisis, from which they recover and acquire indefinite growth potential.

*Enhancer gene(s).* Early viral gene(s) the expression of which results in an increased frequency of transformation.

*Initiation vs maintenance gene(s).* Viral gene(s) involved in the initiation of transformation are not required for the maintenance of a transformed phenotype and may be lost with cell passage. Maintenance gene(s) are essential for the expression of a transformed phenotype.

*Latent infection.* Persistent infection characterized by intermittent acute episodes of disease due to virus replication. Between these episodes the virus is usually not demonstrable.

*Antigen-driven immune responses.* Responses that require the continuous exposure of the immune system to antigen. They can be humoral (antibody) or cell-mediated.

*Seroconversion.* Defines the acquisition by a hitherto naive (non-immune) host, of specific immunity to an antigen.

REFERENCES

1. Evans AS: Causation and Disease: The Henle-Koch Postulates Revisited. Yale J Biol Med 49:175–195, 1976.
2. Koch R: Über bakteriologische Forschung. In: Verh X Int Med Congr Berlin, 1890, p 35, 1892.
3. Rivers TM: Viruses and Koch's Postulates. J Bacteriol 33:1, 1937.
4. Huebner RJ: The Virologist's Dilemma. Ann NY Acad Sci 67:430, 1957.
5. Weil R: Viral 'Tumor Antigens'. A novel type of mammalian regulator protein. Biochem Biophys Acta 516:301–388, 1978.
6. Beswick TSL: The origin and the use of the word herpes. Med Hist 6:214–232, 1962.
7. Bateman T: 'Herpes'. In: A Practical Synopsis of Cutaneous Disease According to the Arrangement of Dr Willan, 3rd ed. London: Longman, Hurst, Orme and Brown, 1814, pp 209–225.
8. Hutfield DS: Herpes genitalis. Brit J Vener Dis 42:263–268, 1966.
9. Kieff ED, Bachenheimer SL, Roizman B: Size, composition, and structure of the deoxyribonucleic acid of herpes simples virus subtypes 1 and 2. J Virol 8:125–132, 1971.
10. Sheldrick P, Berthelot N: Inverted repetitions in the chromosome of herpes simples virus. Cold Spring Harbor Symp Quant Biol 39:667–679, 1975.
11. Kieff E, Hoyer B, Bachenheimer SL, Roizman B: Genetic relatedness of type 1 and type 2 herpes simplex viruses. J Virol 9:738–745, 1972.
12. Buchman TG, Roizman B, Adams G, Stover H: Restriction endonuclease finger printing

of herpes simplex DNA: a novel epidemiology tool applied to a nosocomial outbreak. J Inf Dis 138:488–498, 1978.
13. Cassai EN, Sarmiento M, Spear PG: Comparison of the virion proteins specified by herpes simplex virus types 1 and 2. J Virol 16:1327–1331, 1975.
14. Strnad BC, Aurelian L: Proteins of herpesvirus type 2. I. Virion, nonvirion, and antigenic polypeptides in infected cells. Virology 69:438–452, 1976.
15. Cohen GH, Katze M, Hydrean-Stern C, Eisenberg RJ: Type-common CP-1 antigen in herpes simplex virus is associated with a 59,000 molecular weight envelope glycoprotein. J Virol 27:172–181, 1978.
16. Ching CY, Lopez C: A type-specific antiserum induced by a major herpesvirus type 1 glycoprotein. J Immunol Methods 32:383–391, 1980.
17. Killington RA, Yeo JM, Honess RW, Watson DH, Duncan BE, Halliburton IW, Mumford J: Comparative analysis of the proteins and antigens of five herpesviruses. J Gen Virol 37:297–310, 1977.
18. Smith CC, Aurelian L: Proteins of herpesvirus type 2. VI. Two high molecular weight proteins immunogenic in human infections. In press.
19. Heilman CJ Jr, Zweig M, Stephenson JR, Hampar B: Isolation of a nucleocapsid polypeptide of herpes simplex virus types 1 and 2 possessing immunologically type-specific and cross-reactive determinants. J Virol 29:34–42, 1979.
20. Aurelian L, Smith MF, Cornish JD: IgM antibody to a tumor-associated HSV-2 induced antigen (AG-4): Its use in locating the antigen in infected cells. JNCI 56:471–477, 1976.
21. Josey WE, Nahmias AJ, Naib ZM: Genital herpes simplex in historical perspective. Bull NY Acad Med 52:935–943, 1976.
22. Kaufman RH, Gardner HL, Rawls WE, Dixon RE, Young RL: Clinical features of herpes genitalis. Cancer Res 33:1446–1451, 1973.
23. Smith IW, Peutherer JF, Robertson DH: Characterization of genital strains of herpesvirus hominis. Br J Ven Dis 49:385–390, 1973.
24. Kawana T, Shinkai K, Yoshino K: Typing of herpes simplex virus strains of genital and nongenital origins. Japan J Microbiology 18:235–241, 1974.
25. Roizman B: The role of hormones in viral infections I. Expression of viral adsorption and penetration in cells treated with thyroid hormones in vitro. Proc Nat Acad Sci 48:973–977, 1962.
26. Roizman B: An inquiry into the mechanisms of recurrent herpes infections of man. In: Perspectives in Virology IV, M Pollard, ed. New York: Harper and Row, 1965, pp 283–304.
27. Donnenberg AD, Chaikof E, Aurelian L: Immunity to herpes simplex virus type 2: Cell-mediated immunity in latently infected guinea pigs. Inf Imm 30:99–109, 1980.
28. Barringer RJ: Herpes Simplex Virus in human sensory ganglia. In: Oncogenesis and Herpesviruses II. G deThe, Epstein MA, zurHausen H, eds. pp 73–77, 1975.
29. Scriba M: Extraneural localization of herpes simplex virus in latently infected guinea pigs. Nature 267:531, 1977.
30. Schwartz J, Whetsell WO, Elizan TS: Latent herpes simplex virus infection of mice. Infectious virus in homogenates of latently infected dorsal root ganglia. J Neuropath and Exp Neurol 37:45–55, 1978.
31. Barringer RJ, Swoveland P: Persistent HSV infection in rabbit trigeminal ganglia. Lab Invest 30:230–240, 1974.
32. Galloway DA, Fenoglio C, Shevchuk M, McDougall JK: Detection of herpes simplex RNA in human sensory ganglia. Virology 95:265–268, 1979.
33. Buddingh G, Schrum D, Lanier J, Guidry D: Studies of the natural history of herpes simplex infections. Pediatrics 11:595–612, 1953.

34. Douglas RG, Couch RB: A prospective study of chronic herpes simplex virus infection and recurrent herpes labialis in humans. J Immunol 104:289-295, 1970.
35. Adam E, Kaufman RH, Mirkovic RR, Melnick JL: Persistence of virus shedding in asymptomatic women after recovery from herpes genitalis. Obst Gynec 54:171-173, 1979.
36. Kaufman HE, Brown DC, Ellison ED: Herpesvirus in the lacrimal gland, conjunctiva and cornea of man. A chronic infection. Amer J Ophtal 65:32-35, 1968.
37. Centifanto JM, Drylie DM, Deardourff SL, Kaufman HL: Herpesvirus type 2 in male genitourinary tract. Science 178:318-319, 1972.
38. O'Reilly RJ, Chibburo A, Anger E, Lopez C: Cell-mediated immune respones in patients with recurrent herpes simplex infections. II. Infection associated deficiency of lymphokine production in patients with recurrent herpes labialis or herpes progenitalis. J Immunol 118:1095-1102, 1977.
39. Deardourff SL, Deture FA, Drylie DM, Centifanto J, Kaufman H: Association between herpes hominis type 2 and the male genitourinary tract. J Urol 112:126-127, 1974.
40. Jeansson S, Molin L: Genital herpes infection and non-specific urethritis. Brit Med J 3:247, 1971.
41. Goodwin CS, Gostling JVT, Pead PJ: Genital herpes. Brit Med J 4:558-559, 1970.
42. Gordon HL, Miller DH, Rawls WE: Viral studies in patients with non-specific prostatourethritis. J Urol 108:299-300, 1972.
43. Traub RG, Madden DL, Fucillo DA, McLean TW: The male as a reservoir of infection with cytomegalovirus, herpes and mycoplasma. New Engl J Med 289:697, 1973.
44. Poste G, Hawkins DF, Thomlinson J: Herpesvirus hominis infection of the female genital tract. Obst Gynec 40:871-890, 1972.
45. Naib ZM, Nahmias AJ, Josey WE, Kramer JH: Genital herpetic infection. Association with cervical dysplasia and carcinoma. Cancer 23:940-945, 1969.
46. Jeansson S, Molin L: Genital herpesvirus hominis infection and venereal disease. Lancet I:1064-1065, 1970.
47. Kleger B, Prier JE, Rosato DJ, McGinnis AE: Herpes simplex infection of the female genital tract. I. Incidence of infection. Am J Obst Gyn 102:745-748, 1968.
48. Duenas A, Adam E, Melnick JL, Rawls WE: Herpesvirus type 2 in a prostitute population. Am J Epid 95:483-489, 1972.
49. Centifanto JM, Hildebrandt RJ, Held B, Kaufman HE: Relationship of herpes simplex genital infection and carcinoma of the cervix: Population studies. Am J Obst Gyn 110:690-692, 1971.
50. Kessler II: Human cervical cancer as a venereal disease. Cancer Res 36:783-791, 1976.
51. Nahmias A, Josey WE, Naib ZM, Luce CF, Guest BA: Antibodies to herpesvirus hominis types 1 and 2 in humans. II. Women with cervical cancer. Amer J Epid 91:547-552, 1970.
52. Rawls WE, Gardner HL, Flanders RW, Lowry SP, Kaufman RH, Melnick JL: Genital herpes in two social groups. Am J Obstet Gynecol 110:682-689, 1971.
53. Munyon W, Kraiselburd E, Davis D, Mann J: Transfer of thymidine kinase to thymidine kinaseless L cells by infection with UV-irradiated herpes simplex virus. J Virol 7:813-820, 1971.
54. Camacho A, Spear PG: Transformation of hamster embryo fibroblasts by a specific fragment of the herpes simplex virus genome. Cell 15:993-1002, 1978.
55. Leiden J, Frenkel N: Mapping of the herpes simplex virus sequences in transformed cells. In: Herpesvirus DNA: Recent Studies of the Viral Genome. Y Becker *et al.*, eds. In press.
56. Reyes GR, LaFemina R, Hayward, SD, Hayward GS: Morphological transformation by

DNA fragments of human herpesviruses: evidence for two distinct transforming regions in herpes simplex virus types 1 and 2 and lack of correlation with biochemical transfer of the thymidine kinase gene. Cold Spring Harbor Symp Quant Biol 44:629–641, 1979.
57. Jariwalla RJ, Aurelian L, Ts'o POP: Tumorigenic transformation induced by a specific fragment of herpes simplex virus type 2 DNA. Proc Nat Acad Sci 77:2279–2283, 1980.
58. Galloway DA, Copple CD, McDougall JK: Analysis of viral DNA sequences in hamster cells transformed by herpes simplex virus type 2. Proc Nat Acad Sci 77:880–884, 1980.
59. Berenblum J: Carcinogenesis as a biological problem. In: Frontiers of Biology. A Neuberger, Tatum EL, eds. Amsterdam: North Holland Pub Co., p. 115, 1974.
60. Kimura S, Flannery VL, Levy B, Schaffer PA: Oncogenic transformation of primary hamster cells by herpes simplex virus type 2 (HSV-2) and an HSV-2 temperature sensitive mutant. Int J Cancer 15:786–798, 1975.
61. Manak M, Aurelian L, Ts'o POP: Focus formation and neoplastic transformation by herpes simplex virus type 2 inactivated intracellularly by BUdR+nUV light. In press.
62. Aurelian L, Manak M, Ts'o POP: Mechanism of neoplastic transformation of cultured mammalian cells by herpes simplex virus type 2 or chemical carcinogenesis. A unified hypothesis. In: Biological Carcinogenesis. MA Rich, Furmanski P, eds. New York: Marcel Dekker, pp 229–261, 1982.
63. Preston C, Newton A: The effects of HSV-1 on cellular DNA-dependent RNA polymerase activities. J Gen Virol 33:471–482, 1976.
64. Constanzo F, Campadelli-Fiume G, Foa-Tomas L, Cassai E: Evidence that herpes simplex virus DNA is transcribed by cellular RNA polymerase II. J Virol 21:996–1101, 1977.
65. Kucera L, Edwards I: HSV type 2 functions expressed during stimulation of human cell DNA. J Virol 29:83–90, 1979.
66. Frenkel N, Locker H, Cox B, Roizman B, Rapp F: Herpes simplex virus DNA in transformed cells: Sequence complexity in five hamster cell lines and one derived hamster tumor. J Virol 18:885–893, 1976.
67. Preston V, Davison A, Marsden H, Timbury M, Subak-Sharpe J, Wilkie N: Recombinants between herpes simplex virus types 1 and 2: Analyses of genome structures and expression of immediate early polypeptides. J Virol 28:499–517, 1978.
68. Flannery VL, Courtney RJ, Schaffer PA: Expression of an early, nonstructural antigen of herpes simplex virus in cells transformed *in vitro* by herpes simplex virus. J Virol 21:284–291, 1977.
69. Kucera LA, Gusdon JP, Edwards I, Herbst G: Oncogenic transformation of rat embryo fibroblasts with photoinactivated herpes simplex virus: Rapid *in vitro* cloning of transformed cells. J Gen Virol 35:473–485, 1977.
70. MacNab JCM, Visser L, Jamieson AT, Hay AJ: Specific viral antigens in rat cells transformed by herpes simplex virus type 2 and in rat tumors induced by inoculation of transformed cells. Cancer Res 40:2074–2079, 1980.
71. Simmons D, Martin M, Mora P, Chang C: Relationship among Tau antigens isolated from various lines of simian virus 40-transformed cells. J Virol 34:650–657, 1980.
72. McCormick F, Harlow E: Association of a murine 53,000 dalton phosphoprotein with simian virus 40 large-T antigen in transformed cells. J Virol 34:213–224, 1980.
73. Graessman M, Graessman A: 'Early' simian-virus-40 specific RNA contains information for tumor antigen formation and chromatin replication. Proc Nat Acad Sci 73:366–370, 1976.
74. Gaudray P, Rassoulzadegan M, Cuzin F: Expression of simian virus 40 early genes in transformed rat cells is correlated with the maintenance of the transformed phenotype. Proc Nat Acad Sci 75:4987–4991, 1978.
75. Graessman A, Graessman M, Tjian R, Topp W: Simian virus 40 small-t protein is required for loss of actin cable networks in rat cells. J Virol 33:1182–1191, 1980.

76. Koss LG: Concept of genesis and development of carcinoma of the cervix. Obst Gynec Survey 24:860–860, 1969.
77. Koss LG, Stewart FW, Foote FW, Jordan MJ, Bader GM, Day E: Some histological aspects of behavior of epidermoid carcinoma *in situ* and related lesions of the uterine cervix. A long term prospective study. Cancer 16:1160–1211, 1963.
78. Stern E, Neely PM: Carcinoma and dysplasia of the cervix: A comparison of notes for new and returning populations. Acta Cytol 7:357–361, 1963.
79. Richart RM: Natural history of cervical intraepithelial neoplasia. Clin Obst Gynec 5:748–794, 1968.
80. Munoz N: Effect of herpesvirus type 2 and hormonal imbalance on the uterine cervix of the mouse. Cancer Res 33:1504–1508, 1973.
81. Rapp R, Reed C: Experimental evidence for the oncogenic potential of herpes simplex virus. Cancer Res 36:800–806, 1976.
82. Nastac E, Athanasiu P, Stoian M, Hozoc M, Morfei A: Appearance of uterine leiomyosarcoma in the rabbit following *in situ* inoculation of a nucleic acid extract from HSV-2 infected cell cultures. Rev Roum Med Virol 26:149, 1975.
83. Palmer AE, London WT, Nahmias AJ, Naib ZM, Tunca JT, Fucillo DA, Ellenberg JH, Sever JL: A preliminary report on investigation of oncogenic potential of herpes simplex virus type 2 in Cebus monkeys. Cancer Res 36:807–809, 1976.
84. Strnad BC, Aurelian L: Proteins of herpesvirus type 2. III. Isolation and immunologic characterization of a large molecular weight viral protein. Virol 87:401–415, 1978.
85. Aurelian L, Davis HJ, Julian CG: Herpesvirus type 2 induced tumor specific antigens in cervical carcinoma. Am J Epidem 98:1–9, 1973.
86. Smith CC, Aurelian L: Proteins of herpesvirus type 2. V. Isolation and immunologic characterization of two viral proteins in a virus specific antigenic fraction. Virol 98:255–260, 1979.
87. Smith CC, Aurelian L, Gupta PK, Frost JK, Rosenshein NB, Klacsmann K, Geddes S: An evaluation of herpes simplex virus antigenic markers in the study of established and developing cervical neoplasia. Analytical and Quantitative Cytology 2:131–143, 1980.
88. Dreesman GR, Burck J, Ada E, Kaufman RH, Melnick JL, Powell KL, Purifoy DJ: Expression of herpesvirus induced antigens in human cervical cancer. Nature 283:591–593, 1980.
89. Melnick JL, Adam E, Lewis R, Kaufman RH: Cervical cancer lines containing herpesvirus markers. Intervirol 12:111–114, 1979.
90. Tarro G, Flaminio G, Cocchiera R, DiGioia M, Geraci D: An immune enzymatic asay for purified tumor associated antigen of herpes simplex virus. Cell Mol Biol 25:329–333, 1979.
91. Gall SA, Haines HG: Cervical carcinoma antigen and the relationship to HSV-2. Gynecol Onc 2:451–459, 1974.
92. McDougall JK, Galloway DA, Fenoglio CM: Cervical carcinoma: Detection of herpes simplex virus RNA in cells undergoing neoplastic change. Int J Cancer 25:1–8, 1980.
93. Simard R, Kessous A, Bibor-Hardy V, Suh M, Audet-Lapointe P, Cormier A, Vauclair R: Herpesvirus and cancer of the uterine cervix. Union Med Can 109:103–108, 1980.
94. Frenkel N, Roizman B, Cassai E, Nahmias AJ: A DNA fragment of herpes simplex 2 and its transcripts in human cancer tissue. Proc Nat Acad Sci 69:3784–3789, 1972.
95. Pagano JS: Disease and mechanisms of persistent DNA virus infection: Latency and cellular transformation. J Inf Dis 132:209–223, 1975.
96. Roizman B, Frenkel N, Kieff ED, Spear PG: The structure and expression of human herpesvirus DNAs in productive infection and in transformed cells. In: Origin of Human Cancer. Hiatt HH, Watson JD, Winsten JA, eds. Cold Spring Harbor Conf on Cell Proliferation, Vol. 4, pp. 1069–1111, 1977.

97. Aurelian L: Virions and antigens of herpes virus type 2 in cervical carcinoma. Cancer Res 33:1539–1547, 1973.
98. Aurelian L, Strandberg JD: Biologic and immunologic comparison of two HSV-2 variants: One an isolate from cervical tumor cells. Archiv für die gesamte Virusforschung 45:27–38, 1974.
99. Posevaya TA, Shubladze AK, Grigoriev VV, Ugriumov EP, Kitsak VI, Moisiadi MA, Grebeniuk VN, Shuvaeva NI, Barinskii IF: Role of herpes simplex virus in the etiology of cancer of the cervix uteri. Vopr Virusol 6:611–615, 1979.
100. Denoyel GA, Cloppet H, Gaspar A: Isolation of a herpes simples virus type 2 (HSV-2) from a human cervical cancer by means of cell co-cultivation. Nouv Presse Med 19:253–254, 1980.
101. Srivannaboon S: Cytological study of herpes simplex infection and dysplasia in the female genital tract. J Med Assoc Thai 62:201–207, 1979.
102. Lauchlan SC: Latent herpes cervicitis and mixed cervical carcinoma. Am J Obst Gynec 131:109–110, 1978.
103. Vaczi L, Boldogh I, Gonczol E: Activation of herpes specific antigens Activation of herpes specific antigens and infectious virus in a hamster cell line transformed by HSV-2. Archiv gesamte Virusforsch 44:62–69, 1974.
104. Aurelian L, Kessler II, Rosenshein NB, Barbour G: Viruses and Gynecologic Cancers. Herpesvirus protein (ICP 10/AG-4), a cervical tumor antigen that fulfills the criteria for a marker of carcinogenicity. Cancer. In press.
105. Heise ER, Kucera LS, Raben M, Homesley H: Serological response to patterns to herpesvirus type 2 early and late antigens in cervical carcinoma patients. Cancer Res 39:4022–4026, 1979.
106. Khoo SK, Mackay E, Daumter B: Dinitro-chlorobanzene reactivity of women with cancer of the ovary, cervix and corpus uteri. Int J Gynecol Obst 17:58–62, 1979.
107. Vos GH, Hammond MG, Marascotti G: Changeable lymphocytotoxic antibody activity in patients with cervical carcinoma. Vox Sang 28:285–292, 1975.
108. Anzai T, Dreesman GR, Courtney RJ, Adam E, Rawls WE, Benyesh-Melnick M: Antibody to herpes simplex virus type 2 induced non-structural proteins in women with cervical cancer and control groups. J Nat Cancer Inst 54:1051–1059, 1975.
109. Bell RB, Aurelian L, Cohen GH: Proteins of herpesvirus type 2. IV. Leukocyte inhibition responses to type common antigen(s) in cervix cancer and recurrent herpetic infections. Cell Immunol 41:86–102, 1978.
110. Rivera ES, Hersh EM, Bowen JM, Barnett JW, Wharton T, Murphy SG: Leukocyte migration inhibition assay for tumor immunity in patients with cervical squamous cell carcinoma. Cancer 43:2297–2305, 1979.
111. Thiry L, Sprecher-Goldberger S, Hannecart-Pokorni E, Gould T, Bossens M: Specific nonimmunoglobulin G antibodies in cell-mediated response to herpes simplex virus antigens in women with cervical carcinoma. Cancer Res 37:1301–1306, 1977.
112. Ito H, Kurihara S, Nishimura C: Antibody to herpes simplex virus type 2-induced early antigens and its radioimmunoassay with sera of cervical carcinoma patients. Kitasato Arch Exp Med 51:1–13, 1978.
113. Ito H, Tsutsui F, Kurihara S, Akabayashi T, Tobe T, Nishimura C: Serum antibodies to herpesvirus early antigens in patients with cervical carcinoma as determined by anti-complement immunofluorescence technique. Int J Cancer 18:557–563, 1976.
114. Christenson B: Complement-dependent cytotoxic antibodies in the course of cervical carcinoma. Int J Cancer 20:694–701, 1977.
115. Christenson B: Antibody-dependent cell mediated cytotoxicity to herpes simplex virus type 2 infected target cells in the course of cervical carcinoma. Am J Epid 108:126–135, 1978.

116. Dent PB, Bienenstock J: Absence of IgA antibody to herpesvirus in cervicovaginal secretions of patients with carcinoma of the cervix. Clin Immunol Immunopathol 3:171-177, 1974.
117. Gilman SC, Docherty JJ, Clarke A, Rawls WE: Reaction patterns of herpes simplex virus type 1 and type 2 proteins with sera of patients with uterine cervical carcinoma and matched controls. Cancer Res 40:4640-4647, 1980.
118. Hollinshead AC, Chretien PB, Lee OB, Tarpley JL, Kerney S, Silverman NA, Alexander JC: *In vivo* and *in vitro* measurements of the relationship of human squamous carcinomas to herpes simplex virus tumor-associated antigens. Cancer Res 36:821-828, 1976.
119. Rawls WE, Adam E: Herpes Simplex Viruses and Human Malignancies. In: Origins of Human Cancer Book B. Mechanisms of Carcinogenesis. Hiatt HH, Watson JD, Winsten JA, eds. Cold Spring Harbor Conferences on Cell Proliferation, Vol. 4, CSH, 1979, pp. 1133-1155.
120. Rawls WE, Clarke D, Smith KO, Docherty JJ, Gilman SC, Graham S: Specific antibodies to herpes simplex virus type 2 among women with cervical cancer. In: Viruses in Naturally Occurrring Cancers. Essex M, Todaro G, zurHausen H, eds. Cold Spring Harbor Conference on Cell Proliferation, Vol. 7, CSH, 1980, pp. 117-133.
121. Kessler II: Perspectives on the Epidemiology of cervical cancer with special reference to the herpesvirus hypothesis. Cancer Res 34:1091-1110, 1974.
122. Skinner GRB, Whitney JE, Hartley C: Prevalence of type-specific antibody against type 1 and type 2 herpes simplex virus in women with abnormal cervical cytology. Evidence towards pre-pubertal vaccination of seronegative female subjects. Arch Virol 54:211-221, 1977.
123. Jacobs RP, Aurelian L, Cole GA: Cell-mediated immune response to herpes simplex virus: Type-specific lymphoproliferative responses in lymph nodes draining the site of primary infection. J Immunol 116:1520-1525, 1976.
124. Smith JW, Torres JE, Holmquist ND: Association of herpes simplex virus (HSV) with cervical cancer by lymphocyte reactivity with HSV-2 and HSV-2 antigens. Am J Epid 110:141-147, 1979.
125. Fucillo DA, Sever JL, Moder FL, Chen TC, Catalano L, Johnson LD: Cytomegalovirus antibody in patients with carcinoma of the uterine cervix. Obst Gyn 38:599-601, 1971.
126. Naib ZM, Nahmias AJ, Josey WE, Zolis SA: Relation of cytohistopathology of genital herpesvirus infection to cervical anaplasia. Cancer Res 33:1452-1463, 1973.
127. Catalano LW Jr, Johnson LH: Herpesvirus antibody and carcinoma *in situ* of the cervix. J Am Med Assoc 217:447-450, 1971.
128. Nahmias AJ, Naib ZM, Josey WE, Franklin E, Jenkins R: Prospective studies of the association of genital herpes simplex infections and cervical anaplasia. Cancer Res 33:1491-1497, 1973.
129. Thomas DB, Rawls WE: Relationship of herpes simplex virus type 2 antibodies in squamous dysplasia to cervical carcinoma *in situ*. Cancer 42:2716-2725, 1978.
130. Naib ZM, Nahmias AJ, Josey WE: Cytology and histopathology of cervical herpes simplex infection. Cancer 19:1026-1031, 1966.
131. Pacsa AS, Kummerlander L, Pejtsik B, Simon M, Pali K: Herpes simplex virus antigens in normal cervical cells. Lancet I:597, 1976.
132. Rigoni-Stern D: Fatti Statistici Relativi alle Malatie Cancerose. Giorn Servire Progr Pathol Terap 2:507-517, 1842.
133. Rotkin ID: Adolescent coitus and cervical cancer: Associations of related events with increased risk. Cancer Res 27:603-617, 1967.
134. Aurelian L: Possible role of herpesvirus hominis type 2 in human cervical cancer. Fed Proc 31:1651-1659, 1972.

135. Freedman RS, Joosting AC, Ryan JT, Nkoni S: A study of associated factors including genital herpes in black women with cervical carcinoma in Johannesburg. S Afr Med J 48:1747–1752, 1974.
136. Schneweiss KE, Haag A, Lehmkoster A, Koenig U: Sero-immunological investigations in patients with cervical cancer: Higher rate of HSV-2 antibodies than in syphilis patients and evidence of IgM antibodies to an early HSV-2 antigen. Oncogenesis and Herpesviruses II, part 2, pp. 53–57, IARC publications, 1975.
137. Adam E, Rawls WE, Melnick JL: The association of herpesvirus type 2 infection and cervical carcinoma. Prev Med 3:122–141, 1974.
138. Reid BL, Frenck PW, Sugar A, Hogan BE, Coppleson M: Sperm basic proteins in cervical carcinogenesis: Correlation with socioeconomic class. Lancet II:60–62, 1978.
139. Kunkel M, Dberender H, Gartner L, Hofmann R, Ratz KH, Heise H: Antibodies to herpes simplex virus type 2 in husbands of patients with cervical carcinoma. Lancet II:585–586, 1978.
140. Swan SH, Brown WL: Vasectomy and cancer of the cervix. New Engl J Med 301:46, 1979.
141. Aurelian L: The herpesvirus hypothesis. In: Cervical Cancer: Past, Present and Future. Kessler II, ed. Springer-Verlag. In press.
142. Syrjanen KJ: Morphologic survey of the condylomatous lesions in dysplasia and neoplastic epithelium of the uterine cervix. Arch Gynec 227:153–161, 1979.
143. Meisels A, Marin C, Casas-Cordero M, Braun L, Shah KV, Roy M, Fortier M: The peroxidase antiperoxidase technique and human papillomavirus (HPV) infection of the cervix. Abstracts Ann Meeting Am Soc Cytol Nov, 1980, pp. 46.
144. Woodruff JD, Braun L, Cavalieri R, Gupta PK, Pass F, Shah KV: Immunological identification of papillomavirus antigen in paraffin-processed condyloma tissue from the female genetical tract. Ob Gyn 56:727–732, 1980.
145. deGraaff-Guilloud-Gentenaar JC, Fox CH, Brown MW: Quantitative features of cells from classical dysplasia and from condylomatous lesions of the uterine cervix. Anal Quant Cytol 2:294, 1980.
146. Aurelian L, Tyrer HW, Gupta PK, Frost JK, Adams LA, Tiffany SM: Microfluorometric quantitation of size deoxyribonucleic acid and viral antigenic determinants in cells productively infected with HSV-2. Anal Quant Cytol 1:207–216, 1979.
147. Strnad BC, Aurelian L: Proteins of herpesvirus type 2. II. Studies demonstrating a correlation between a tumor-associated antigen (AG-4) and a virion protein. Virology 73:244–258, 1976.
148. Smith CC, Aurelian L, Cohen GH, Eisenberg R, Schaffer PA: Proteins of herpesvirus type 2. VII. Further characterization of viral protein ICP 10 and its relationship to viral DNA polymerase. In press.
149. Spear PG, Roizman B: Herpes simplex viruses. In: Molecular Biology of Tumor Viruses. Part 2. Tooze J, ed. Cold Spring Harbor Lab Pub, pp. 615–745, 1980.
150. Aurelian L, Gupta PK, Frost JK, Rosenshein NB, Smith CC, Tyrer HW, Mantione JM, Albright CH: Fluorescence activated separation of cervical abnormal cells uding herpesvirus antigenic markers. Analytical and Quantitative Cytology 1:89–102, 1979.
151. Deinhardt F, Deinhardt J: Comparative aspects: Oncogenic animal herpesviruses. In: The Epstein-Barr Virus. Epstein MA, Achong BG, eds. Berlin: Springer Verlag, 1979, pp 373–400.
152. Hampar B, Boyd AL, Derge JG, Zweig M, Eader L, Showalter SD: Comparison of properties of mouse cells transformed spontaneously by UV light irradiated herpes simplex virus or by Simian virus 40. Cancer Res 40:2213–2222, 1980.
153. deThe G: Demographic studies implicating the virus in the causation of Burkitt's Lym-

phoma; prospects for nasopharyngeal carcinoma. In: The Epstein-Barr Virus. Epstein MA, Achong BG, eds. Berlin: Springer Verlag, 1979, pp. 417–435.
154. Aurelian L, Strandberg JD, Davis HJ: HSV-2 antigens absent from biopsied cervical tumor cells: a model consistent with latency. Proc Soc Exp Biol Med 140:404–408, 1972.
155. Pacsa AS, Kummerlander L, Pejtsik B, Krommer K, Pali K: Herpes simplex virus-specific antigens in exfoliated cervical cells from women with and without cervical anaplasia. Cancer Res 36:2130–2132, 1976.
156. Adelusi B, Osunkoya BO, Fabiyi A: Herpes type 2 virus antigens in human cervical carcinoma. Obstet and Gynecol 47:545–548, 1976.
157. Minhui G, Yuexin P, Xuejun J, Wenxian Z: Detection of herpes simplex virus type 2 (HSV-2) antigen in the cells of human cervical carcinoma by the indirect immunofluorescence method. Chinese J Oncol 1:255–259, 1979.
158. Athanasiu P, Nastac E, Stoian M, Predescu E, Hozoc M: Immunofluorescence study of the presence of herpes type 1 and 2 antigens in patients with cancer of the uterine cervix. Rev Roum Med Virol 29:251–253, 1978.
159. Melnick JL: In: The Virus Cancer Program Progress Report No. 15, 1978, p. 159.
160. Arsenakis M, Georgiou GM, Welsh JK, Cauchi MN, May JT: AG-4 complement-fixing antibodies in cervical cancer and herpes infected patients using local herpes simplex cirus type 2. Int J Cancer 25:67–71, 1980.
161. Kawana T, Cornish JD, Smith MF, Aurelian L: Frequency of antibody to a virus-induced, tumor-associated antigen (AG-4) in Japanese sera from patients with cervical cancer and controls. Cancer Res 36:810–820, 1976.
162. Kawana T, Sakamoto S, Kasamatsu T, Aurelian L: Frequency of anti-AG-e antibody in patients with uterine cervical cancer and controls. Gann 69:589–591, 1978.
163. Heise ER, Kucera LS: Antibodies in human carcinoma to herpes simplex virus type 2 (HSV-2) induced antigens. Proc Am Soc Microbiol, p. 217, 1976.
164. Notter MFD, Docherty JJ: Comparative diagnostic aspects of herpes simplex virus tumor associated antigens. J Nat Cancer Inst 57:483–488, 1976.
165. Aurelian L, Royston I, Davis HJ: Antibody to genital herpesvirus: Association with cervical atypia and carcinoma *in situ*. J Nat Cancer Inst 45:455–464, 1970.
166. Rawls WE, Tompkins WAF, Melnick JL: The association of herpesvirus type 2 and carcinoma of the uterine cervix. Am J Epid 89:547–554, 1969.
167. Adam E, Kaufman RH, Melnick JL, Levy AH, Rawls WE: Seroepidemiologic studies of herpesvirus type 2 and carcinoma of the cervix. III. Houston, Texas. Am J Epid 96:427–442, 1972.
168. Plummer G, Masterson JG: Herpes simplex virus and carcinoma of the cervix. Am J Obst Gyn 3:81–84, 1971.
169. Munoz N, deThe G, Aristizabal N, Yee C, Rabson A, Pearson G: Antibodies to herpesviruses in patients with cervical cancer and controls. In: Oncogenesis and Herpesviruses II. deThe G, Epstein MA, zurHausen H, eds. Lyon, France: IARC publications, pp. 45, 1975.
170. Skinner GRB, Thoules ME, Jordan JA: Antibodies to type 1 and type 2 herpes virus in women with abnormal cervical cytology. J Obstet Gyn Br Commonw 78:1031–1038, 1971.
171. Vestergaard BF, Hornsleth A, Pedersen SN: Occurrence of herpes and adenovirus antibodies in patients with carcinoma of the cervix uteri. Cancer 30:68–74, 1972.
172. Sprecher-Goldberger S, Thiry L, Cattoor JP, Hooghe R, Pestcan J: Herpesvirus type 2 infection and carcinoma of the cervix. Lancet II:266, 1970.
173. Christenson B, Epsmark A: Long-term follow-up studies on herpes simplex antibodies in

the course of cervical cancer. II. Antibodies to surface antigen of herpes simplex virus infected cells. Int J Cancer 17:381-325, 1976.
174. Kessler II, Kulcar Z, Rawls WE, Smerdel S, Strnad M, Lilienfeld AM: Cervical cancer in Yougoslavia. I. Antibodies to genital herpesvirus in cases and controls. J Nat Cancer Inst 52:369-376, 1974.
175. Pacsa AS, Kummerlander L, Pejtsik B, Pali K: Herpesvirus antibodies and antigens in patients with cervical anaplasia and in controls. J Nat Cancer Inst 55:775-781, 1975.
176. Janda Z, Kanka J, Vonka V, Svoboda B: A study of herpes simplex type 2 antibody states in groups of patients with cervical neoplasia in Czechoslovakia. Int J Cancer 12:626-630, 1973.
177. Menczer J, Leventon-Kriss S, Modan M, Oelsner G, Gerichter CB: Antibodies to herpes simplex virus in Jewish women with cervical cancer and in healthy Jewish women of Israel. J Nat Cancer Inst 55:3-6, 1975.
178. Adelusi B, Osunkoya BO, Fabiyi A: Antibodies to herpesvirus type 2 and carcinoma of the cervix uteri in Ibadan, Nigeria. Am J Obst Gynec 123:758-761, 1975.
179. Kao CL, Chen YH, Tang MC, Wen HK, Hsca S: Association of herpes simplex type 2 virus with cervical cancer of the uterus. J Formosan Med Assoc 73:122-127, 1974.
180. Kawana T, Yoshino K, Yasamatsui T: Estimation of specific antibody to type 2 herpes simplex virus among patients with carcinoma of the uterine cervix. GANN 65:439-445, 1974.
181. Ory HW, Jenkins R, Byrd JG, Nahmias AS, Tyler CW, Allen DT, Conger SB: The epidemiology and interrelationship of cervical dysplasia and type 2 herpesvirus in a low-income housing project. Am J Obst Gynec 123:269-274, 1975.
182. Seth P, Prakash SS, Ghosh D: Antibodies to herpes simplex virus types 1 and 2 in patients with squamous-cell carcinoma of uterine cervix in India. Int J Cancer 22:708-714, 1978.
183. Anderson K, Costa R, Holland L, Wagner E: Characterization of herpes simplex virus type 1 RNA present in the absence of de novo protein synthesis. J Virol 34:9-27, 1980.
184. Morse LS, Buchman TG, Roizman B, Schaffer PA: Anatomy of herpes simplex virus DNA IX. Apparent exclusion of some parental DNA arrangements in the generation of intertypic (HSV-1 and HSV-2) recombinants. J Virol 24:231-248, 1977.
185. Chartrand P, Crumpacker C, Schaffer P, Wilkie N: Physical and genetic analysis of herpes simplex virus DNA polymerase locus. Virology 103:311-326, 1980.

# 2. Tumor Markers in Gynecologic Malignancies

JOHN R. VAN NAGELL

## 1. INTRODUCTION

For practical purposes, a tumor marker can be defined as a substance which is selectively produced by a tumor and then released into the circulation in detectable amounts. An ideal marker is tumor-specific, i.e. produced only by tumor cells. Elevated serum levels of such a marker would, therefore, indicate the presence of a tumor and its absence following therapy would signify the lack of viable malignant cells. Unfortunately, no truly tumor-specific markers have been detected in gynecologic cancers. Rather, several nonspecific oncofetal and hormonal markers have been shown to be quantitatively increased both in the tumor tissue and sera of patients with gynecologic malignancies. Also, a small number of tumor-associated antigens have been described in ovarian and cervical cancers. Although elevated plasma and tumor concentrations of these biochemical markers have been confirmed by a number of investigators, there remains considerable skepticism concerning their usefullness in clinical medicine.

In the present review, an attempt will be made to describe in some detail the current knowledge concerning those markers which have been studied most completely in patients with gynecologic cancer. A conceptual model will be defined in which immunohistochemical techniques can be utilized to help identify which markers will be most useful in an individual tumor. Also, the role of tumor-associated antigens as targets for radiolabeled antibodies used in radioimmunodetection and radioimmunotherapy experiments will be presented. Specific sections will be devoted to carcinoembryonic antigen, human chorionic gonadotropin, alpha feto-protein, and both ovarian and cervical cancer-associated antigens.

*Griffiths, C. T. and Fuller, A. F. (eds.), Gynecologic Oncology.*
© *1983, Martinus Nijhoff Publishers, Boston. ISBN 0-89838-555-5.*
*Printed in The Netherlands.*

## 2. CARCINOEMBRYONIC ANTIGEN

Carcinoembryonic antigen (CEA) is a glycoprotein with a molecular weight of approximately 200,000 daltons which was originally described as a tumor-specific antigen in adenocarcinoma of the colon [1]. This antigen is soluble in perchloric acid and has beta-globulin mobility on electrophoresis [2]. Since its initial description, CEA has been detected in the tumors and plasma of patients with a variety of gynecologic cancers [3-9]. Plasma levels of CEA are elevated (>2.5 ng/ml) in approximately 50% of patients with invasive gynecologic malignancies and in 11% of healthy volunteers (Table 1). The observation that CEA levels are elevated in a significant number of patients with diverse gynecologic malignancies emphasizes that this antigen can be produced by tumors of nonendodermal origin. Nevertheless, the lack of specificity of CEA has severely limited its diagnostic efficacy. Goldenberg [10] has reported that 47% of patients with granulomatous colitis and 70% of patients with alcoholic cirrhosis have elevated plasma CEA titers. Similarly, CEA levels have been shown to be abnormal in 18% of patients with benign gynecologic diseases [11]. It should be pointed out, however, that plasma CEA concentrations fall between 2.5 ng/ml and 10.0 ng/ml in the majority of patients with benign inflammatory diseases. Therefore, a plasma CEA concentration in excess of 20 ng/ml in the presence of a pelvic tumor is highly suggestive of ovarian malignancy.

Plasma CEA concentration is related to the stage or extent of disease, tumor CEA concentration, and antigen metabolism. In cervical cancer, plasma CEA is elevated in approximately 35% of patients with Stage Ib disease as opposed to 60% in patients with advanced (Stages III and IV) disease [6-8]. There is also a general relationship between plasma antigen levels and the total tumor CEA content. Shuster and colleagues [12] have demonstrated that circulating plasma CEA concentration is inversely related

Table 1. Plasma carcinoembryonic antigen levels in patients with gynecologic cancer and in healthy volunteers.

| Diagnosis | Patients | Plasma CEA (ng/ml) | |
|---|---|---|---|
| | | <2.5 | ≥2.5 |
| Healthy volunteers | 176 | 157 (89%) | 19 (11%) |
| Benign gynecologic disease | 95 | 78 (82%) | 17 (18%) |
| Cervical intraepithelial neoplasia | 100 | 71 (71%) | 29 (29%) |
| Invasive cervical cancer | 542 | 256 (47%) | 286 (53%) |
| Ovarian cancer | 109 | 58 (53%) | 51 (47%) |
| Endometrial cancer | 125 | 70 (56%) | 55 (44%) |

Data obtained from DiSaia et al. [4], Donaldson et al. [30], and van Nagell et al. [45-9].

to hepatic function in experimental animals, and this finding has been more recently confirmed in human subjects [13].

In ovarian and cervical cancer, plasma and tumor CEA levels have been shown to be associated with specific cell types (see Chapter 6, Section 2.1). The cyst fluid of mucinous cystadenocarcinomas has been reported to contain mean CEA concentrations in excess of 7500 ng/ml compared to less than 200 ng/ml in the cyst fluid of serous cystadenocarcinomas [11]. Similarly, elevated plasma CEA levels have been noted in 53% of serous carcinomas. In cervical cancer, plasma and tissue CEA levels have been most consistently increased in patients with endocervical adenocarcinomas and keratinizing squamous cell carcinomas [9, 14].

The major clinical role for CEA determinations is in the follow-up of patients whose tumors or plasma contain high antigen levels prior to treatment. The value of serial plasma CEA determinations in the follow-up of patients with CEA-producing gynecologic cancers has been emphasized by several investigators. Barrelet and Mach [15] noted that plasma CEA levels rapidly returned to normal following curative therapy in patients with cervical, ovarian, and endometrial cancer. Khoo and MacKay [3] first reported that elevated plasma CEA concentrations fell to normal within 8 weeks following complete surgical excision of ovarian and cervical cancers, and this observation has been confirmed by many investigators. The decline in plasma CEA concentrations in cervical cancer patients undergoing radiation therapy may take considerably longer. Donaldson and colleagues [16] reported that plasma CEA titers often did not return to normal until 3 months following completion of radiation therapy. Presumably, this delay may be the result of prolonged release of antigen from the cell membrane of radiation damaged tumor cells. Conversely, van Nagell and co-workers [9] reported that progressively rising plasma CEA levels were predictive of recurrent disease in over 80% of cervical cancer patients whose tumors contained detectable amounts of antigen by immunohistochemical staining. Rising plasma CEA titers preceded clinical evidence of recurrence by up to 6 months in selected cases. In contrast, a positive correlation between elevated plasma CEA concentrations and clinical disease status could be found in only 28% of patients whose tumors were apparently devoid of CEA.

Khoo and co-workers [17, 18] studied the accuracy of serial CEA values in predicting clinical disease status in 213 patients with ovarian cancer. Serial CEA values when initially elevated accurately reflected disease status in over 95% of patients who had minimal residual disease after initial tumor debulking. Predictive accuracy fell to only 62% when tumor excision was incomplete and the patient was left with a significant tumor burden.

The cellular location of CEA has been studied using a variety of different techniques. Immunofluorescent and electron-microscopic studies have indicated that CEA is localized on the surface of cells lining the glands in colonic adenocarcinoma [17, 18] and this location has been confirmed in mucinous cystadenocarcinomas of the ovary [6, 7, 8]. Investigation of the localization of CEA within gynecologic tumor specimens has been greatly facilitated by the perfection of a triple-bridge, indirect, peroxidase-antiperoxidase method for the detection of CEA in tissue specimens processed for histopathology [19, 10]. Using this technique, van Nagell and co-workers [6, 7, 8] reported that CEA was detectable in a significantly greater percent of mucinous ovarian carcinomas than in serous ovarian malignancies. In most gynecologic tumors, CEA appears to be a cell membrane component. Moreover, its presence within glandular lumena and in the mucinous glycocalyx has led several investigators to postulate that CEA is a secretory product rather than a structural component of the cell [20]. Wahlstrom and colleagues [14], using a modification of this method, reported that adenocarcinomas of the endocervix could be differentiated from endometrial adenocarcinomas on the basis of CEA production. These investigators demonstrated CEA staining in 131 of 163 endocervical adenocarcinomas (80%) as opposed to only 11 of 137 endometrial adenocarcinomas (8%), and suggested that immunohistochemical staining could provide information of practical significance to the clinician.

Carcinoembryonic antigen has also been used as a target for radiolabeled antibodies in tumor scintiscanning experiments (see Chapter 6, Section 2.3). Goldenberg and colleagues [21] reported that diverse CEA-producing cancers could be localized using radiolabeled anti-CEA antibodies and a gamma scintillation camera. These tumors included four ovarian cancers and five cervical cancers. Scans were negative in control patients without tumors and in patients whose tumors did not contain CEA by immunohistochemical techniques. Endogenous circulating antigen levels of up to 350 ng/ml did not inhibit successful tumor imaging. Using this technique, van Nagell and co-workers [22] reported the successful localization of all 13 malignant ovarian tumors scanned. In addition, 6 of 9 sites of metastatic ovarian cancer were identified, some of which were not detected by rigorous application of other diagnostic methods, such as CT scanning, ultrasonography, and angiography. The major limitation of radioimmunodetection was that it failed to localize lesions less than 2 cm in diameter.

## 3. HUMAN CHORIONIC GONADOTROPIN

Human chorionic gonadotropin (hCG) is a trophoblastic glyocprotein with a molecular weight of 39,000. Two dissimilar subunits, the alpha and beta chains are noncovalently linked. The alpha chain of human luteinizing hormone (hLH) thyroid stimulating hormone (TSH), and hCG are similar; the C-terminal residues of the beta chains of these hormones are different. In 1972, Vaitukaitis and co-workers [23] reported the development of a specific radioimmunoassay for hCG based on the immunologic characteristics of its beta subunit. This assay distinguished between low concentrations of hLH and hCG, and allowed further evaluation of threshold levels of hCG as a tumor marker.

An early observation concerning the possible clinical role of hCG as a tumor marker was made by Li and Hertz [24]. These investigators noted increased amounts of hCG in the urine of patients with choriocarcinoma, and found that hCG concentrations decreased with successful treatment of these tumors [25] (See Chapter 5). Furthermore, the magnitude of response to chemotherapy was inversely related to the initial hCG titer. In the strictest sense of the definition, hCG is an antigen only in heterologous species and is not a tumor-specific product of trophoblastic neoplasia. Nevertheless, it is quantitatively increased in these tumors and its presence in the serum closely correlates with the number of viable trophoblastic tumor cells. In 1969, Patillo and co-workers [26] established a cell line of trophoblastic cells which produced hCG in tissue culture. The rate of production of hCG in choriocarcinoma cell lines has varied from 120 ng to 1000 ng per $10^6$ cells per day [27], and immunocytochemical studies have indicated that up to 70% of all trophoblastic cells in a stimulated state are producing hCG [28]. In normal pregnancy, hCH is produced by the trophoblast of the blastocyst, and is usually undetectable in the serum until 9–10 days after ovulation. Following implantation, serum concentrations increase rapidly with a doubling time of approximately 2.0 days. Peak hCG levels up to 100,000 mIU/ml occur between 60 and 90 days after last menses. Although a single elevated hCG value cannot reliably differentiate trophoblastic disease from pregnancy, a progressive rise in serum hCG after 90 days of gestation (the time at which hCG would plateau in a normal pregnancy) is highly suggestive of trophoblastic neoplasia. An absolute hCG titer in excess of 300,000 mIU/ml in the presence of a low serum hPL concentration is indicative of trophoblastic disease.

The selective production of hCG by trophoblastic cells has enabled the clinician to make a diagnosis of persistent trophoblastic disease without resorting to invasive methods. Complicated trophoblastic disease has been defined as (1) failure of serum hCG levels to decrease to normal within 8 weeks of uterine evacuation (2) plateau in serum hCG levels for two or more weeks after definitive therapy, or (3) rise in serum hCG values at any time following therapy. Serum hCG concentrations have so accurately reflected the number of viable trophoblastic tumor cells that the determination has become a paradigm of markers for neoplastic disease. Consequently, thera-

*Table 2.* Serum levels of human chorionic gonadotropin in patients with non-trophoblastic gynecologic cancers.

| Diagnosis | Patients | Elevated hCG |
|---|---|---|
| Healthy volunteers | 317 | 9 ( 3%) |
| Cervical cancer | 318 | 111 (35%) |
| Endometrial cancer | 167 | 26 (16%) |
| Ovarian cancer | 81 | 28 (35%) |

Data from Dash *et al.*, Donaldson *et al.* [30], Fishman *et al.*, (1975), Goldstein (1974), Rosen (1975), and Rutanen and Seppala [31].

peutic decisions have been made on the basis of hCG concentration alone. For example, a serum hCG concentration in excess of 40,000 mIU/ml in the presence of metastatic disease places a patient in the 'poor prognosis' category, thereby necessitating treatment with combination chemotherapy [29]. Conversely, the absence of detectable hCG in the serum is a reliable indicator of complete response to therapy. The current definition of remission in complicated trophoblastic disease is the absence of circulating levels of hCG for three consecutive weeks.

With the increased sensitivity of the beta subunit assay for hCG [23], elevated serum levels of this hormone have been detected in patients with nontrophoblastic gynecologic malignancies (Table 2). Serum hCG levels have been consistently elevated in about 35% of patients with ovarian and cervical malignancies [30, 31]. These observations are consistent with *in vitro* studies demonstrating hCG production by both ovarian and cervical cancer cell lines [27]. The absolute levels of this marker are considerably lower than those reported in patients with trophoblastic disease. Rutanen and Seppala [31], for example, noted that elevated serum hCG concentrations in 276 gynecologic cancer patients varied between 7 and 66 mIU/ml (mean 16.3 mIU/ml). The presence of detectable amounts of hCG in the serum of normal patients has prevented the use of this hormone as a tumor marker in patients with nontrophoblastic gynecologic tumors with the exception of ovarian germ cell malignancies such as dysgerminomas and embryonal cell carcinomas (see Chapter 4).

Immunohistochemical staining methods have indicated that hCG is present in virtually all embryonal cell carcinomas, and serum hCG concentrations have been shown to be elevated prior to surgical excision of these tumors [32]. Also, with the known production rates of hCG in tissue culture, it is quite likely that hCG will be a reliable clinical marker in ovarian choriocarcinoma [33].

Clinical detection of human cancers by radioimmunolocalization using radiolabeled anti-hCG antibodies has been reported by Goldenberg and colleagues [34]. After intravenous administration of $^{131}$I-labeled anti-hCG antibodies, images of the chest and abdomen by a gamma scintillation camera localized all three hCG-producing tumors. One patient with a hydatidiform mole had both pre-evacuation and post-evacuation scintigrams which demonstrated a sufficient concentration of antibodies to produce a clear photoscan image prior to therapy, but an insufficient concentration for a post-evacuation image (see Chapter 5, Section 5.8).

4. ALPHA FETO-PROTEIN

Alpha feto-protein (AFP) is a 10,000 molecular weight glycoprotein [35] with alpha$_1$-globulin mobility on electrophoresis. Abelev [36] first described its presence in the sera of newborn mice and in the sera of adult mice bearing transplantable hepatocellular carcinomas. Human AFP can be detected in fetal serum as early as 4 weeks gestation and reaches a peak concentration at a gestational age of about 100 days [37]. This oncofetal protein has been detected in highest concentrations in the sera and tumors of patients with hepatocellular carcinomas and malignant germ cell tumors of the testis and ovary [36, 38, 39]. Furthermore, embryonic hepatic and yolk sac cells have produced detectable amounts of AFP in tissue culture [37]. With the development of a specific radioimmunoassay for AFP [35], small amounts of this protein have been identified in a number of tumors including squamous cell carcinoma of the cervix and epithelial tumors of the ovary [30]. The absolute concentrations of AFP in the sera of these patients are usually not high (<100 ng/ml) and the presence of this marker in the sera of patients with a variety of benign inflammatory conditions of the liver has prevented its use as a reliable immunodiagnostic test.

For practical purposes, the clinical use of AFP in gynecologic cancer is confined to ovarian endodermal sinus tumors, embryonal cell carcinomas, and mixed germ cell tumors containing these specific cellular elements (see Chapter 4). Immunohistochemical staining methods have demonstrated AFP in every endodermal sinus tumor studied [40, 41]. These investigations have suggested, in fact, that endodermal sinus tumors can be reliably differentiated from embryonal cell carcinomas on the basis of marker production. Endodermal sinus tumors were found to produce only AFP, whereas embryonal cell carcinomas contained both AFP and hCG. Serial serum AFP determinations have reflected clinical disease status in patients whose ovarian germ cell tumors initially contained high AFP levels [39, 42]. Talerman and co-workers [39] noted that elevated serum levels of AFP were present in all patients with germ cell tumors of the ovary which contained endodermal sinus elements. Serum AFP concentrations fell to normal 5-7 weeks after tumor excision and rose prior to the clinical detection of recurrent disease. Similarly, Sell and colleagues [42] reported that serum AFP concentrations correlated closely with tumor regression or progression in patients undergoing chemotherapy for ovarian endodermal sinus tumors.

The use of radiolabeled antibodies to AFP for the detection of AFP-producing cancers by photoscan localization has been reported by Goldenberg and colleagues [43]. This technique accurately localized both primary and metastatic AFP-producing tumors in 83% of the cases. The most remarkable radiolocalizations occurred in two patients with embryonal cell carcinoma of the testis; circulating levels of AFP exceeded 750 ng/ml in these patients, and photoscanning successfully localized both primary and metastatic lesions.

## 5. TUMOR – ASSOCIATED ANTIGENS (see Chapter 6, Section 2.2)

With the refinement of analytic techniques for antigen isolation, much work has been devoted to the search for more specific tumor-associated antigens. Tumor-associated antigens may be newly expressed at the time of malignant transformation or they may represent normal tissue antigens which are quantitatively increased through enhanced production by tumor cells. Like other markers, tumor-associated antigens must be produced by a significant percentage of cells within a tumor, and then released into the circulation in sufficient concentrations to be measured by conventional techniques.

Since Witebsky and co-workers [44] first reported the isolation of antisera to tissue components of ovarian cancer, numerous investigators have detected what they consider to be specific antigens for either squamous cell carcinoma of the cervix or epithelial ovarian cancer. The techniques for isolation of these antigens have usually involved injection of cultured tumor cells or extracts of tumor tissue homogenates into animal hosts which develop antibodies to these extracts. The antiserum is then absorbed with corresponding normal tissue and blood components and tested by immunodiffusion against cancer tissue extracts. The presence of a common precipitin line is indicative of a specific antigenic component. Final steps in the preparation of specific antisera include antigen purification and the development of a specific radioimmunoassay. Although a relatively large number of tumor-associated antigens has been isolated from patients with gynecologic malignancies, rigorous purification of these antigens has permitted the development of radioimmunoassays for only three (Table 3).

The first of these antigens is the ovarian cystadenocarcinoma antigen (OCAA) reported by Bhattacharya and Barlow [45, 46]. This antigen is a

Table 3. Tumor-associated antigens undergoing clinical trials in patients with gynecologic cancer.

| Antigen | Investigator | Biochemical classification | Tumor |
|---|---|---|---|
| OCAA | Bhattacharya and Barlow, 1972, 1975 [45-46] | Mucoprotein | ovarian carcinoma |
| OCA | Knauf and Urbach, 1974, 1977, 1978 [49-51] | glycoprotein | ovarian carcinoma |
| TA-4 | Kato and Torigoe, 1977, 1979 [52, 54] | glycoprotein | cervical carcinoma |

high molecular weight mucoprotein which has β-electrophoretic mobility, and appears to be of cytoplasmic origin by immunofluorescence studies. It is composed of approximately 60% protein and 40% carbohydrate [47]. This antigen is immunologically distinct from CEA, AFP and normal histocompatibility antigens, and is not present in normal ovarian tissue. Ouchterlony double diffusion experiments indicated that OCAA was present in 26 of 37 serous cystadenocarcinomas and in all 7 mucinous cystadenocarcinomas, but was absent in germ cell and stromal tumors of the ovary. Likewise, OCAA was not detectable in any other gynecologic cancers. With development of a radioimmunoassay for OCAA [48], a serum level of 10 ng/ml was established as the upper limit of normal. Using this criterion, elevated serum levels of OCAA were observed in 66% of patients with Stages II and III ovarian cancer and in 80% of patients with Stage IV disease. Initial serum OCAA concentrations were related to total tumor burden, and usually returned to normal approximately three weeks following tumor excision [48]. Circulating antigen levels correlated quite well with response to therapy. Patients responding to treatment had OCAA levels less than 10 ng/ml, whereas a rise in serum antigen concentrations was indicative of tumor recurrence. The presence of cross-reacting substances in the sera of patients with other advanced stage malignancies has precluded the use of this antigen as a reliable diagnostic marker. When initially elevated, however, it has been effective as a biochemical marker of disease status in monitoring patients with serous and mucinous cystadenocarcinomas of the ovary.

The second tumor-associated antigen for which there is a radioimmunoassay is the ovarian cancer antigen (OCA) reported by Knauf and Urbach [49, 50, 51]. This antigen is a high molecular weight glycoprotein which is soluble in perchoric acid and immunologically distinct from CEA. Immunodiffusion experiments indicated that this antigen was present in serous cystadenocarcinomas, but was not detectable in normal ovary or normal human serum. With the use of a double-antibody radioimmonoassay, a plasma value in excess of 1.9 ng/ml was considered abnormally elevated [51]. Serum OCA levels were elevated in 66 of 126 patients (52%) with ovarian cancer as compared to 5 of 61 normal patients. Serum levels of CEA were elevated (>2.5 ng/ml) in only 28% of these patients. The specificity of OCA, although higher than CEA, was not sufficient to allow its use as a diagnostic method for ovarian cancer. However, serial levels of OCA correlated quite well with clinical disease status in patients whose tumors or plasma contained high antigen levels.

The final gynecologic tumor-associated antigen that has been subjected to clinical trials is the cervical cancer antigen (TA-4) initially described by Kato and Torigoe [52]. This antigen is a glycoprotein with a molecular weight of approximately 48,000. Normal cervical tissue extracts showed an inhibition effect in the radioimmunoassay suggesting the presence of TA-4 in normal cervical tissue [52]. In serum, however, 27 of 35 patients with cervical squamous cell carcinoma had elevated TA-4 levels as compared to none of the patients in the normal control group. In a subsequent clinical trial using patients from the NCI-Mayo Clinic Serum Bank [53] 13 of 25 cervical cancer patients had positive serum TA-4 levels as opposed to only one of 58 control patients. Serum TA-4 levels were elevated in all patients with advanced disease and accurately reflected status of disease following therapy (see Chapter I, Section 5).

## 6. CLINICAL APPLICATION OF TUMOR MARKERS

Although there have been many advances in the science of tumor immunology and antigen chemistry, indications for the proper clinical use of tumor markers have not been fully defined. On the basis of presently available data, it is clear that tumor markers provide information essential to the management of patients with trophoblastic disease and germ cell tumors of the ovary. The potentially useful markers for several tumor types are presented in Table 4. The clinical value of serum hCG determinations in the management of patients with trophoblastic disease has been well established. Similarly, hCG levels have reliably predicted disease status in germ cell ovarian tumors containing either choriocarcinoma or embryonal cell elements. Alpha feto-protein is a valuable marker in endodermal sinus tumor of the ovary, embryonal cell carcinoma, and in mixed germ cell tumors containing these elements. Finally, CEA is a reliable marker for mucinous cystadenocarcinoma of the ovary and for endocervical adenocarcinomas.

A fundamental and yet unanswered question is how to determine the optimal markers for the majority of tumors for which there are no unique

*Table 4.* Clinical use of markers in gynecologic cancer according to tumor type.

| Marker | Tumor type |
| --- | --- |
| hCG | Trophoblastic disease |
|  | Ovarian choriocarcinoma |
|  | Embryonal cell carcinoma |
| AFP | Endodermal sinus tumor |
|  | Embryonal cell carcinoma |
| CEA | Mucinous cystadenocarcinoma of the ovary |
|  | Adenocarcinoma of the endocervix |
| OCAA | Serous and mucinous cystadenocarcinomas of the ovary |
| OCA | Serous and mucinous cystadenocarcinomas of the ovary |
| TA-4 | Squamous cell carcinoma of the cervix |

associated antigens. Included in these tumors are most ovarian and cervical carcinomas, endometrial cancer, and vulvar cancer. A previous approach to the development of a strategy for the evaluation of markers has been the measurement of a battery of different serum antigens with the intent of discovering an elevation of one or more of these markers in a particular patient. The concentration of this antigen was then followed serially and correlated with the clinical response to therapy. Unfortunately, this approach has been costly and often inaccurate. Serum marker concentration is related both to antigen concentration in tumor tissue and to the extent of disease. Consequently, a patient with an extensive tumor may have increased serum levels of a particular antigen prior to therapy, but this antigen may not be measurable in the presence of a small tumor recurrence. For a specific marker to accurately reflect clinical disease status, it must be present within the tumor itself and be shed into the circulation. What is needed, therefore, is a tissue screening test which can reliably identify the antigenic profile of each tumor. Radioimmunoassay of tumor extracts has not proven practical as a tissue antigen screening method since much of the tumor must be processed for histopathology. Likewise, production rates of markers in cultured tumor cells often does not correlate with *in vivo* synthesis rates.

In 1966, Nakane and Pierce [51] reported a technique for the histochemical localization of antigens using enzyme-labeled antibodies. In this method, antibodies are labeled with peroxidase and after incubation the antigenic site is identified by a histochemical reaction. Primus and co-workers [19, 55] reported a modification of this method for the detection of CEA in formalin-fixed specimens prepared routinely for histopathology. This technique has successfully localized many oncofetal, hormonal and tumor-associated antigens (see Chapter 4).

The clinical importance of the immunoperoxidase technique is that it can identify those markers which should most accurately reflect disease status. For example, van Nagell and co-workers [9] reported that serial plasma CEA values correlated with clinical disease in over 80% of cervical cancer patients whose tumors contained CEA by immunohistochemical staining. In contrast, plasma CEA levels accurately reflected disease status in only 28% of patients whose cervical tumors were devoid of antigen. A potential source of error in this method is incomplete sampling of a heterogeneous tumor. In tumors of mixed histologic patterns, every effort must be made to stain multiple areas within the tumor so that the appropriate marker can be identified. Furthermore, characterization of a tumor simply as antigen-positive or antigen-negative is insufficient because the number and distribution of antigen-producing cells within each tumor is important. Protocols should be developed in which both the initial serum marker concentration and the relative number of marker-producing cells within each tumor are used to predict which patients will benefit from serial marker determinations after therapy. It is apparent that serum antigen determinations will most accurately reflect the number of viable tumor cells within a host if the majority of these cells produce and shed the antigen being measured. This is the case in trophoblastic disease where almost all tumor cells produce hCG. Therefore, histochemical staining should be used when possible to identify those markers that are highly concentrated within the tumor. Conversely, if a marker is absent from tumor tissue, it is highly unlikely that serial marker determinations will provide clinically important information.

Two areas for the possible clinical application of markers are (1) radioimmunodetection of both primary and metastatic tumors and (2) antibody-directed therapy. In 1953, Pressman [56] reported the successful localization of rat lymphosarcomas using radiolabeled antilymphosarcoma antibodies. More recently, Goldenberg and co-workers [21] reported successful photoscan localization of diverse CEA-producing tumors using $^{131}$I-labeled goat IgG prepared against CEA. Using this same technique, van Nagell and colleagues [22] reported the successful detection of both primary and metastatic ovarian cancer. Tumor localization has also been reported using radiolabeled antibodies to AFP and hCG. In general, this method has not yet proven superior to conventional imaging techniques such as ultrasonography and CT scanning in the diagnosis of pelvic tumors. However, with the identification of more specific tumor antigens and the development of improved computed scanning techniques, it is likely that the resolution of radioimmunodetection procedures will improve (see Chapter 5, Section 5.8).

The use of antibodies to direct chemotherapeutic agents or radionuclides to antigen-producing tumor cells has obvious clinical advantages. Since therapy is directed specifically at marker-producing malignant cells, normal cells are spared and systemic drug toxicity is reduced. For this approach to be successful, antibodies must be produced which have high specificity for tumor cells and minimal affinity for normal cells. The cytotoxic activity of the therapeutic agent must be preserved until it is bound to the tumor cell and the specificity of the antibody must not be modified by adding the agent. In 1967, Spar and co-workers [57], reported the use of $^{131}$I-labeled antifibrin antibodies in the treatment of fibrin containing human tumors. Although remissions were observed, autoradiographs indicated variable distribution of radiolabeled antibodies within the tumors, and regrowth was observed in all cases. More recently, Ghose and co-workers [58] were able to demonstrate regression of malignant melanomas using chlorambucil-bound antimelanoma globulins, and these observations have been confirmed in experimental animal models [59, 60]. To date, antibody-directed therapy has not been utilized in the treatment of gynecologic malignancies.

A proposed system for the clinical use of tumor markers is illustrated in Figure 1. In this model, immunohistochemical staining defines the marker profile for each tumor. The most appropriate marker can then be used for radioimmunodetection and antibody-directed therapy. Finally, the response to therapy can be monitored with the appropriate serial marker determinations. Many questions concerning antigen purification and specificity remain to be answered before such a model can become operational. Nevertheless, tumor associated markers presently provide information of clini-

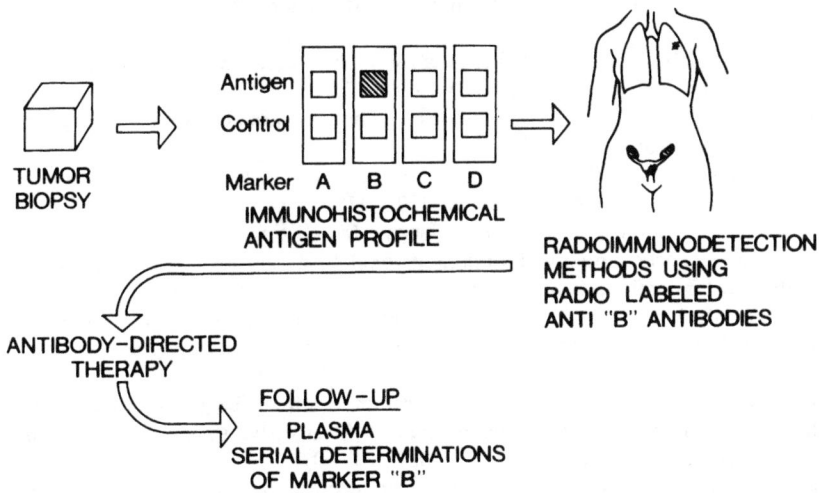

*Figure 1.* Conceptual scheme for clinical use of tumor markers.

cal importance to many cancer patients and their potential use is even more promising.

REFERENCES

1. Gold P, Freedman SO: Demonstration of tumor specific antigens in human colonic carcinoma by immunological tolerance and absorption techniques. J Exp Med 121:439–462, 1965.
2. Krupey J, Gold P, Freedman SO: Purification and characterisation of carcinoembryonic antigens of the human digestive system. Nature (London) 215:67–68, 1967.
3. Khoo SK, MacKay EV: Carcinoembryonic antigen in cancer of the female reproductive system. Sequential levels and effects of treatment. Aust New Zealand J Obstet Gynecol 13:1–7, 1973.
4. DiSaia PJ, Haverback BJ, Morrow CP: Carcinoembryonic antigen in patients with gynecologic malignancies. Am J Obstet Gynecol 121:159–166, 1975.
5. van Nagell JR, Donaldson ES, Wood EG, Sharkey RM, Goldenberg DM: The prognostic significance of carcinoembryonic antigen in the plasma and tumors of patients with endometrial adenocarcinoma. Am J Obstet Gynecol 128:308–313, 1977.
6. van Nagell JR, Donaldson ES, Gay EC, Sharkey RM, Rayburn P, Goldenberg DM: Carcinoembryonic antigen in ovarian epithelial cystadenocarcinomas: Prognostic value of serial plasma determinations. Cancer 41:2335–2340, 1978.
7. van Nagell JR, Donaldson ES, Wood EC, Goldenberg DM: The clinical significance of carcinoembryonic antigen in the plasma and tumors of patients with gynecologic malignancies. Cancer 42:1527–1532, 1978.
8. van Nagell JR, Donaldson ES, Gay EC, Rayburn P, Powell DF, Goldenberg DM: Carcinoembryonic antigen in carcinoma of the uterine cervix. 1. The prognostic value of serial plasma determinations. Cancer 42:2428–2434, 1978.
9. van Nagell JR, Donaldson ES, Gay EC, Hudson S, Sharkey RM, Primus FJ, Powell DF, Goldenberg DM: Carcinoembryonic antigen in carcinoma of the uterine cervix. 2. Tissue localization and correlation with plasma antigen concentration. Cancer 44:944–948, 1979.
10. Goldenberg DM, Sharkey RM, Primus FJ: Carcinoembryonic antigen in histopathology: Immunoperoxidase staining of conventional tissue sections. J Natl Cancer Inst 57:11–21, 1976.
11. van Nagell JR, Meeker W, Parker JC, Harralson JD: Carcinoembryonic antigen in patients with gynecologic malignancy. Cancer 35:1372–1376, 1975.
12. Shuster J, Silverman M, Gold P: Metabolism of human carcinoembryonic antigen in xenogeneic animals. Cancer Res 33:65–68, 1973.
13. Lurie BB, Oweinstein MS, Zamcheck N: Elevated carcinoembryonic antigen levels and biliary tract obstruction. JAMA 233:326–330, 1975.
14. Wahlstrom T, Lindgren J, Korhonen M, Seppala M: Distinction between endocervical and endometrial adenocarcinoma with immunoperoxidase staining of carcinoembryonic antigen in routine histological tissue specimens. Lancet 24:1159–1160, 1979.
15. Barrelet V, Mach J: Variations of the carcinoembryonic antigen level in the plasma of patients with gynecologic cancers during therapy. Am J Obstet Gynecol 121:164–168, 1975.
16. Donaldson ES, van Nagell JR, Wood EG, Pletsch Q, Goldenberg DM: Carcinoembryonic antigen in patients treated with radiation therapy for invasive squamous cell carcinoma of the uterine cervix. Am J Roentgenol 127:829–831, 1976.
17. Gold P, Krupey J, Ansari H: Position of the carcinoembryonic antigen of the human digestive system in ultrastructure of tumor cell surface. J Natl Cancer Inst 45:219–225, 1970.

18. Tappeiner G, Denk H, Eckerstorfer R, Holzner JH: Vergleichende Untersuchungen über Auftreten und Lokalisation des carcinoembryonalen Antigens (CEA) und eines normalen perchlorsaure-extrahierbaren Dickdarmschleimhautantigens (NC) in Carcinomen und Polypes des Dickdarmes. Virchows Arch Path Anat 360:129–140, 1973.
19. Primus FJ, Wang RH, Sharkey RM, Goldenberg DM: Detection of carcinoembryonic antigen in tissue sections by immunoperoxidase. J Immunol Methods 8:267–276, 1975.
20. Huitric E, Laumonier R, Burtin P, Kleist S, von Chevanel G: An optical and ultrastructural study of the localization of carcinoembryonic antigen (CEA) in normal and cancerous human rectocolonic mucosa. Lab Invest 34:97–107, 1976.
21. Goldenberg DM, DeLand F, Kim E, Bennett S, Primus FJ, van Nagell JR, Estes N, De Simone PJ, Rayburn P: Use of radiolabeled antibodies to carcinoembryonic antigen for the detection and localization of diverse cancers by external photoscanning. N Engl J Med 298:1384–1388, 1978.
22. van Nagell JR, Kim E, Casper S, Primus FJ, Bennett S, DeLand FH, Goldenberg DM: Radioimmunodetection of primary and metastatic ovarian cancer using radiolabeled antibodies to carcinoembryonic antigen. Cancer Res 40:502–506, 1980.
23. Vaitukaitis JL, Braunstein GP, Ross GT: A radioimmunoassay which specifically measures human chorionic gonadotropin in the presence of human luteinizing hormone. Am J Obstet Gynecol 113:751–756, 1972.
24. Li MC, Hertz R, Bergenstral DM: Therapy of choriocarcinoma and related trophoblastic tumors with folic acid and purine antagonists. N Engl J Med 259:66–70, 1958.
25. Hertz R, Lewis J, Lipsett MB: Five years' experience with the chemotherapy of metastatic choriocarcinoma and related trophoblastic tumors in women. Am J Obstet Gynecol 82:631–637, 1961.
26. Pattillo RA, Grey GO: The establishment of a cell line of human hormone synthesizing trophoblastic cells *in vitro*. Cancer Res 24:1231–1236, 1968.
27. Kanabus J, Braunstein GD, Emry PK, DiSaia PJ, Wade ME: Kinetics of growth and ectopic production of human chorionic gonadotropin by an ovarian cystadenocarcinoma cell line maintained *in vitro*. Cancer Res 38:765–770, 1978.
28. Yorde DE, Hussa RO, Garancis JC, Pattillo RA: Immunocytochemical localization of human choriogonadotropin in human malignant trophoblast: Model for human choriogonadotropin secretion. Lab Invest 40:391–398, 1979.
29. Hammond CB, Weed JC, Currie JL: The role of operation in the current therapy of gestational trophoblastic disease. Am J Obstet Gynecol 136:844–858, 1980.
30. Donaldson ES, van Nagell JR, Pursell S, Kashmiri R, Meeker WR, van de Voorde J, Gay EC: Multiple Biochemical markers in patients with gynecologic malignancies. Cancer 45:948–953, 1980.
31. Rutanen EM, Seppala M: The hCG-subunit radioimmunoassay in non-trophoblastic gynecologic tumors. Cancer 41:692–696, 1978.
32. Kurman RJ, Norris HJ: Embryonal carcinoma of the ovary: A clinico-pathological entity distinct from endodermal sinus tumor resembling embryonal carcinoma of the adult testes. Cancer 38:2420–2433, 1976.
33. Kohler PO, Bridson WE, Hammond J, Weintraub B, Kirschner MA, Van Thiel DH: Clonal lines of human choriocarcinoma cells in culture. In: Diczfalusy E, ed.: Karolinska Symposia on Research Methods in Reproductive Endocrinology, Denmark, 1971, Bogtry Keriet Forum, pp. 137–153.
34. Goldenberg DM, Kim E, DeLand FH, van Nagell JR, Javadpour N: Clinical radioimmunodetection of cancer using radioactive antibodies to human chorionic gonadotropin. Science 208:1284–1286, 1980.
35. Ruoslahti E, Seppala M: Studies of carcino- fetal proteins. III. Development of a radioim-

munoassay for α-fetoprotein in serum of healthy human adults. Int J Cancer 8:374–383, 1971.
36. Abelev GI: Study of the antigenic structure of tumors. Acta Un Intern Cancer 19:80–92, 1963.
37. Seppala M, Ruoslahti E: Alpha-fetoprotein: Physiology and pathology during pregnancy and application to antenatal diagnosis. J Perinat Med 1:104–113, 1973.
38. Tatarinov JS: Presence of embryonal α-globulin in the serum of a patient with primary hepatocellular carcinoma. Vop Med Khim 1:90–91, 1964.
39. Talerman A, Haije WG, Beggerman L: Serum alpha-fetoprotein (AFP) in diagnosis and management of endodermal sinus (yolk-sac) tumor and mixed germ cell tumor of the ovary. Cancer 41:272–278, 1978.
40. Kurman RJ, Norris HJ: Endodermal sinus tumor of the ovary. Cancer 38:2404–2419, 1976.
41. Gallion H, van Nagell JR, Powell DF, Donaldson ES, Hanson M: Therapy of endodermal sinus tumor of the ovary. Am J Obstet Gynecol 135:447–451, 1979.
42. Sell A, Sogaard H, Horgaard-Pedersen B: Serum alpha feto-protein as a marker for the effect of post-operative radiation therapy and/or chemotherapy in eight cases of ovarian endodermal sinus tumour. Int J Cancer 18:574–580, 1976.
43. Goldenberg DM, Kim E, DeLand F, Spermulli E, Nelson MO, Cockerman JP, Primus FJ, Corgan RL, Alpert E: Clinical studies on the radioimmunodetection of tumors containing alpha-fetoprotein. Cancer 45:2500–2505, 1980.
44. Witebsky E, Rose NR, Schulman S: Studies of normal and malignant tissue antigens. Cancer Res 16:831–841, 1956.
45. Bhattacharya M, Barlow JJ: Immunologic studies of human serous cystadenocarcinoma of ovary. Cancer 31:588–595, 1972.
46. Bhattacharya M, Barlow JJ: A tumor-associated antigen from cystadenocarcinomas of the ovary. Natl Cancer Inst Monog 42:25–32, 1975.
47. Bhattacharya M, Barlow JJ: Tumor markers for ovarian cancer. Int Adv Surg Oncol 2:155–176, 1979.
48. Bhattacharya M, Barlow JJ: Ovarian tumor antigens. Cancer 42:1616–1620, 1978.
49. Knauf S, Urbach EI: Ovarian tumor-specific antigens. Am J Obstet Gynecol 119:966–970, 1974.
50. Knauf S, Urbach GI: Purification of human ovarian tumor-associated antigen and demonstration of circulating tumor-antigen in patients with advanced ovarian malignancy. Am J Obstet Gynecol 127:705–711, 1977.
51. Knauf S, Urbach GI: The development of a double-antibody radioimmunoassay for detecting ovarian tumor-associated antigen fraction OCA in plasma. Am J Obstet Gynecol 131:780–786, 1978.
52. Kato H, Torigoe T: Radioimmunoassay for tumor antigen of human cervical squamous cell carcinoma. Cancer 40:1621–1628, 1977.
53. Kato H, Miyauchi F, Morioka H, Fujino T, Torigoe T: Tumor antigen of human cervical squamous cell carcinoma. Correlation of circulating levels with disease progress. Cancer 43:585–590, 1979.
54. Nakane PK, Pierce GB: Enzyme labeled antibodies: Preparation and application for the localization of antigens. J Histochem Cytochem 14:929–931, 1966.
55. Primus FJ, Sharkey RM, Hansen HJ, Goldenberg DM: Immunoperoxidase detection of carcinoembryonic antigen: An overview. Cancer 42:1540–1545, 1978.
56. Pressman D, Koringold L: The *in vivo* localization of anti-Wagner osteogenic sarcoma antibodies. Cancer 6:619–623, 1953.
57. Spar JL, Bale WF, Marrack D, Dewey WC, McCardle RJ, Harper PV: Labeled antibodies to human fibrinogen. Diagnostic studies and therapeutic trials. Cancer 20:865–870, 1967.

58. Ghose T, Norvell ST, Guclu A, Bodurtha A, Tai J, MacDonald AS: Immunochemotherapy of malignant melanoma with chlorambucil-bound antimelanoma globulins and preliminary results in patients with disseminated disease. J Natl Cancer Inst 58:845–852, 1977.
59. Harwitz E, Schecter B, Arnon R, Sela M: Binding of anti-tumor immunoglobulins and their daunomycin conjugates to the tumor and its metastases. *In vitro* and *in vivo* studies with Lewis lung carcinoma. Int J Cancer 24:461–470, 1979.
60. Latif ZA, Lozzio BB, Wust CJ, Krauss S, Aggio MC: Evaluation of drug antibody conjugates in the treatment of human myelosarcomas transplanted in nude mice. Cancer 45:1326–1333, 1980.

# 3. Hormonal Receptors in Endometrial and Ovarian Neoplasia

GEORGE S. RICHARDSON and DAVID T. MACLAUGHLIN

## 1. INTRODUCTION

Estrogen stimulates proliferation of the ductal tissue in the breast, of the glands and stroma of the endometrium, and of the granulosa cells in the ovary. Habit has settled oncologists with the idea that estrogen is directly mitogenic; after all, it has been defined from the beginning by bioassays (vaginal exfoliation and uterotropic response) that depend on mitotic activity. Moreover, its action on normal human endometrium is assessed by finding glandular and stromal mitoses [1]. The mitogenic action of estrogen has never been satisfactorily demonstrated *in vitro*, however, and the possibility exists that its mitogenic action may be indirect [2, 3, 4].

The endocrinologist, on the other hand, does not think in terms of mitosis, but focuses instead on how hormones direct the genome to make new protein. This habit is based on the evolution of molecular biology and its preoccupation, since the work of Beadle and Tatum, with the association of a single gene with a single enzyme. It is now well established that the necessary first step in steroid hormone action is binding of the hormone to a receptor, a protein of the cytoplasm that (1) exists only in target cells, (2) binds hormonal steroids with an affinity greater than that of plasma binders, (3) binds them with an affinity proportional to their biological activity, (4) undergoes a process of temperature-dependent transformation (activation) that allows it to carry the steroid into the nucleus (translocation), (5) binds to 'acceptor' sites on chromatin, and (6) activates the transcription of DNA into protein-synthesizing message (mRNA) [5].

With the last two steps, the receptor makes its contribution to the action of steroid hormones on target cells. These steps have been worked out in considerable detail for the chick oviduct where the binding of the receptor-steroid complex to chromatin appears to increase the number of initiation sites for DNA transcription in a dose-related manner. While this mecha-

*Griffiths, C. T. and Fuller, A. F. (eds.), Gynecologic Oncology.*
© *1983, Martinus Nijhoff Publishers, Boston. ISBN 0-89838-555-5.*
*Printed in The Netherlands.*

nism is clearly applicable to the production of hormone-dependent products, as in the example of ovalbumin production by the chick oviduct, its relation to mitotic events is not at all clear. If one were to restrict the term 'receptor' to cases in which a relation has been demonstrated between binding to cytosol protein, activation, and translocation, on the one hand, and the transcription of DNA on the other, none of the 'receptors' described in this chapter would qualify. For this reason Jensen has consistently used the term 'estrophilin' for what others have termed 'estrogen receptor'.

To return to the problem of steroid hormones and mitotic events, or growth: receptors of lower affinity that are associated with the nucleus (nuclear Type II receptors) may be concerned with mitotic events, whereas the high-affinity receptors of the cytosol, which have been the focus of so much oncological research, are not [6, 7]. The presence of receptors that have somehow arrived in the nucleus without their cargo of steroid hormone or have appeared there endogenously suggests that the cells that contain them may be continuously stimulated in the absence of estrogen. Originally demonstrated in cultured breast cancer cells whose growth was estrogen-independent but was blocked by anti-estrogens [8] these receptors have now been found in nonmalignant tissues [9, 10] including normal human endometrium [11, 12, 13].

So far at least, the clinical usefulness of assays for estrogen and progesterone binding proteins in breast cancer has allowed oncologists to ignore these questions. It is now generally agreed that for breast cancer (1) the presence of estrogen receptors correlates with good prognosis, independent of other prognostic factors such as stage and grade of the tumor, and (2) only tumors that contain estrogen receptors respond to hormonal manipulations [14]. This last observation is surprising, since the hormones that the oncologist administers are only effective in doses that far exceed the maximum capacity of any receptor. The effect has no physiological parallel in the tissue that is parent to the tumor. In view of this observation, the physiology of the endometrium and ovary with respect to steroid 'receptors' may or may not be relevant to neoplasia, but the few known facts can be reviewed.

*1.1. The physiology of steroid receptors in normal endometrium*

Estrogen increases the level of the progesterone receptor in the cytoplasm of the endometrial cell. Progesterone, on the other hand, counteracts the effect of estrogen in four ways: (1) like the anti-estrogens, it inhibits replenishment of the estrogen receptor; (2) it shortens the duration of estrogen retention on the nuclear acceptor; (3) it decreases the level of its own receptor; and (4) it increases the level of the enzyme that converts estradiol to the less active metabolite, estrone [15–17]. It follows from these observations that the levels of total estrogen and progesterone receptor in normal endometrium tend to parallel the serum estrogen concentrations. Because of translocation, the level of unoccupied cytosolic estrogen receptor begins to fall before the estrogen peak is reached [18] whereas the level of nuclear estrogen receptor and the level of cytosolic progesterone receptor tend to parallel the serum estrogen concentration [19]. The presence of the progesterone receptor is in itself evidence of the ability of the tissue to respond to estrogen. If we take the level of nuclear estrogen receptor (ERn) as a measure of the degree of stimulation by estrogen, and the level of cytosolic progesterone receptor (PRc) as the degree of response, then the level of PRc per unit ERn can be taken as a measure of the sensitivity of the tissue to estrogen. On this basis, King [20] has estimated that the estrogenic sensitivity of adenomatous hyperplasia is greater than that of cystic glandular hyperplasia and both are greater than that of normal proliferative or postmenopausal endometrium. This concept, unfortunately, has not been tested in enough cases to be accepted without reservation and has not been systematically applied to the study of endometrial cancer.

There is evidence for the presence of an androgen receptor in human endometrium, but its function is unknown [21].

*1.2. The physiology of steroid receptors in normal ovary*

The granulosa cells of the ovarian follicle are stimulated to proliferate by estrogen, which increases the amount of its own receptor and sensitizes the cells to a further proliferative stimulus provided by FSH [22, 23]. Androgens are apparently the physiological stimulus for follicular atresia [24] and may be promoters of progesterone biosynthesis [25]. Other compartments of the normal ovary are not known to be targets of steroid hormones. The monolayer of mesothelium (so-called 'germinal epithelium') on the surface of the ovary responds to the hormones of pregnancy with deciduation – as does the peritoneal mesothelium with which it has a common origin in the coelomic epithelium – and it is this tissue, after all, which is thought to give rise to the common epithelial cancers of the ovary. Sex steroid receptor-like proteins have been described in bovine [27], rabbit [28], and rodent ovaries [29], and only recently in normal human ovaries [30–32]. In these experiments the entire ovary was assayed, so that the binding cannot be assigned to any specific ovarian compartment. There is no obvious physiological reason for the normal human ovary to contain a progesterone receptor, but one has been described [31]. Testosterone competes for this binder, albeit at the disadvantage of a binding affinity that is an order of magnitude less. The observations suggest that this protein is the receptor that mediates androgen-induced atresia, and that progesterone is the physiological antagonist.

## 2. METHODS

What follows is a synopsis of the considerations that are important for the evaluation of data of the kind that is presented in this review. For a detailed consideration of various methods for the assay of receptors, the reader should consult the review by G.C. Chamness and W.L. McGuire [33].

### 2.1. Preparation and preservation of tissue

Receptors, especially the progesterone receptor, are labile and the tissue must be kept cold and processed within hours, or frozen, preferably in liquid nitrogen, and stored at $-70\,°C$. While the choice of buffers is not controversial, the use of a thiol reagent to protect sulfhydryl groups and the use of glycerol, especially in the preparation of the progesterone receptor, is not universal but these reagents are probably important. Molybdate stabilizes receptors [34] but has not been used in the studies reported here.

### 2.2. Specificity of labeled ligand

Diethylstilbestrol (DES), unlike the natural estrogens, binds to the estrogen receptor, but not to sex hormone binding globulin (SHBG). Estradiol dissociates only very slowly from its receptor and is the most commonly used ligand for ER, perhaps because it is the physiological compound. DES is often used in parallel incubations to displace the ligand from receptor sites while leaving it attached to binders that are not receptors. Specific binding is estimated by subtracting these values. The synthetic progestins R5020 and ORG2058, unlike progesterone, bind to the receptor but not to cortisol binding globulin (CBG). An additional advantage of these compounds as ligands is that they dissociate far more slowly from the receptor than does progesterone, and are bound with comparable affinity. The fact that R5020 has a higher affinity for albumin than progesterone does is a potential source of problems, since an unknown fraction of labeled R5020 may fail to be removed from albumin with charcoal extraction, and albumin-bound R5020 can give a labeled peak in the 4S region of sucrose density gradients [35].

Androgen receptors have commonly been measured using $5\alpha$-dihydrotestosterone as the ligand, but this compound binds to SHBG which can confound the assay [36].

### 2.3. Specificity of the binding protein

Cytosols are invariably contaminated with serum proteins, so that the binding of estrogens and androgens must be presumed to include binding by SHBG; likewise the binding of progesterone must be presumed to include binding by CBG and both must be presumed to include binding by albumin.

One approach, as noted, is to saturate the nonreceptor binders with other ligands, such as DES or cortisol. Another is to separate the receptor protein from the rest of the mixture. This can be accomplished (1) by sucrose density gradient centrifugation (SDG), (2) by adsorption of the receptor onto hydroxylapatite (HAP) [37] or DEAE filters, or (3) by agar gel electrophoresis [38].

## 2.4. Separation of bound from unbound ligand

After incubation until equilibrium, dextran-coated charcoal (DCC) is most often used to extract unbound ligand from cytosol without removing significant amounts of receptor protein. The DCC assay for estrogen receptor (ER) measures only the portion that is found as 8S protein on sucrose density gradients [39]. High salt concentrations that convert the binder to the 4-5S form are associated with a progressive decrease in binding as detected by the DCC assay.

## 2.5. Occupied vs unoccupied receptors

Receptors bind to their ligands with high affinity. The equilibrium constant of dissociation (Kd) is of the order of $10^{-9} M$, that is, the receptor is half-saturated when the free hormone is at nanomolar concentration. This level of estradiol is reached during the normal menstrual cycle well before the midcycle peak, and the level of progesterone in midluteal phase far exceeds it. The preponderance of evidence indicates that only the cytosolic estrogen receptor (ERc) that is unoccupied by estradiol exchanges with labeled estradiol during an 18-hour incubation at 4°C [33]. Data have been brought forward, however, that indicate that estrogen receptor, if present, is detected with reasonable accuracy in most assays regardless of the plasma estrogen concentration [40, 41]. Even so, ERc-negative breast cancers have been observed to become positive after prior treatment with dextran-coated charcoal [42]. With a shorter incubation at higher temperatures (20°C) full exchange takes place and total ERc can be measured [43], but the loss of ERc by degradation during the incubation period can occur and is best identified by means of a control incubation. Exchange assays have long been used for the estimation of nuclear estrogen receptor (ERn) in many situations, and have been successfully applied to endometrial cancer for the measurement of both ERn [44] and PRn [45]. The progesterone receptor is very heat-labile, but the ligand dissociates rapidly and exchange takes place under most assay conditions [16, 46]. When progesterone is at its highest concentration in the luteal phase, it is also at high concentration in the tissue and incomplete exchange can result in an underestimation of the concentration of receptor [31, 40]. Under these conditions, prior incubation with DCC to remove excess endogenous free hormone can correct the situation [31]. This preliminary step has been often used in assays for both estrogen and progesterone receptors in the cases reported here [31, 47–50]. The existence of unoccupied ERn has been alluded to above.

*2.6. Estimation of binding affinity and the heterogeneity of receptors*

It has long been assumed that only high-affinity (Type I) binding is clinically relevant. The presence of variable amounts of lower affinity steroid-specific (Type II) binding means that a multiple point assay is required in order to measure both types. The conventional method for this purpose is the DCC assay, corrected for nonspecific binding, and a Scatchard plot of the data that yields both the number of binding sites and their affinity constants. The possible involvement of Type II nuclear binders in mitotic events [6] suggests that it may be important to obtain accurate assays for them as well [7]. It is of interest that the postmenopausal human uterus contains only the high-affinity (Type I) binder, suggesting that the continuous presence of estrogen may be required to maintain Type II [51].

*2.7. The problem of tumor sampling*

Endometrial curettings that contain carcinoma may also contain variable amounts of normal or hyperplastic tissue [52]. Since the normal endometrium of cycling women always contains some receptor, and hyperplastic tissue usually contains high levels, the receptor detected in a cancer sample may in some instances be due to the presence of these nonmalignant elements. Where the volume of tissue is limited, most of it should be sent for pathological examination, leaving only a small amount available for receptor assay. Under these conditions it may be possible to do only a single point saturation assay and risk confusion between high and low affinity (Type I and Type II) receptors. Endometrial cancers that yield abundant curettings often consist in part of tissue that has outgrown its blood supply and become necrotic with loss of receptor. Such tissue could readily yield false-negative results. An interesting additional variable in endometrial sampling arises from the fact that at all phases of the cycle the amount of the receptor present in normal endometrium varies, depending upon the location within the endometrial cavity from which the sample is obtained. Specifically, the cytosolic receptors are most numerous in cells from the region of the fundus, falling progressively in number toward the cervix. The nuclear receptors exhibit a gradient in the opposite direction [53, 54]. Ovarian carcinomas pose even greater sampling problems than do endometrial carcinomas. They are commonly bulky and contain much extracellular material in the form of mucin. In many instances, the stroma adjacent to the tumor exhibits luteinization, and in any given instance it may be the stroma that contains the receptor.

## 2.8. Pathological evaluation of tumors

The distinction between atypical hyperplasia of the endometrium and cancer is not sharp, and pathologists from different institutions are apt to apply somewhat different criteria. The methods are divided broadly between the evaluation of nuclear abnormalities and mitotic activity, on the one hand, and of architectural abnormalities on the other. The criteria used in the many reports of receptor levels have not been spelled out in detail, and there is unquestionably a great deal of variation between reports from different centers. An example of what might be done in the case of endometrial cancer is the report by Robboy and Bradley [55], who assessed 17 histological variables: (1) histological type of tumor, (2) grade, (3) depth of invasion, (4) percent of squamous component, (5) intracellular and extracellular mucin, (6) presence of ciliated cells, (7) growth pattern (tubular, papillary, solid, mixed), (8) intercellular bridges, (9) individual cell keratinization, (10) pearls composed of squamous cells, (11) intraluminal cellular buds, (12) cytoplasmic eosinophilials ('pink cells'), (13) glycogen content, (14) foam cells in stroma, (15) tumor necrosis, (16) mitotic index, and (17) cyclic phase of adjacent benign endometrium. These workers identified 6 microscopic patterns of tumor: adenocarcinoma, adenoacanthoma, atypical adenoacanthoma, adenosquamous carcinoma, clear cell adenocarcinoma and undifferentiated carcinoma. The histological assessment of ovarian cancers is far more complicated, even when the study is confined to the common epithelial neoplasms.

## 2.9. Endocrine status of the patient

The dependence of receptor levels on the presence of serum hormone is so great that a meaningful evaluation of one requires some knowledge of the other. In the case of the premenopausal woman one would at least like to know the phase of the menstrual cycle in which the cancer sample was obtained. The perimenopausal patient may or may not have significant continuing levels of unopposed estrogen. The postmenopausal patients would be expected to have low hormone levels and therefore low receptor levels; of course, it is this group in whom the majority of cancer occurs. In all instances, one would like to know about the use of exogenous hormones, such as oral contraceptives, or estrogens for the treatment of menopausal symptoms.

## 3. RESULTS

### 3.1. Estrogen receptors in endometrial cancer

Table 1 shows that cytosolic estrogen receptor (ERc) was present in 75%

Table 1. Frequency of cytosolic estrogen receptor (ERc) in endometrial carcinoma: correlation with the degree of differentiation and presence of cytosolic progesterone receptor (PRc).

| Author | Method | Well-differentiated | | Mod. differentiated | | Undifferentiated | | Total | | PRc also present | |
|---|---|---|---|---|---|---|---|---|---|---|---|
| | | # | % | # | % | # | % | # | % | # | % |
| Friberg, 1978 [38] | 1 | 12/18[a] | 67 | 9/22[a] | 41 | 2/10[a] | 20 | 23/50 | 46 | | |
| Martin, 1979 [48] | 2 | 13/13 | 100 | 18/18 | 100 | 8/8 | 100 | 39/39 | 100 | | |
| Soutter, 1979 [44] | 2 | 1/1 | 100 | 5/5 | 100 | – | – | 7/8 | 88 | | |
| Spona, 1979 [72] | 2 | 9/10 | 90 | 3/3 | 100 | 4/5 | 80 | 16/18 | 89 | 16/18 | 89 |
| Grilli, 1977 [73] | 2 | 7/7 | 100 | 4/5 | 80 | – | – | 11/12 | 92 | 5/12 | 42 |
| Prodi, 1979 [21] | 2 | 13/13 | 100 | 8/10 | 80 | 0/1 | 0 | 15/18 | 83 | | |
| McCarty, 1979 [49] | 2 | 19/20[a] | 95 | 12/17[a] | 71 | 4/8[a] | 38 | 35/45 | 78 | 28/45 | 62 |
| McCarty, 1979 [43] | 3 | 18/20 | 90 | 6/17 | 35 | 2/8 | 25 | 26/45 | 58 | 22/45 | 49 |
| Young, 1979 [74] | 2 | 4/7 | 57 | 7/11 | 64 | 0/4 | 0 | 12/22 | 58 | | |
| Ehrlich, 1981 [56] | 2 | 18/22 | 82 | 31/37 | 84 | 5/9 | 56 | 54/68 | 79 | 36/68 | 53 |
| Hunter, 1980 [57] | 2 | 18/27 | 67 | 15/22 | 68 | 8/11 | 73 | 52/73 | 71 | | |
| Total | | 114/138[b] | 83 | 112/150[b] | 75 | 31/56[b] | 55 | 264/353 | 75 | 85/143 | 59 |

1. Agar gel electrophoresis.
2. Dextran-coated charcoal.
3. Sucrose density gradient. Not included in total.
[a] $p < 0.05$ by $G$ test.
[b] $p < 0.005$ by $\chi^2$ test.

of cases reported in 10 studies (range 46–100%). The table shows a tendency for receptor to be present more frequently in well-differentiated than in poorly-differentiated tumors. This is significant when data from the different sources are pooled. This association is not significant, however, in the 2 largest series reported [56, 57]. Less than one fifth are poorly-differentiated tumors, as might be expected, and more than half of these are receptor positive. Almost 80% of ERc positive cases are also PRc positive. The data in 3 other reports in which the cases were not analyzed according to grade are corroborative [58–60].

The overall incidence of cytosolic progesterone receptor (PRc) in Table 2 is 62% (range 33–89 in 10 reports), not lower than the frequency of ERc. The relation to tumor grade is clearer for PRc than for ERc, and is significant not only for the pooled data but also for the largest series [56]. One third of the small number of undifferentiated tumors are PRc positive.

Nuclear estrogen receptors (ERn) were evaluated in 3 reports: 3 of 3 [12], 7 of 8 [44], and 4 of 4 [13] cancers were positive. In 12 of these 15 cases ERc was also measured and was positive. As previously noted, the presence of ERn does not mean that there is appreciable circulating estrogen and translocation of receptor from cytosol to nucleus. Nuclear progesterone receptor (PRn) was found in one study to correlate with tumor grade [45]. It was positive in 11 of 11 well-differentiated tumors, 11 of 15 moderately-differentiated tumors, and none of 3 undifferentiated tumors.

In several studies the level as well as the prevalence of ERc and PRc have been found to be proportional to the degree of differentiation of the tumor [49, 56, 57]. A better correlation is obtained with PRc than ERc [49]. (One report, however, finds a tendency for ERc to be more abundant in the more anaplastic cancers, rather than the reverse [18]!) The level of PRn has been found to be lowest in undifferentiated cancers and metastases. In addition, the PRn of cancers may be different from that of normal tissue since it dissociates more rapidly and is more labile [45].

Receptor levels do not correlate with the extent of the tumor (myometrial invasion, extrauterine disease) [57, 61] but the behavior of receptor positive tumors seems to be less aggressive [61].

Relatively few patients with endometrial carcinoma are premenopausal, and it is therefore not surprising that correlations between serum estrogen and progesterone concentrations and receptor levels in premenopausal patients are not detectable in the cancer group [49, 50, 58]. In one study, however, only one of ten patients under 55 had ERc or PRc levels below 10 femtomoles/mg of cytosol protein, whereas almost half of the older patients had these low levels (the exception was a Grade 3 cancer) [49]. Estrogen production rate in postmenopausal women is related to body weight, but neither weight nor number of years beyond the menopause have been

Table 2. Cytosolic progresterone receptor (PRc) in endometrial carcinoma: correlation with degree of differentiation.

| Author | Method | Well-differentiated | | Mod. differentiated | | Undifferentiated | | Total | |
|---|---|---|---|---|---|---|---|---|---|
| | | # | % | # | % | # | % | # | % |
| MacLaughlin, 1976 [16] | 1 | 2/3 | 66 | 2/8 | 25 | 0/1 | – | 4/12 | 33 |
| Martin, 1979 [48] | 1 | 11/11[a] | 100 | 11/18[a] | 61 | 3/8[a] | 38 | 25/37 | 68 |
| Spona, 1979 [72] | 1 | 9/10 | 90 | 3/3 | 100 | 4/5 | 80 | 16/18 | 89 |
| Grilli, 1977 [73] | 1 | 4/17 | 57 | 1/5 | 20 | – | – | 5/12 | 42 |
| Prodi, 1979 [71] | 1 | 10/11 | 91 | 4/6 | 67 | 0/1 | 0 | 14/18 | 78 |
| McCarty, 1979 [49] | 1 | 17/20 | 85 | 12/17 | 71 | 4/8 | 50 | 33/45 | 73 |
| McCarty, 1979 [49] | 2 | 17/20 | 85 | 10/17 | 59 | 3/8 | 38 | 30/45 | 67 |
| Young, 1979 [74] | 1 | 6/7[a] | 86 | 6/11[b] | 55 | 0/4[a] | 0 | 12/22 | 55 |
| Ehrlich, 1981 [56] | 1 | 17/22[b] | 77 | 21/37[b] | 57 | 1/9[b] | 11 | 39/68 | 57 |
| Hunter, 1980 [57] | 1 | 3/7 | 43 | 8/16 | 50 | 1/3 | 33 | 12/26 | 46 |
| Total | | 79/98[b] | 81 | 68/121b[b] | 56 | 13/39[b] | 33 | 160/258 | 62 |

1. Dextran-coated charcoal.
2. Sucrose density gradient. Not included in total.
[a] $p < 0.05$ by $G$ test.
[b] $p < 0.005$ by $\chi^2$ test.

correlated with PRc [50]. When ERc levels are high, however, PRc levels are also high ($r = 0.7$, $p<0.001$) [58], as expected; in most reports PRc is seldom present in the absence of ERc [49, 58].

The administration of a progestin such as medroxyprogesterone acetate (MPA) brings about a fall in receptor levels that is greatest in well-differentiated and least in undifferentiated cancer [18, 48, 58]. PRc seems to be a more sensitive predictor than ERc [58]. Masking of PRc by circulating MPA as a cause of apparently low PRc levels seems to have been ruled out [58]. Progestin therapy for a 4-week period also brings about 'secretory or acanthomatous' morphology in the responsive patient [48]. Estrogen administration increases the level of PRc [18] and might be used to improve tumor response to progestins except for concern for its mitogenic effect.

The limited amount of available data on the relation between PRc levels and clinical response to progestin therapy is summarized in Table 3. PRc positivity seems clearly related to a favorable response to treatment. Of the responding PRc-positive patients whose tumor grade was reported, 14 of 28 had higher than Grade 1 tumors [48, 58, 59] and in Ehrlich's series [56] 3 of 7 were Grade 3, suggesting that the presence of PRc predicts responsiveness to progestin therapy independent of tumor grade. In the same series a threshold level for PRc of $>50$ femtomoles/mg cytosol protein was used as a criterion of positivity, whereas most other groups have considered $>10$ femtomoles/mg to be sufficient [48, 49, 58].

A reverse relation between PRc and response to combination chemotherapy has been reported [60]. Whereas 7 of 10 patients who had ERc or PRc levels *less than* 30 femtomoles/mg experienced complete or partial remissions, only 1 of 5 with higher levels of both receptors responded. The receptor measurements were performed prior to treatment with cytotoxic drugs.

*Table 3.* Frequency of response of advanced-recurrent endometrial cancer in the presence of PRc.

| Author | PRc+ | % | PRc− | % | $P^d$ |
|---|---|---|---|---|---|
| Martin, 1979 [48] | 13/13[a] | 100 | 1/5 | 7 | <0.05 |
| McCarty, 1979 [49] | 4/5[a] | 80 | 0/8 | 0 | <0.05 |
| Benraad, 1980 [59] | 5/6[b] | 33 | 0/5[c] | 0 | <0.05 |
| Ehrlich, 1981 [56] | 7/8 | 88 | 1/16 | 6 | <0.001 |
| Total | 29/32 | 91 | 2/34 | 6 | |

[a] ERc also positive.
[b] ERc also positive, 2/3 of ERc+, PRc− patients also responded.
[c] ERc also negative.
[d] Fisher's exact test.

The drugs used were doxorubicin, cyclophosphamide, 5-fluorouracil and vincristine. All cases had received MPA initially as adjuvant therapy before advanced or recurrent disease required a more vigorous approach.

*3.2. Estrogen, progesterone and androgen receptors in ovarian carcinoma*

The common epithelial carcinomas of the ovary are derived from coelomic epithelium, and differentiate into Mullerian-like tissue. They have more in common with the endometrium than they do with functional elements of the normal ovary or with tumors derived from sex-cords or stroma. For this reason, it might be expected that these tumors would contain receptors for steroid hormones, and they do, as shown in Table 4. The earliest report listed in the table records the presence of ERc in 2 of 5 patients but does not give pathological or clinical details. In the second [38], estrogen receptors were found in 2 of 8 ovarian tumors, both a cystadenofibroma in a 73-year old woman and a papillary ovarian cancer in a 74-year old woman. Dihydrotestosterone receptors were found in 4 of 8 tumors, three 'mucinous cystadenomas', Stages IA, IIB, and IIC in patients aged 22, 32 and 60 and a papillary cancer in a 62-year old woman. The method used (agar gel electrophoresis) excludes confusion with CBG and SHBG. Holt et al. [63] reported 16 cases, 8 of which contained ERc, while 3 of these 8 contained PRc as well: one of these last was a Grade i-ii adenocarcinoma while the other two were papillary cystadenocarcinomas with metastases. Of 6 cases of ERc-positive tumors and metastases available for test, ERc was found in the metastases of 2 of the 6 patients. In 8 patients with recurrent disease, ERc was found in the metastases of 4: in metastases to lung and omentum in 2 cases and in metastases to bowel in 2 others. No receptor was

*Table 4.* Frequency of cytosolic estrogen receptor (ERc), cytosolic progesterone receptor (PRc), and nuclear estrogen receptor (ERn) in common epithelial cancers of the ovary.

| Author | ERc | % | PRc | % | Both | % | ERn | % |
|---|---|---|---|---|---|---|---|---|
| Kiang, 1977 [62] | 2/5 | 40 | | | | | | |
| Friberg, 1978 [38] | 2/8 | 25 | | | | | | |
| Holt, 1979 [63] | 8/16 | 47 | 8/16 | 47 | 3/16 | 20 | | |
| Janne, 1980 [64] | 15/21 | 71 | 8/21 | 38 | 8/21 | 38 | | |
| Holt, 1981 [65] | 15/17 | 88 | | | | | 12/14 | 86 |
| Holt, 1981 [65][a] | 9/12 | 75 | | | | | 3/9 | 33 |
| Galli, 1981 [67] | 7/10 | 70 | 6/10 | 60 | 6/10 | 60 | | |
| Hamilton, 1981 [68] | 5/12 | 42 | | | | | | |
| Bergqvist, 1981 [69] | 8/11 | 73 | 3/8 | 38 | 3/8 | 38 | | |
| Hähnel, 1982 [70] | 10/23 | 43 | 3/16 | 19 | 3/23 | 19 | | |
| Total | 81/135 | 60 | 28/71 | 39 | 23/78 | 29 | 15/23 | 65 |

[a] Recurrent and metastatic tumors.

found in 3 colon and 4 gastric cancers metastatic to the ovary, and none was found in 7 of 8 benign ovarian tumors (the exception was PRc in a thecoma). The methods used appear impeccable, but so do those of the Janne et al. [64] who compared 21 malignant tumors (6 serous, 1 mucinous, 6 endometrioid, 8 undifferentiated) with 29 benign tumors (8 serous, 18 mucinous, 1 Brenner's, 2 fibromas) and 28 'tumor-like lesions' (13 endometriomas, 13 functional cysts, 2 polycystic ovaries). The incidence of both receptors was higher in the malignancies than those previously reported. Both receptors were more prevalent and present in higher levels in the malignant tumors than in the benign lesions. With the exception of high levels of PRc in endometriosis and luteal cysts, the frequency and level of receptors was lowest of all in the tumor-like lesions. Receptor levels were elevated in all 3 groups, however. A second report by Holt et al. [65] utilizing a single-point saturation assay shows a still higher level of ERc than the others, both for primary and recurrent or metastatic ovarian lesions. The report includes 30 control tissues, of which all but 2, a thecoma and a granulosa cell tumor, were receptor-negative. The list of control tissues consists of 11 dermoids, 3 thecomas, 4 granulosa cell tumors, 1 struma ovarii and 11 'gut carcinomas' metastatic to ovary. ERn was measured by a single-point saturation assay after adsorption on HAP and was found to be present in 86% of the primary tumors, in 33% of their metastases, and in all 5 benign cystadenomas. Peroxidase was measured and found to be present in many of these tumors [65] an observation of some interest since peroxidase has been shown to be estrogen-inducible in target tissues [66].

The report by Galli et al. [67] includes 10 epithelial tumors, and 13 disease-free ovaries from women of varying age. ERc and PRc were measured together with receptors for androgens (ARc) and glucocorticoids (GRc). Receptor levels were if anything higher in the cancers, but the normal ovaries exhibited a high frequency of binding across the board: ERc 46%, PRc 54%, ARc 85%, GRc 92%. The method for assaying ARc by displacement of labeled $5\alpha$-dihydrotestosterone with $5\beta$-dihydrotestosterone is said to eliminate participation of SHBG, but this method has not been widely used by other workers. Other assays in the report were standard, with Scatchard estimates of affinity and appropriate controls.

Hamilton et al. [68] found ERc in 5/12 ovarian carcinomas (4/6 papillary or serous, 1/1 borderline) and ARc in 8/8 (5 papillary or serous, 1 mucinous, 1 endometrioid, 1 borderline). Bergqvist et al. include grading as well as histology in their report [69], but no pattern emerges: both ERc and PRc were present in a Grade 3 serous 'cystocarcinoma', a Grade 3 serous papillary adenocarcinoma, and a Grade I mucinous cystadenocarcinoma.

The report of Hahnel et al. [70] includes menopausal status, staging and grading as well as histology. ERc was present in 5/10 serous, 1/4 mucinous, and 3/6 endometrioid carcinomas; 2/8 serous (Grades 3 and 4), and 1/4 endometrioid (Grade 2) tumors contained PRc as well. Of the ERc positive tumors 3 were Grade 2, 4 were Grade 3, and 3 were Grade 4 cancers.

## 4. DISCUSSION

Are receptor assays likely to prove valuable as a means of choosing treatment in endometrial cancer? Available reviews do not provide a clear answer to this question [74–78]. Experience with endometrial cancer indicates that less than one third of patients treated with progestin for recurrent-metastatic cancer are responsive to the treatment [79–82]. Favorable responses are associated with the younger patient, the well-differentiated tumor, a long interval between original treatment and recurrence, pulmonary metastasis as opposed to recurrence elsewhere, and, for recurrences in other locations, the absence of prior irradiation. The data in Tables 1 and 2 indicate that a majority of endometrial cancers are receptor-positive, 75% for ERc and 62% for PRc, and even the undifferentiated tumors are positive with surprising frequency – 55% for ERc and 33% for PRc. The potential clinical value of the receptor assay is greatest in this last group of patients, since these are the ones that are most likely to develop recurrences or

*Table 5.* Problems with receptor assays in endometrial cancer.

| Problems | Remedies |
| --- | --- |
| Too many false-positives: | |
| normal endometrium, endometrial hyperplasia in sample [52] | a) histological check on assay sample<br>b) test recurrences, metastases only |
| CBG, SHBG included in measurement | choose appropriate ligand or competitor |
| Type II (low affinity) receptors included | multiple-point assay with Scatchard plot |
| Receptors may be nonfunctional | a) accept only if ERc, PRc both positive?<br>b) accept only if PRc >50 fm/mg protein (56)?<br>c) test for PRn (45)?<br>d) test second sample after treating patient with hormone?? |
| Some false-negatives: | |
| mishandled tissue | fresh tissue, prompt storage at $-70\,°C$ |
| masking of binding sites by circulating hormone | a) test serum samples for estradiol, progesterone levels in premenopausals<br>b) check history of hormone treatment<br>c) preincubate samples with charcoal |
| tumor necrosis, or no tumor in sample | histological check on assay sample |

metastases and to be considered as candidates for hormone therapy. If we can use experience with breast cancer as a model, we would expect none of the receptor-negative and about one half of the receptor-positive group to be hormone-responsive. Receptor determinations are useless if they merely provide information that is already available from clinical and pathological assessment. Unfortunately, the data summarized in Table 4 are too meager to document the usefulness of the assay in this respect, and we can only note that some of Ehrlich's receptor-positive responders had Grade iii tumors.

The main problems associated with receptor assays in endometrial cancer are summarized in Table 5. First and foremost is the tissue sample itself, which may fail to contain tumor, or may contain only necrotic tumor, or may be a mixture of normal endometrium and endometrial hyperplasia with tumor. Since the clinical usefulness of receptors measurements is limited to patients with recurrent or metastatic disease it would probably be wisest at the present time to limit our tests to samples of recurrences or metastases. The methodological problems have been discussed, and are readily overcome. The problem of the nonfunctional receptor reminds us that we do not have a test for hormonal responsiveness, but only a test for one step in the chain that leads to the response. An assay that requires obtaining a second sample of tissue for testing after a brief period of treatment is simply impractical in most clinical situations. The best-documented quantitative response of endometrial tissue to progestins, *in vivo* and *in vitro*, is the 17β-hydroxysteroid dehydrogenase assay: this, unfortunately, has not proved to be useful for testing endometrial cancers [83, 84]. Other tests are required that will establish the presence of full-fledged responsiveness. This goal may be attained through the measurement of hormone-directed endometrial products [85], or through some breakthrough in research that will define the relation of hormones to mitotic events.

The finding of a higher response rate to chemotherapy in patients who lack receptor [60] requires confirmation. Similar claims with respect to breast cancer [86] have met with mounting contrary evidence [87-91].

An understanding of receptors and hormonal mechanisms could lead to a more rational and effective mode of hormonal therapy for patients with endometrial cancer. Robel's suggestion is a good example of this [92]: he reported that tamoxifen increased progesterone receptor levels without stimulating tumor growth in patients with endometrial cancer. Specifically, ornithine decarboxylase, a growth-related enzyme that is stimulated by estrogen, was used as a marker: it was not stimulated by tamoxifen. On this basis Robel suggested that tamoxifen would potentiate progestin action, a concept made all the more persuasive with evidence that tamoxifen alone is an effective agent against endometrial cancer [93, 94].

Evidence that the common epithelial cancers of the ovary can respond to hormonal therapy is interesting but limited [69, 95–. Until further evidence is forthcoming, results from receptor assays will seem only to be curiosities. Unfortunately, the data on the ovary is equivocal with respect to the presence or absence of receptor in normal controls. Two reports emphasize the absence of receptor in 'gut tumors', and yet in a recent paper on human colon cancer [98], 10 tumors (4 males, 6 females) of 30 cases examined were positive for estrogen receptors, and of these 6 of the 23 assayed contained receptors for progesterone and dihydrotestosterone as well. Continuing research on receptors in ovarian cancers is clearly worthwhile in order to determine the relation between the presence of receptor and response to various therapies. The presence of receptor has proven to be an independent prognostic factor in cancer of the breast [14], and perhaps the same may prove to be true for ovarian cancers.

It is unfortunate that the available reports about both types of cancer do not include enough clinical and pathological data to make it possible to evaluate the relation between receptor levels and the many factors that might be included in a multivariate analysis. The more recent publications are apt to include more detail, and it is to be hoped that this trend will continue.

## REFERENCES

1. Noyes AT, Hertig AT, Rock J: Dating the endometrial biopsy. Fertil Steril 1:3, 1950.
2. Sonnenschein C, Soto AM: The mechanism of estrogen action: the old and a new paradigm. In: Estrogens in the Environment. McLachlan JA (ed), Elsevier-North Holland, 1980.
3. Sonnenschein C, Soto AM: But ... are estrogens per se growth-promoting hormones? J Natl Cancer Inst 64:211–215, 1980.
4. Sirbasku DA, Leland SE, Benson RH: Properties of a growth factor activity present in crude extracts of rat uterus. J Cell Physiol 107:345–358, 1981.
5. Baxter JD, Funder JW: Hormone receptor. N Engl J Med 301:1149–1161, 1979.
6. Markaverich BM, Upchurch S, McCormack SA, Glasser SR, Clark JH: Differential stimulation of uterine cells by nafoxidine and clomiphene: relationship between nuclear estrogen receptors and Type II estrogen binding sites and cellular growth. Biol Reprod 24:171–181, 1981.
7. Markaverich BM, Williams M, Upchurch S, Clark JH: Heterogeneity of nuclear estrogen-binding sites in rat uterus: a simple method for the quantitation of Type I and Type II sites by $^3$H-estradiol exchange. Endocrinol 109:62–29, 1981.
8. Zava DT, McGuire WL: Estrogen receptor. Unoccupied sites in nuclei of breast tumor cell line. J Biol Chem 252:3703–3708, 1977.
9. Jungblut PW, Kallweit E, Sierralta W, Truitt AJ, Wagner RK: The occurrence of steroid-free, 'activated' estrogen receptor in target cell nuclei. Hoppe-Seyler's Z Physiol Chem 359:1259–1268, 1978.
10. Carlson RA, Gorski J: Characterization of a unique population of unfilled estrogen-binding sites associated with the nuclear fraction of immature rat uterus. Endocrinol 106:1776–1785, 1980.

11. Levy C, Mortel R, Eychenne B, Robel P, Baulieu EE. Unoccupied nuclear oestradiol-receptor sites in normal human endometrium. Biochem J 185:733-738, 1980.
12. Fleming H, Gurpide E: Available estradiol receptors in nuclei from endometrium. J Steroid Biochem 13:3-11, 1980.
13. Geier A, Beery R, Levran D, Menczer J, Lunenfeld B: Unoccupied nuclear receptors for estrogen in human endometrial tissue. J Clin Endocrinol Metab 50:541-545, 1980.
14. Consensus Meeting on Steroid Receptors in Breast Cancer, Bethesda, MD, June 27-29, 1979.
15. Hsueh AJW, Peck EJ Jr, Clark JH: Control of uterine estrogen receptor levels by progesterone Endocrinol 98:428-444, 1976.
16. MacLaughlin DT, Richardson GS: Progesterone binding by normal and abnormal human endometrium. J Clin Endocrinol Metab 42:667-678, 1976.
17. Tseng L, Gurpide E: Induction of human endometrial estradiol dehydrogenase by progestins. Endocrinol 97:824-833, 1974.
18. Pollow K, Schmidt-Gollwitzer M, Pollow B: Progesterone- and estradiol-binding proteins from normal human endometrium and endometrial carcinoma: a comparative study. In: Steroid Receptors and Hormone Dependent Neoplasia. Wittliff Jl, Dapunt O (eds), Innsbruck, 1978.
19. Levy C, Robel P, Gautray JP, Debrux J, Verma U, Descomps B, Baulieu EE: Estradiol and progesterone receptors in human endometrium: normal and abnormal menstrual cycles and early pregnancy. Am J Obstet Gynecol 136:646-651, 1980.
20. Richardson GS, MacLaughlin DT (eds): Hormonal Biology of Endometrial Carcinoma, Geneva, UICC Technical Report Vol 42, 1978, p 152.
21. MacLaughlin DT, Richardson GS: Specificity of medroprogesterone binding in human endometrium: interaction with testosterone and progesterone binding sites. J Steroid Biochem 10:371-377, 1979.
22. Richards JS: Hormonal control of ovarian follicular development: a 1978 perspective. Rec Prog Hormone Res 35:343-373, 1979.
23. Richards JS, Midgley AR Jr: Protein hormone action: a key to understanding ovarian and follicular luteal cell development. Biol Reprod 14:82-94, 1976.
24. Hillier SG, Reichert LE Jr, Van Hall EV: Control of preovulatory follicular estrogen biosynthesis in the human ovary. J Clin Endocrinol Metab 52:847-856, 1981.
25. Hillier SG, Knazek RA, Ross GT: Androgenic stimulation of progesterone production by granulosa cells from preantral follicles: further in vitro studies using replicate cell cultures. Endocrinol 100:1539-1549, 1977.
26. Jacobs BR, Smith RG: Evidence for a receptor-like protein for progesterone in bovine ovarian cytosol. Endocrinol 106:1276-1282, 1980.
27. Wilcox DL, Thorburn GD: Progesterone binding protein in the bovine corpus lutem. J Steroid Biochem 14:841-850, 1981.
28. Scott RS, Rennie PIC: An estrogen receptor in the corpus luteum of the pseudopregnant rabbit. Endocrinol 89:297-301, 1971.
29. Richards JS: Content of nuclear estradiol complex in rat corpora lutea during pregnancy-relationship to estrogen concentration and cytosol receptor availability. Endocrinol 96:227-230, 1975.
30. Punnonen R, Kouvonen I, Lovgren T, Rauramo L: Uterine and ovarian estrogen receptor levels in climacteric women. Acta Obstet Gynecol Scand 58:389-391, 1979.
31. Jacobs BR, Suchocki S, Smith RG: Evidence for a human ovarian progesterone receptor. Am J Obstet Gynecol 138:332-336, 1980.
32. Milwidsky A, Younes MA, Besch NF, Besch PK, Kaufman RH: Receptor-like binding proteins for testosterone and progesterone in the human ovary. Am J Obstet Gynecol 138:93-98, 1980.

33. Chamness GC, McGuire WL: Steroid receptor assays in human breast cancer. In: Steroid Receptors and the Management of Cancer, Thompson EB, Lippman ME (eds), CRC Press, 1979, p 3.
34. Anderson KM, Phelan J, Marogil M, Hendrickson C, Economou S: Sodium molybdate increases the amount of progesterone and estrogen detected in certain human breast cancer cytosols. Steroids 35:273–280, 1980.
35. Siiteri PK: Steroid hormones and endometrial cancer. Cancer Res 38:4360–5366, 1978.
36. Mainwaring WIP: Androgen receptors in the future management of carcinoma of the prostate. In: Steroid Receptors and the Management of Cancer, Thompson EB, Lippman ME (eds), CRC Press, 1979, p 99.
37. Garola RE, McGuire WL: A hydroxylapatite micromethod for measuring estrogen receptor in human breast cancer. Cancer Res 38:2216–2220, 1978.
38. Friberg LG, Kullander S, Persijn JP, Korsten CB: On receptors for estrogens ($E_2$) and androgens (DHT) in human endometrial carcinoma and ovarian tumours. Acta Obstet Gynecol Scand 57:265–271, 1978.
39. Peck EJ, Clark JH: Effect of ionic strength on charcoal adsorption assays of receptor-estradiol complexes. Endocrinol 101:1034–1043, 1977.
40. Saez S, Martin PM, Chouvet CG: Estradiol and progesterone receptor levels in human breast adenocarcinoma in relation to plasma estrogen and progesterone levels. Cancer Res 38:3468–3473, 1978.
41. Edery M, Goussard J, Dehennin L, Scholler R, Reiffsteck J, Drosdowsky MA: Endogenous oestradiol-17β concentration in breast tumours determine by mass fragmentography and by radioimmunoassay: relationship to receptor content. Eur J Cancer 17:115–120, 1981.
42. Sarrif AM, Durant JR: Evidence that estrogen-receptor-negative, progesterone-receptor-positive breast and ovarian carcinomas contain estrogen receptor. Cancer 48:1215–1220, 1981.
43. Garcia M, Rochefort H: Evidence and characterization of the binding of two $^3$H-labeled androgens to the estrogen receptor. Endocrinol 104:1797–1804, 1979.
44. Soutter WP, Hamilton K, Leake RE: High affinity binding of oestradiol-17β in the nuclei of human endometrial cells. J Steroid Biochem 10:529–534, 1979.
45. Feil P, MannW Jr, Mortel R, Bardin CW: Nuclear progestin receptors in normal and malignant human endometrium. J Clin Endocrinol Metab 48:327–334, 1979.
46. Janne O, Kontula K, Vihko R: Progestin receptors in human tissues: concentration and binding kinetics. J Steroid Biochem 7:1061–1068, 1976.
47. Smith RG, Clarke SG, Zalta E, Taylor RN: Two estrogen receptors in reproductive tissue. J Steroid Biochem 10:31–35, 1979.
48. Martin PM, Rolland PH, Gammerre M, Serment H, Toga M: Estradiol and progesterone receptors, histopathological examinations and clinical responses under progestin therapy. Int J Cancer 23:321–329, 1979.
49. McCarty KS Jr, Barton TK, Fetter BF, Creasman WT, McCarty KS: Correlation of estrogen and progesterone receptors with histologic differentiation in endometrial adenocarcinoma. Am J Pathol 96:171–184, 1979.
50. Rodriquez J, Sen KK, Seski JC, Meno M, Johnson TR, Menon KMJ: Progesterone binding by human endometrial tissue during the proliferative and secretory phase of the menstrual cycle and by hyperplastic and carcinomatous endometrium. Am J Obstet Gynecol 133:660–665, 1979.
51. Gibbons W, Buttram V Jr, Besch P, Smith R: Estrogen-binding proteins in human postmenopausal uterus. Am J Obstet Gynecol 135:799–803, 1979.
52. Horwitz RI, Feinstein AR, Vidone RA, Sommers SC, Robboy SJ: Histopathologic distinctions in the relationship of estrogens and endometrial cancer. JAMA 246:1425–1427, 1981.

53. Tsibris JCM, Cazenave CR, Cantor B, Notelovitz M, Kalra PS, Spellacy WN: Distribution of cytoplasmic estrogen and progesterone receptors in human endometrium. Am J Obstet Gynecol 132:449–454, 1978.
54. Tsibris JCM, Fort FL, Cazenave CR, Cantor B, Bardawil WA, Notelovitz M, Spellacy WN: The uneven distribution of estrogen and progesterone receptors in human endometrium. J Steroid Biochem 14:997–1003, 1981.
55. Robboy SJ, Bradley R: Changing trends and prognostic features in endometrial cancer associated with exogenous estrogen therapy. Obstet Gynecol 54:269–277, 1979.
56. Ehrlich CE, Young PCM, Cleary RE: Cytoplasmic progesterone and estradiol receptors in normal, hyperplastic and carcinomatous endometria: therapeutic implications. Am J Obstet Gynecol 141:539–546, 1981.
57. Hunter RE, Longcope C, Jordan VC: Steroid hormone receptors in adenocarcinoma of the endometrium. Gynecol Oncol 10:152–161, 1980.
58. Janne O, Kauppila A, Kontula K, Syrjala P, Vihko R: Female sex steroid receptors in normal hyperplastic and carcinomatous endometrium. The relationship to serum steroid hormones and gonadotropins and changes during medroxyprogesterone acetate administration. Int J Cancer 24:545–554, 1979.
59. Benraad ThJ, Friberg LG, Koenders AJM, Kullander S: Do estrogen and progesterone receptors ($E_2R$ and PR) in metastasizing endometrial cancers predict the response to gestogen therapy? Acta Obstet Gynecol Scand 59:155–159, 1980.
60. Kauppila A, Janne O, Kujansuu E, Vihko R: Treatment of advanced endometrial adenocarcinoma with a combined cytotoxic therapy. Cancer 46:2162–2167, 1980.
61. Creasman WT, McCarty KS, Barton TK, McCarty KS: Clinical correlates of estrogen- and progesterone-binding proteins in human endometrial adenocarcinoma. Obstet Gynecol 55:363–370, 1980.
62. Kiang DT, Kennedy BJ: Estrogen receptor assay in the differential diagnosis of adenocarcinoma. JAMA 238:32–34, 1977.
63. Holt JA, Caputo TA, Kelly KM, Greenwald P, Chorost S: Estrogen and progestin binding in cytosols of ovarian adenocarcinoma. Obstet Gynecol 53:50–58, 1979.
64. Janne O, Kauppila A, Syrjala P, Vihko R: Comparison of cytosol estrogen and progestin receptor status in malignant and benign tumors and tumor-like lesions of human ovary. Int J Cancer 25:175–179, 1980.
65. Holt JA, Lyttle CR, Lorincz MA, Stem SD, Press MA, Herbst AL: Estrogen receptor and peroxidase activity in epithelial ovarian carcinomas. J Natl Cancer Inst 67:307–318, 1981.
66. Lyttle CR, DeSombre ER: Uterine peroxidase as a marker for estrogen action. Proc Natl Acad Sci USA 74:3162–3166, 1977.
67. Galli MC, DeGiovanni C, Nicoletti G, Grilli G, Nanni P, Prodi G, Gola G, Rocchetta R, Orlandi C: The occurrence of multiple steroid hormone receptors in disease-free and neoplastic human ovary. Cancer 47:1297–1302, 1981.
68. Hamilton TC, Daview P, Griffiths K: Androgen and oestrogen binding in cytosols of human ovarian tumours. J Endocrinol 90:421–431, 1981.
69. Bergqvist A, Kullander S, Thorell J: A study of estrogen and progesterone cytosol receptor concentration in benign and malignant ovarian tumors and a review of malignant ovarian tumors treated with maeroxyprogesterone acetate. Acta Obstet Gynecol Scand Supp 101:75–81, 1981.
70. Hähnel R, Kelsall GRH, Martin JD, Masters AM, McCartney AJ, Twaddle E: Estrogen and progesterone receptors in tumors of the human ovary. Gynecol Oncol 13:145–151, 1982.
71. Prodi G, DeGiovanni C, Galli MC, Gola G, Grilli S, Rocchetta R, Orlandi C: 17β-Estradiol, 5α-dihydrotestosterone, progesterone and cortisol receptors in normal and neoplastic human endometrium. Tumori 65:241–253, 1979.

72. Spona J, Ulm R, Bieglmayer C, Husslein P: Hormone serum levels and hormone receptor contents of endometria in women with normal menstrual cycles and patients bearing endometrial carcinoma. Gynecol Obstet Invest 10:71-80, 1979.
73. Grilli S, Ferreri A, Gola G, Rocchetta R, Orlandi C, Prodi G: Cytoplasmic receptors for 17β-estradiol, 5α-dihydrotestosterone and progesterone in normal and abnormal human uterine tissues. Cancer Letters 2:247-258, 1977.
74. Young PCM, Ehrlich CE: Progesterone receptors in human endometrial cancer. In: Steroid Receptors and the Management of Cancer, Vol I, Thompson EB, Lippman ME (eds), Boca Raton, Florida, CRC Press, 1979, p 135-160.
75. Siiteri PK: Steroid hormone and endometrial cancer. Cancer Res 38:4360-4366, 1978.
76. Hoffman PG, Siiteri PK: Sex steroid receptors in gynecologic cancer. Obstet Gynecol 55:648-652, 1980.
77. Gurpide E: Hormone receptors in endometrial cancer. Cancer 48:638-641, 1981.
78. Janne OA, Kontula KK: Hormone receptors and target cell responsiveness. Ann Clin Res 12:174-191, 1980.
79. Kelley RM, Baker WH: Progestational agents in the treatment of carcinoma of the endometrium. N Engl J Med 264:216-222, 1960.
80. Malkasian G, Decker D, Mussey E, Johnson C: Progestagen treatment of recurrent endometrial carcinoma. Am J Obstet Gynecol 110:15-23, 1971.
81. Reifenstein EC: The treatment of advanced endometrial cancer with hydroxyprogesterone caproate. Gynecol Oncol 3:377, 1974.
82. Rozier J, Underwood P: Use of progestational agents in endometrial carcinoma. Obstet Gynecol 44:60-64, 1974.
83. Holinka CF, Deligdisch L, Deppe G, Fleming H, Namit C, de la Pena MM, Gurpide, E: Evaluation of in vivo and in vitro responses of endometrial adenocarcinoma to progestins. In: Hormones and Cancer. Advances in Experimental Medicine and Biology, Vol 138. WW Leavitt (ed), Plenum Press, 1982, p 365.
84. Satyaswaroop PG, Mortel R: Failure of progestins to induce estradiol dehydrogenase activity in endometrial carcinoma, in vitro. Cancer Res 42:1322-1325, 1982.
85. MacLaughlin DT, Richardson GS: The specificity of the endometrial response to estrogens and progestins. In: Steroid Receptors and the Management of Cancer. Thompson EB, Lippman ME (eds), CRC Press, 1979, p 161.
86. Lippman ME, Allegra JC, Thompson EB, Simon R, Barlock A, Green L, Hoff KK, Do HMT, Aitken SC, Warren R: The relation between estrogen receptors and response rate to cytotoxic chemotherapy in metastatic breast cancer. N Engl J Med 298:1223-1228, 1978.
87. Kiang DT, Frenning DH, Goldman AI, Ascensao VF, Kennedy BJ: Estrogen receptors and responses to chemotherapy and hormonal therapy in advanced breast cancer. N Engl J Med 299:1330-1334, 1978.
88. Webster DJT, Bronn DG, Minton JP: Estrogen receptors and response of breast cancer to chemotherapy. N Engl J Med 299:604, 1978.
89. Samal B, Singhakowinta A, Brooks SC, Vaitkevicius VK: Estrogen receptors and response of breast cancer to chemotherapy. N Engl J Med 299:604, 1978.
90. Greenspan EM: Estrogen receptors and response of breast cancer to chemotherapy. N Engl J Med 299:604, 1978.
91. Paone JF, Abeloff MD, Ettinger DS, Arnold EA, Baker RR: The correlation of estrogen and progesterone receptor levels with response to chemotherapy for advanced carcinoma of the breast. Surg Gynecol Obstet 152:70-74, 1981.
92. Robel P, Levy C, Wolff JP, Nicolas JP, Baulieu EE: Réponse à un anti-oestrogène comme critère d'hormono-sensibilité du cancer de l'endomètre. CR Acad Sci Paris 287:1353-1356, 1978.

93. Bonte J, Ide P, Billiet G, Synants P: Tamoxifen as a possible chemotherapeutic agent in endometrial adenocarcinoma. Gynecol Oncol 11:140–161, 1981.
94. Swenerton KD, Shaw D, White GW, Boyes DA: Treatment of advanced endometrial carcinoma with tamoxifen. N Engl J Med 301:105, 1979.
95. Tobias JS, Griffiths CT: Management of ovarian carcinoma. Current concepts and future prospects. N Engl J Med 294:877–882, 1976.
96. Guthrie D: The treatment of advanced cystadenocarcinoma of the ovary with gestronol and continuous oral cyclophosphamide. Brit J Obstet Gynecol 86:497–500, 1979.
97. Myers AM, Moore GE, Major FJ: Advanced ovarian carcinoma: response to antiestrogen therapy. Cancer 48:2368–2370, 1981.
98. Alford TC, Do HMT, Geelhoed GW, Tsangaris NT, Lippman ME: Steroid hormone receptors in human colon cancers. Cancer 43:980–984, 1979.

# 4. Germ Cell Tumors of the Ovary: Pathology, Behavior and Treatment

ROBERT J. KURMAN and EDMUND S. PETRILLI

## 1. INTRODUCTION

Germ cell tumors of the ovary occur primarily in children and young women and represent 15-20% of all ovarian neoplasms. Approximately 4% of all germ cell tumors are malignant. In patients under 20 years of age nearly 60% of ovarian tumors are of germ cell origin and in children less than 10 years of age, 84% of these are malignant [1, 2]. Within this category are some highly aggressive tumors which until recently were almost uniformly and rapidly fatal.

*Pathogenesis.* There have been two main theories of the pathogenesis of germ cell tumors; origin from a somatic cell or misplaced blastomere and origin from the embryonic germ cell. In the gonad, there has been no evidence in recent years to support the former theory, a view still held for extragonadal germ cell tumors [3]. At present, it is universally acknowledged that gonadal germ cell tumors originate from germ cells. In human species, the germ cells arise in the yolk sac [4] and migrate to the ovary via ameboid action through the celomic cavity, hindgut mesentery and possibly through lymphatic vessels as well. The origin of extragonadal germ cell tumors is thus explained by the neoplastic transformation of primordial germ cells that have been arrested during migration. Germ cells in the mediastinum, retroperitoneum, posterior abdominal wall and sacro-coccygeal region give rise to tumors that are similar in appearance to those of the gonads [5].

Because of their rarity, malignant germ cell tumors in the past were poorly understood. The reported series described small heterogeneous mixtures of different tumors, the diagnostic criteria were not uniform and successful treatment was uncommon. The recognition that pure tumors, unlike mixed cell types, had a characteristic biologic behavior paved the way for an

*Table 1.* Classification of germ cell tumors of the ovary (modification of the 1973 WHO classification [7]).

---

I. Germ cell tumors
  A. Dysgerminoma
  B. Endodermal sinus tumor
  C. Teratomas
    1. Immature (malignant) teratoma
    2. Mature (cystic and solid) teratoma
    3. Monodermal or highly specialized
      (a) Struma ovarii
      (b) Carcinoid
      (c) Strumal carcinoid
      (d) Others
  D. Embryonal carcinoma
  E. Choriocarcinoma
  F. Malignant mixed germ cell tumors
II. Mixed germ cell and stromal tumors
  A. Gonadoblastoma
  B. Mixed germ cell – sex cord stromal tumor

---

improved classification system [6]. The classification of ovarian tumors introduced by the World Health Organization (WHO) in 1973 [7] established standard nomenclature and histologic criteria and imposed order in an area where confusion once reigned. A modification of the WHO classification is shown in Table 1. Coincident with these developments was the discovery that alpha feto-protein (AFP) and human chorionic gonadotropin (hCG) could serve as tumor markers thereby permitting a more accurate means of diagnosis and also providing a highly sensitive method for monitoring the response to therapy.

*Staging.* Recent advances in surgical staging have also played an important role in the development of a rational approach to treatment. The staging system for ovarian cancer as proposed by the FIGO is shown in Table 2. Although most germ cell tumors appear to be limited to one ovary at the time of diagnosis, meticulous surgical staging is required because occult metastatic disease is present in the majority of patients. Adequate staging includes differential peritoneal washings of the pelvis and paracolic gutters for cytologic examination if no ascites is present. In addition, biopsies should be performed from the grossly uninvolved ovary, the omentum, pelvic and para-aortic lymph nodes, adhesions and random areas of the parietal peritoneal surfaces of the pelvis and abdomen. Careful inspection of the liver, large and small bowel and their mesentery and palpation of the undersurface of the diaphragm is also necessary. Only in this way will a diagnosis of Stage I disease be confirmed or occult metastatic tumor be recognized.

*Table 2.* FIGO staging[a].

Stage I: Growth limited to the ovaries.
  Stage Ia: Growth limited to one ovary; no ascites.
    1. No tumor on the external surface; capsule intact.
    2. Tumor present on the external surface or/and capsule raptured
  Stage Ib: Growth limited to both ovaries; no ascites.
    1. No tumor on the external surface; capsule(s) intact.
    2. Tumor present on the external surface or/and capsule(s) ruptured.
  Stage Ic: Tumor either Stage Ia or Stage Ib, but with ascites[b] present or positive peritoneal washings.
Stage II: Growth involving one or both ovaries with pelvic extension.
  Stage IIa: Extension and/or metastases to the uterus and/or tubes
  Stage IIb: Extension to other pelvic tissues.
  Stage IIc: Tumor either Stage IIa or Stage IIb, but with ascites[b] present or positive peritoneal washings.
Stage III: Growth involving one or both ovaries with intraperitoneal metastases outside the pelvis and/or positive retroperitoneal nodes.
Tumor limited to the true pelvis with histologically proved malignant extension to small bowel or omentum.
Stage IV: Growth involving one or both ovaries with distant metastases.
If pleural effusion is present, there must be positive cytology to allot a case to Stage IV.
Parenchymal liver metastasis equals Stage IV.

[a] Based on findings at clinical examination and surgical exploration. Final histology after surgery is to be considered in the staging, as well as cytology as far as effusions are concerned.
[b] Ascites is peritoneal effusion which, in the opinion of the surgeon, is pathologic and/or clearly exceeds normal amounts.

Patients with obvious disease disseminated within the abdomen do not require the elaborate staging procedures described but they may benefit from extensive surgical resection of gross tumor to reduce the tumor volume, potentially enhancing the effectiveness of chemotherapy and increasing the likelihood of prolonged survival and possible cure. Finally, the successful use of adjuvant combination chemotherapy has revolutionized the treatment of patients with these neoplasms [8, 9]. This chapter will emphasize and correlate the respective roles of histogenesis, histopathologic criteria, tumor markers, surgery and chemotherapy in the diagnosis and management of germ cell tumors and mixed germ cell and stromal tumors.

## 2. GERM CELL TUMORS

### 2.1. Dysgerminoma

Dysgerminoma is the most common malignant germ cell tumor of the ovary accounting for nearly one-half of this group and representing 2% of all malignant ovarian neoplasms. Three-quarters of the patients are between 10 and 30 years of age and only 4% of patients are over 40; the median age is 22 years [6, 10]. Dysgerminoma is rare in infancy. It is the most common ovarian malignancy in pregnancy [11] and the most common tumor associated with gonadoblastoma and cryptorchid testis in patients with testicular feminization.

*2.1.1. Histogenesis.* The germinoma (a term used to include both the seminoma of the male and the dysgerminoma of the female) was originally thought to be composed of germ cells having a 46XX chromatin pattern in females and 46XY pattern in males, suggesting that both were derived from diploid germ cells before the first meiotic division. This view is not completely accepted, however, as nuclear chromatin is difficult to identify reliably in dysgerminomas. Since dysgerminoma is sometimes admixed with teratoma, one might expect it to arise by the same process as teratomas. The DNA content of dysgerminoma is almost twice that of the lymphocyte [6] and is equivalent to that of oocytes in prophase arrest, suggesting that dysgerminoma arises from the same developmental stage of germ cell as do teratomas. In contrast to teratomas and all other germ cell tumors, however, dysgerminoma is considered to be arrested at a completely undifferentiated stage of development and is, therefore, functionally inert. This view is supported by the fact that neither AFP or hCG is elaborated by pure dysgerminoma [12].

*2.1.2. Clinical presentation.* The presentation is nonspecific and may include a pelvic or abdominal mass with abdominal enlargement and pain. Approximately 10% of patients are asymptomatic [6]. The duration of symptoms ranges from one month to two years with a median of four months [6]. In two series [6, 11] 15% of dysgerminomas were discovered during pregnancy, usually as an incidental finding or as a cause of dystocia during labor. Menstrual abnormalities are uncommon. About 2% of nonpregnant women have positive pregnancy tests and children may present with precocious puberty. The source of the hCG production in pure dysgerminoma is usually isolated syncytotrophoblastic cells. A mixed germ cell tumor containing elements of choriocarcinoma, however, should be considered since the biologic behavior of such a neoplasm may be more aggressive and also require individualized adjuvant chemotherapy for the nondysgerminomatous component.

It was once thought that dysgerminoma was frequently encountered in intersex individuals and patients with abnormally developed gonads [13]. Most females with dysgerminoma are genetically normal and are capable of bearing children; nonetheless, germinoma is the most common malignant germ cell tumor in intra-abdominal gonads containing a Y chromosome. It occurs in males with cryptorchid testes, and is found in approximately one-half of gonadoblastomas which usually arise in a dysgenetic gonad bearing a Y chromosome. Germinoma develops between the ages of 20-50 years in one-quarter to one-third of patients with testicular feminization [14].

*2.1.3. Gross features.* Dysgerminoma is a solid, fleshy tumor with a smooth exterior surface. Although it may be only a few centimeters in diameter, it tends to be large with a median diameter of 15 cm. The cut surface bulges and has a homogeneous tan to pink appearance. Although there may be focal hemorrhage or necrosis, larger areas of hemorrhage or cystic change suggest the possibility of admixed elements of choriocarcinoma, endodermal sinus tumor, or teratoma. Dysgerminoma contains other germ cell components in up to 20% of cases [19].

*2.1.4. Microscopic features.* The homogeneous appearance of dysgerminoma on gross examination is reflected in its microscopic appearance as well. It is identical to seminoma of the testes and to germinoma arising in sacrococcygeal, mediastinal, and pineal regions. The tumor is composed of aggregates of large polygonal cells with vesicular nuclei containing one or more nucleoli, clear or lightly granular cytoplasm, abundant cytoplasmic glycogen, and prominent cell membranes (Figure 1). The cells resemble primordial germ cells histochemically and ultrastructurally but tend to be smaller [15, 16]. Delicate fibrous septae may create lobulation and if densely fibrous areas are present, a cord-like pattern results. The tumor is often infiltrated by lymphocytes, and foreign body giant cells are present in 20% of the cases [6]. It has been suggested that a prominent chronic inflammatory infiltrate may portend a less aggressive behavior, but to date, a significant statistical difference has not been demonstrated [6].

In some dysgerminomas, giant cells resembling syncytiotrophoblastic giant cells are present and associated hCG has been demonstrated by the immunoperoxidase reaction [12, 17]. Scattered clusters of syncytiotrophoblastic giant cells may produce an elevation of serum hCG but since they lack the dimorphic population of syncytiotrophoblast and cytotrophoblast found in choriocarcinoma, they alone are insufficient for a diagnosis of choriocarcinoma.

In well-fixed tissue, dysgerminoma presents little diagnostic difficulty but poor preservation and fixation causes a shrinkage artifact that gives the impression of gland formation which may mimic a poorly-differentiated

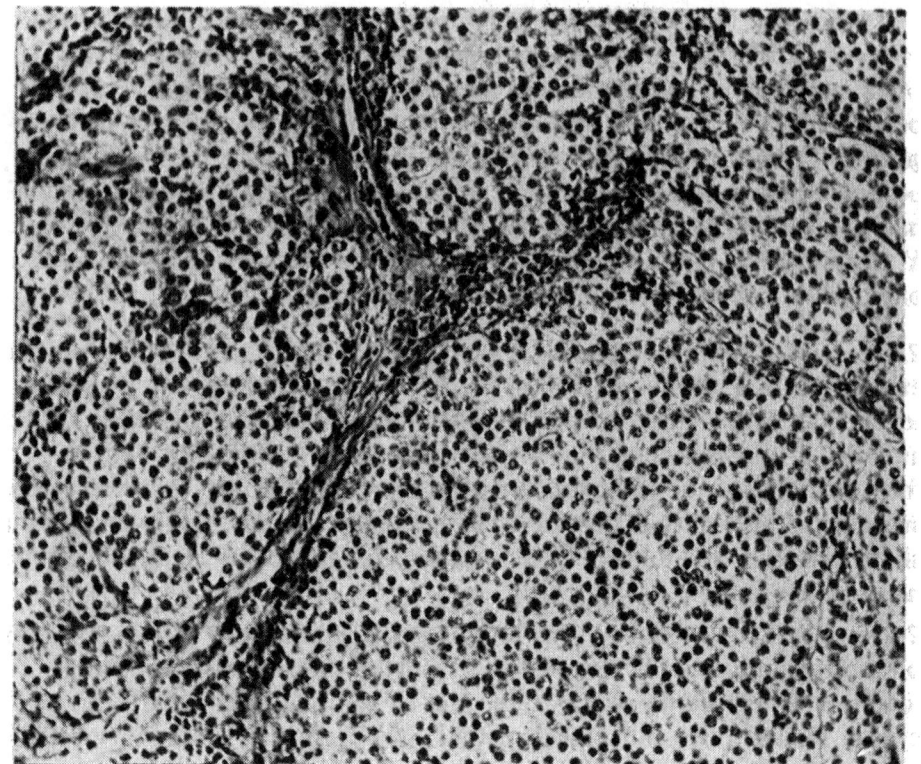

*Figure 1.* Dysgerminoma composed of aggregates of a relatively uniform population of large polygonal cells.

carcinoma. A dysgerminoma comprised of scattered cells in a densely fibrotic stroma may be confused with Hodgkin's disease or a granulomatous reaction, especially if foreign body giant cells are present. A periodic acid-Schiff reaction with diastase control typically reveals intracytoplasmic glycogen in dysgerminoma and may thus aid in the diagnosis. Alkaline phosphatase reactions are also positive in dysgerminoma as they are in primitive germ cells.

*2.1.5. Behavior and therapy.* Although dysgerminoma is less aggressive than other malignant germ cell tumors (Table 3), the disease is lethal and requires effective primary therapy as evidenced by the 45% survival in one series of patients referred with recurrent disease [18].

Adequate surgical staging and complete tumor excision is the initial approach to diagnosis and treatment. Dysgerminoma is unique in that it is a highly radiosensitive tumor and, when indicated, postoperative treatment consists of radiation therapy, whereas the other germ cell malignancies are radioresistant and are best treated by postoperative chemotherapy.

*Table 3.* Actuarial survival by type and stage of tumor in 263 patients with malignant germ cell tumors of the ovary [19].

| Tumor | No. followed | Percent survival Stage I | Percent survival all stages |
|---|---|---|---|
| Dysgerminoma | 98 | 90[a] | 63[a] |
| Endodermal sinus | 67 | 16[c] | 13[c] |
| Immature teratoma | 56 | 75[a] | 63[c] |
| Malignant mixed germ cell | 28 | 50[b] | 46[b] |
| Embryonal carcinoma | 14 | 50[b] | 39[b] |

[a] Disease-free at 10 years.
[b] Disease-free at 5 years.
[c] Disease-free at 3 years.

Most data relating to the stages of germ cell tumors must be viewed with skepticism because adequate surgical staging has only become an accepted practice in recent years. Contemporary studies may subsequently reveal a lower frequency of Stage I disease than the older literature indicates. At the time of laparotomy, nearly three-quarters of patients have Stage I disease but in contrast to the other malignant germ cell tumors, dysgerminoma is the only one that is occasionally bilateral (Stage Ib) (Table 4). Ten percent of these tumors are visibly confined to both ovaries at the time of operation. Five percent of patients with a tumor that appears to be confined to one ovary with a visibly normal contralateral ovary has occult microscopic dysgerminoma in that ovary [19].

Therapy for dysgerminoma can be individualized according to the patient's age, desire for future childbearing and the pathological characteristics and stage of the tumor. In young women unilateral oophorectomy alone may be performed if the tumor is Stage Ia, well encapsulated, less than

*Table 4.* Status of contralateral ovary in 191 patients with Stage I germ cell tumors of the ovary [19].

| Tumor | Stage Ia patients | Stage Ib patients | Stage Ia patients with microscopic spread to opposite grossly normal ovary |
|---|---|---|---|
| Dysgerminoma | 71 | 7 (10%) | 4 (5%) |
| Endodermal sinus tumor | 51 | 0 | 0 |
| Immature teratoma | 40 | 0 | 0 |
| Embryonal carcinoma | 9 | 0 | 0 |
| Mixed germ cell tumor | 19 | 1 (5%) | 1 (5%)[a] |

[a] The primary neoplasm in the opposite ovary contained dysgerminoma and endodermal sinus tumor but the occult involvement in the grossly normal ovary was dysgerminoma only.

*Table 5.* Dysgerminoma. Survival after treatment for recurrent disease.

| Author | Patients with recurrence | Patients surviving after treatment | Percent | Survival duration (months) |
|---|---|---|---|---|
| Asadourian and Taylor [6] | 23 | 10 | 23 | Not specified |
| Krepart *et al.* [11] | 10 | 7 | 70 | >33 |
| Freel *et al.* [18] | 9 | 4 | 44 | 24-252 |
| Boyes *et al.* [129] | 5 | 3 | 60 | 121-196 |
| Alfridi *et al.* [124] | 5 | 4 | 80 | 6-216 |
| Total | 52 | 28 | 54 | |

10 cm in diameter, neither ruptured nor adherent to nearby structures and if ascites is absent [11, 18]. Surgical staging must be adequate to exclude occult, advanced disease. All patients who do not meet the above criteria for conservative surgical treatment should undergo abdominal hysterectomy and bilateral salpingo-oophorectomy, in addition to adequate staging and complete tumor excision followed by abdominal and pelvic irradiation. If para-aortic lymph nodes are positive, the radiation fields should be extended to include the mediastinum and supraclavicular nodal areas in addition to the pelvis, abdomen and para-aortic areas [11, 18]. Patients must be followed closely since 65% of recurrences are evident within two years [6].

The five-year survival rate of patients with dysgerminoma drops from 96% in Stage Ia to 63%, with extra-ovarian spread [6]. Effective primary treatment is important because only about half of the patients treated for recurrence can be expected to survive (Table 5). Recurrences should be treated aggressively with re-exploration, tumor excision, and additional radiotherapy which is possible because of the relatively low doses required to obtain a tumor response. Chemotherapy has been used infrequently in dysgerminoma because of its exquisite radiosensitivity. Encouraging results have been reported in the treatment of recurrent disease using chemotherapeutic regimens similar to those effective for endodermal sinus tumor of the ovary and seminoma of the testes [11, 18, 19-22].

## 2.2. *Endodermal sinus tumor (yolk sac tumor)*

Endodermal sinus tumor is the second most common malignant germ cell tumor of the ovary and represents about one percent of all ovarian malignancies [2]. Originally confused with mesonephroma, Teilum [23] demonstrated its origin from yolk sac endoderm, thereby elucidating its histogenesis and proving that it was a germ cell tumor. The remaining 'mesonephromas' were later renamed clear cell carcinomas by Scully and Barlow when their derivation from the surface epithelium of the ovary was recognised [24].

*2.2.1. Histogenesis.* See embryonal carcinoma.

*2.2.2. Clinical features.* The patients range in age from 14 months to 45 years, with a median age of 19 years [25]. This tumor is rare in patients over the age of 40.

The clinical presentation of endodermal sinus tumor is frequently sudden; half of the patients have symptoms for one week or less. Three-fourths of the patients have abdominal pain and nearly all have a large abdominal or pelvic mass [25]. When the tumor is on the right side, acute symptoms may occasionally mimic acute appendicitis. Young women usually do not have endocrine or menstrual abnormalities and children do not present with precocious puberty. Reports of endodermal sinus tumor associated with hormonal activity probably represent mixed germ cell tumors with unrecognized elements of choriocarcinoma or embryonal carcinoma. In pure endodermal sinus tumor, serum AFP levels are elevated but hCG levels are not [12].

*2.2.3. Gross features.* Endodermal sinus tumors range in diameter from 3 to 30 cm with a median of 15 cm. The exterior is smooth and the cut surface is soft and predominantly solid. Cysts of variable size throughout give it a honeycombed appearance. Large areas of necrosis and hemorrhage are common. Endodermal sinus tumors co-exist with benign cystic teratoma in the ipsilateral ovary in 14% of patients and in the contralateral ovary in 5% of patients.

*2.2.4. Microscopic features.* Endodermal sinus tumors display a wide range of patterns which are frequently admixed. Occasionally one pattern may dominate to the exclusion of the others and in rare instances a tumor may be comprised of only one 'pure' type. Five interrelated growth patterns have been described in detail by Teilum [23, 26]: (1) The most common is the reticular pattern composed of a loose meshwork of spaces and channels lined by flattened or cuboidal cells with scanty cytoplasm and indistinct borders (Figure 2). Hyaline droplets are common in this pattern (Figure 3). (2) The typical endodermal sinus pattern (festoon pattern) is the easiest to identify because it contains abundant perivascular structures (Schiller-Duval bodies) composed of a central capillary core surrounded by a mantle of primitive appearing cells that are pathognomonic of the neoplasm (Figure 4). These structures are thought to recapitulate the endodermal sinuses of the yolk sac. They are not prominent in the human but are readily identified

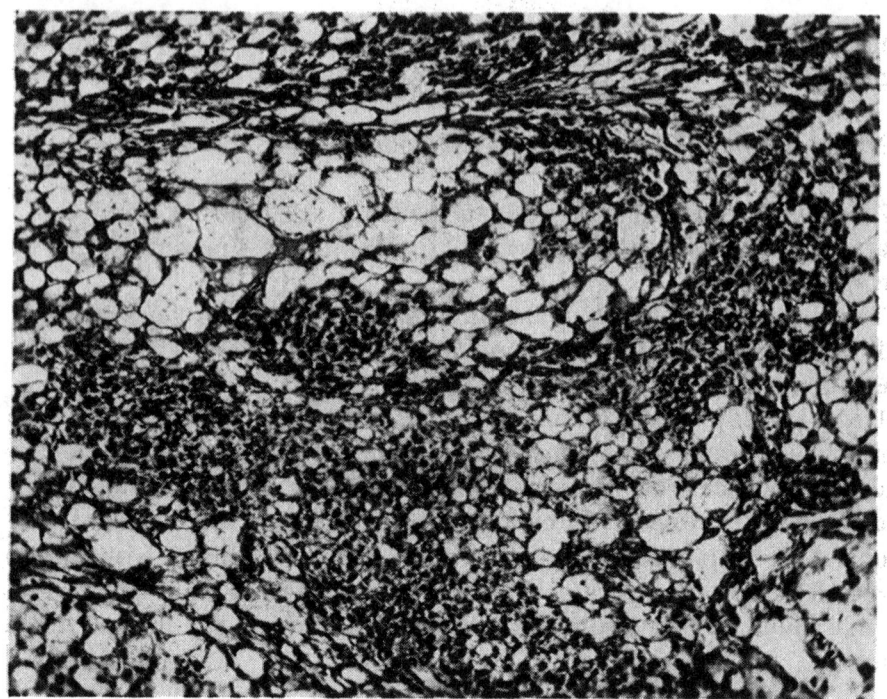

*Figure 2.* Endodermal sinus tumor, showing solid and reticular areas. (From Kurman and Norris: Cancer 38:2404, 1976.)

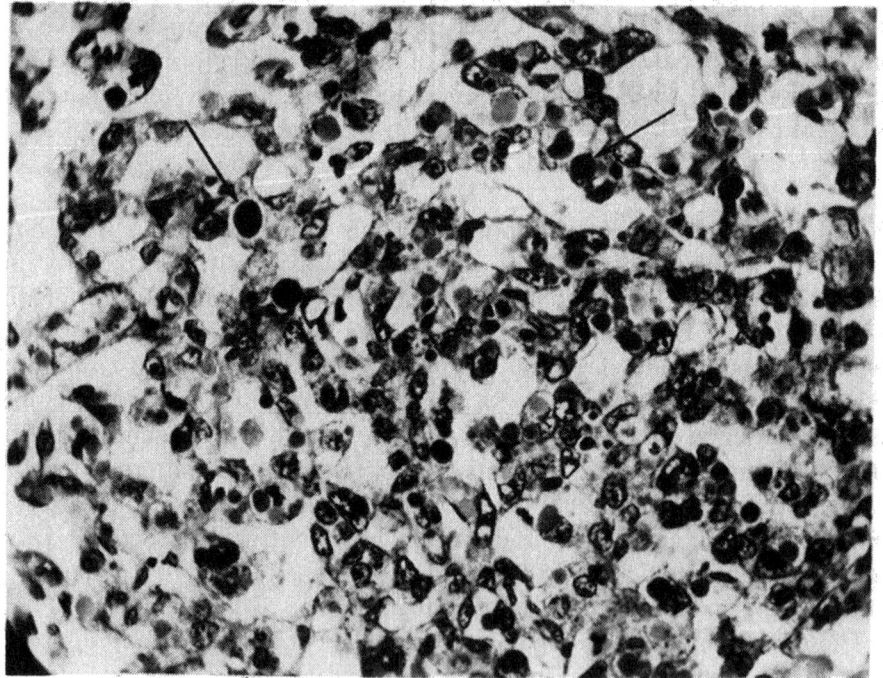

*Figure 3.* Endodermal sinus tumor showing solid and reticular pattern with numerous hyaline droplets (arrows). (From Kurman and Norris: Path Ann 13:291, 1978.)

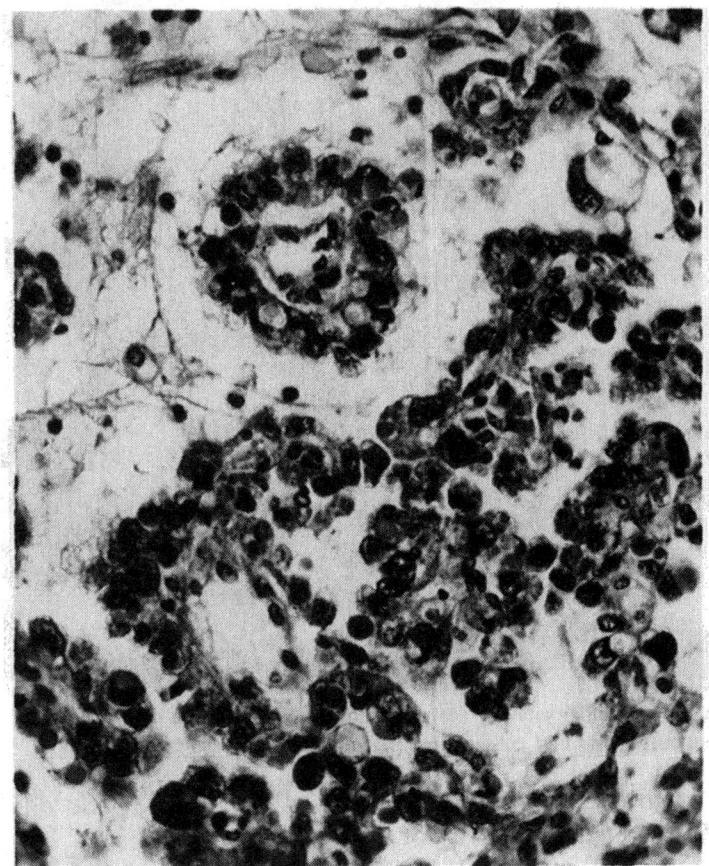

*Figure 4.* A Schiller-Duval body (top of field) pathognomonic of the endodermal sinus tumor. (From Kurman and Norris: Cancer 38:2404, 1976.)

in the rodent. (3) The polyvesicular vitelline pattern is rarer and is characterized by multiple cysts and vesicles with flat columnar epithelial cells which have clear cytoplasm lying in a dense fibroblastic stroma (Figure 5). This pattern is said to reflect the conversion of the primary to the secondary yolk sac and has recently been encountered in a pure form [27]. (4) The alveolar-glandular pattern is comprised of cystic spaces lined by papillary processes covered with cuboidal epithelium (Figure 6). (5) The rarest form is the solid pattern composed of a relatively solid growth of undifferentiated cells resembling embryonal carcinoma (Figure 2). There is no prognostic difference between any of the histologic types.

Schiller-Duval bodies are absent in one-fourth of tumors whereas hyaline droplets, which stain positively with periodic acid-Schiff, reagent are always present [25]. Immunohistochemical studies suggest that the hyaline droplets

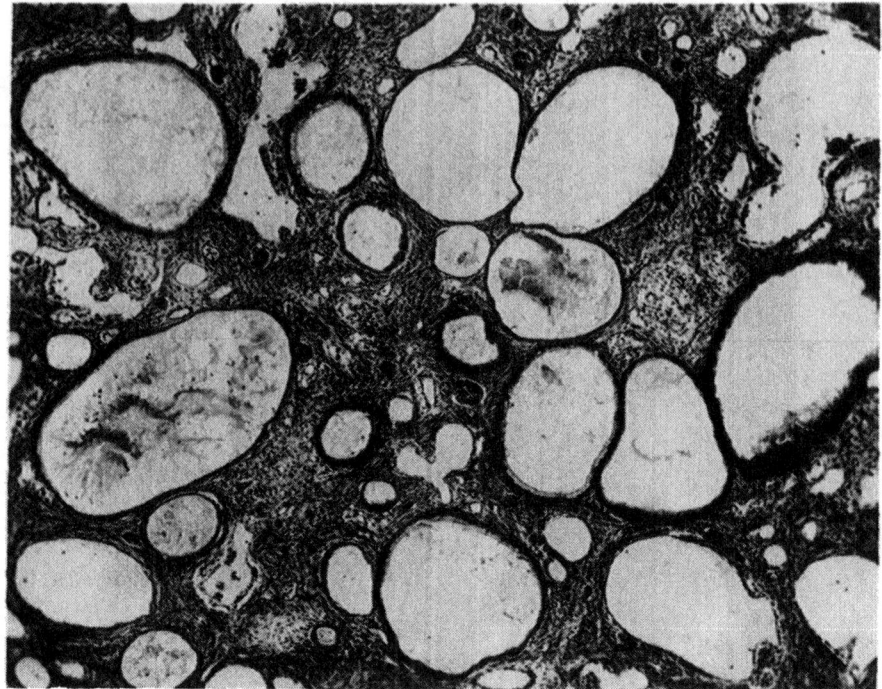

*Figure 5.* The polyvesicular vitelline pattern is characterized by multiple cysts lined by flattened cells and frequently columnar cells containing mucin in a dense spindle stroma.

represent a variety of proteins but mainly AFP [25, 28] and alpha-1-antitrypsin [29] secreted by the tumor.

*2.2.5. Behavior and therapy.* The endodermal sinus tumor is characterized by extremely rapid growth. At the time of primary operation, 71% of the patients appear to have Stage Ia disease; involvement of the contralateral ovary is uncommon except in the presence of disseminated peritoneal spread (Table 4). Six percent of tumors are classified in Stage II and 23% in Stage III. Stage IV neoplasms are rare. About one-fourth of tumors rupture before or during surgical removal.

Ascites is present in a few Stage I patients and in about half of those with metastatic disease at initial laparotomy. This contrasts with the early appearance of ascites in over 90% of patients with recurrences.

Prior to modern chemotherapy, 84% of patients with Stage Ia tumors died, in spite of surgical treatment or the combination of surgical and radiation therapy (Table 6). This result underlines the need for more effective therapy. Although histologic examination of the opposite normal appearing ovary does not disclose microscopic metastases, it is likely that occult metastases, are present at the time of initial diagnosis. For this reason adju-

*Table 6.* Endodermal sinus tumor, Stage I. Survival after surgical treatment alone or operation and radiation therapy.

| Author | Patients | Survivors (2 yrs or more) | Percent |
|---|---|---|---|
| Jimerson and Woodruff [125] | 26 | 2 | 8 |
| Kurman and Norris [25] | 39 | 5 | 13 |
| Smith [126] | 3 | 1 | 33 |
| Total | 68 | 8 | 12 |

vant triple agent chemotherapy is given to patients even in the absence of gross residual disease. It has been shown in animal models that tumors can be eradicated by chemotherapy if the tumor is still small and the dose of the chemotherapeutic agent is adequate [30]. Furthermore, the proportion (growth fraction) of dividing cells (those most sensitive to chemotherapeutic drugs and radiation) is relatively higher when the tumor is small [30, 31]. Although radiation therapy and extensive surgery have not reduced the mortality of patients with endodermal sinus tumor, success has been reported in patients treated with adjuvant triple chemotherapy, utilizing either vincristine, actinomycin-D, and cyclophosphamide (VAC) [25, 32, 33] or methotrexate, actinomycin-D and chlorambucil (MAC) [22, 32]. A survival rate of greater than 70% has been reported in patients with Stage I disease

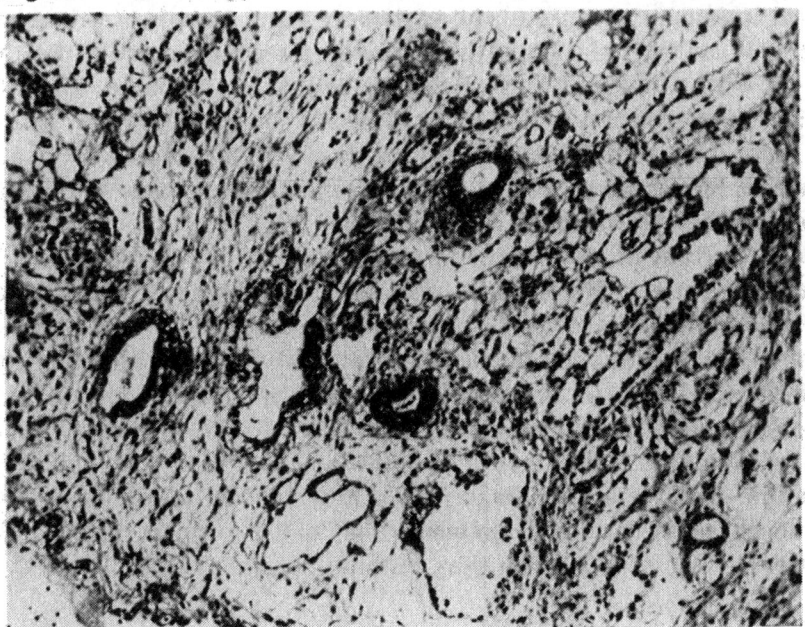

*Figure 6.* Endodermal sinus tumor containing glands (alveolar-glandular pattern) intermixed with a reticular pattern.

Table 7. Endodermal sinus tumor-Stage I. Survival after operation and VAC (vincristine, actinomycin-D, cytoxan).

| Author | Patients | Survivors | Percent | Survival duration (months) |
|---|---|---|---|---|
| Slayton et al. [32] | 11 | 5 | 45 | 14–34 |
| Smith [126] | 7 | 7 | 100 | 4–47 |
| Kurman and Norris [25] | 4 | 3 | 75 | 25–30 |
| Gallion et al. [9] | 1 | 1 | 100 | 24 |
| Cangir et al. [8] | 2 | 2 | 100 | 45–77 |
| Total | 25 | 18 | 72 | |

(Table 7) and in greater than 50% of patients with Stage III and IV disease. Excellent results have been obtained with testicular germ cell tumors using velban, bleomycin and Cis-platinum (VBP) with complete response rates of 76% reported [34]. The preliminary use of this combination in ovarian endodermal sinus tumors and other cell types has yielded favorable results that will probably be similar to the results in testicular tumors because of their similar biologic behavior [35–37]. In general, these drug combinations are used in the primary treatment of all malignant germ cell tumors except dysgerminoma. Radiation therapy is an important modality only in the treatment of dysgerminoma. Chemotherapy should be initiated shortly after surgical treatment because of the extremely rapid growth of the neoplasm. Treatment can start as soon as the second or third postoperative day. Young patients with confirmed Stage I disease should be managed by unilateral salpingo oophorectomy followed by adjuvant chemotherapy. In this situation, there is no need for removal of the uninvolved contralateral ovary and the uterus. Successful pregnancy following unilateral salpingo oophorectomy and chemotherapy has been reported [38].

Ninety percent of recurrences appear within a year of diagnosis. Endodermal sinus tumor metastasizes primarily by intraperitoneal spread and through lymphatics, although hematogeneous spread may occur later in the course of the disease. Autopsy findings reveal that the liver and peritoneum are uniformly involved. Progressive lymphatic spread begins with the retroperitoneal lymph nodes with subsequent extension to mediastinal and cervical lymph nodes. Other metastatic sites include bowel (46%), lungs (41%), omentum (27%), and diaphragm (23%) [25]. The histologic appearance of the metastasis is usually the same as that of the primary tumor although occasionally the solid pattern may become dominant [25].

*2.3. Teratoma*

The vast majority (99%) of ovarian teratomas may be divided into two broad categories depending on whether the component tissues are mature or immature. The remaining 1% of teratomas constitute a group of tumors that display monodermal or a highly specialized form of differentiation. Immaturity reflects the degree to which the neoplastic tissue resembles embryonic tissue and indicates a potential for recurrence. The quantity and grade of immature tissue present indicates the potential for malignant behavior [39-41]. Prior to the WHO introduction of the term immature teratoma, malignant behavior was thought to depend on whether a teratoma was cystic or solid. Generally, cystic teratomas are benign and solid teratomas are malignant. Solid mature teratomas behave in a benign fashion and immature teratomas containing visible cystic areas (one-third of cases) [39] may display malignant behavior. Immaturity must not be confused with malignant transformation occurring in mature teratomas since such neoplasms, although they are malignant, develop within mature tissues.

*2.4. Immature teratoma*

These tumors are the third most common malignant germ cell tumor of the ovary after dysgerminoma and endodermal sinus tumor [2] and represent nearly one-quarter of all ovarian germ cell tumors in children under 15 years of age.

*2.4.1. Histogenesis.* See embryonal carcinoma.

*2.4.2. Clinical features.* The median age is 18 years, and the oldest patients are about 40 years of age; 20% are prepubertal [40]. The symptoms are nonspecific and are usually present for a short duration, but are occasionally acute. Three-quarters of patients have a palpable abdominal or pelvic mass, frequently accompanied by pain.

*2.4.3. Gross features.* Immature teratomas are usually large unilateral tumors with a median diameter of 18 cm. The external surface is smooth and the cut surface is soft, gray to pink, with visible hemorrhage and necrosis and large cysts in a third of the cases. Hair is present in two-fifths of the tumors. Teeth are rare, but bone, cartilage, or calcification are usually evident.

*2.4.4. Microscopic features.* This neoplasm is comprised of varying proportions of immature tissue derived from the three germ layers. The degree of immaturity is graded; the immature neural tissue is the most common element and easiest to grade. In order to assess the degree of differentiation, adequate sampling requires a block of tissue for each centimeter of the tumor diameter. The least differentiated area determines the grade. The most widely used grading system is that of Norris and his associates [40]

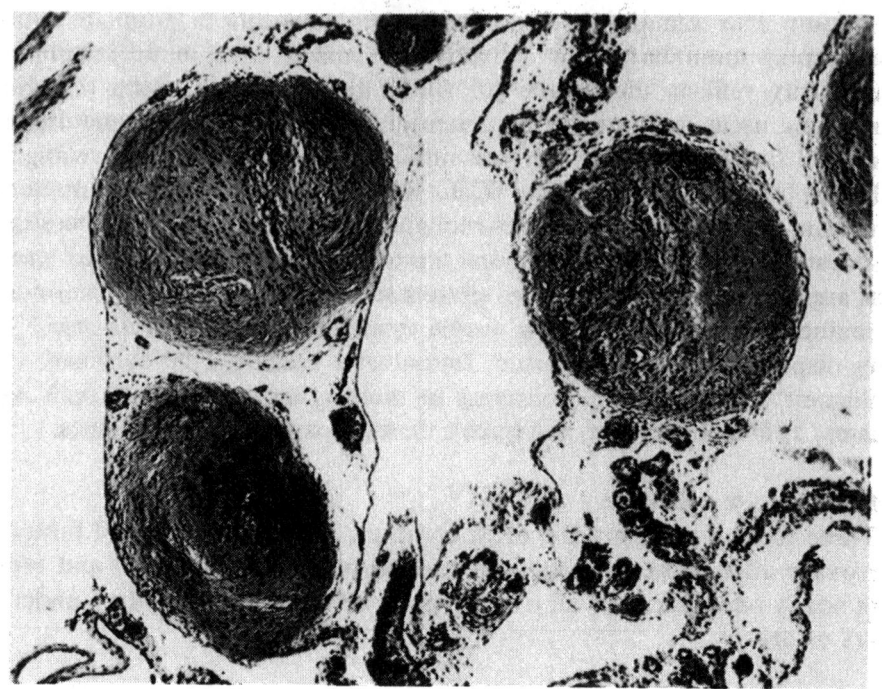

*Figure 7.* Grade O glial implants on the peritoneum from an immature teratoma. (From Kurman and Norris: Path Ann 13:291, 1978.)

which is a modification of that proposed earlier by Robboy and Scully [41].

Grade 0: wholly mature tissue (Figure 7).

Grade 1: abundant mature tissue but some immaturity, mainly glia in a primitive mesenchyme. Mitotic figures are rare and neural epithelium is absent or limited to one low power field (40×) per slide.

Grade 2: more than one low power field of neural epithelium but not exceeding three low power fields per slide (Figure 8).

Grade 3: extensive areas of immaturity are present, neural epithelium is found in four or more low power fields per slide frequently merging with a highly primitive appearing 'sarcomatous' stroma; mitotic activity is common.

Although neural epithelium, often forming tubules or rosettes (Figure 8) and glial tissue are the most frequently encountered ectodermal derivatives, ganglion cells, nerve trunks, ocular structures, skin, sweat glands and hair may also be seen.

Tissue derived from mesoderm includes cartilage, bone, lymphoid tissue and occasionally smooth muscle. Striated muscle is rare and is suggestive of a mixed mesodermal tumor. Endodermal elements include columnar tissue

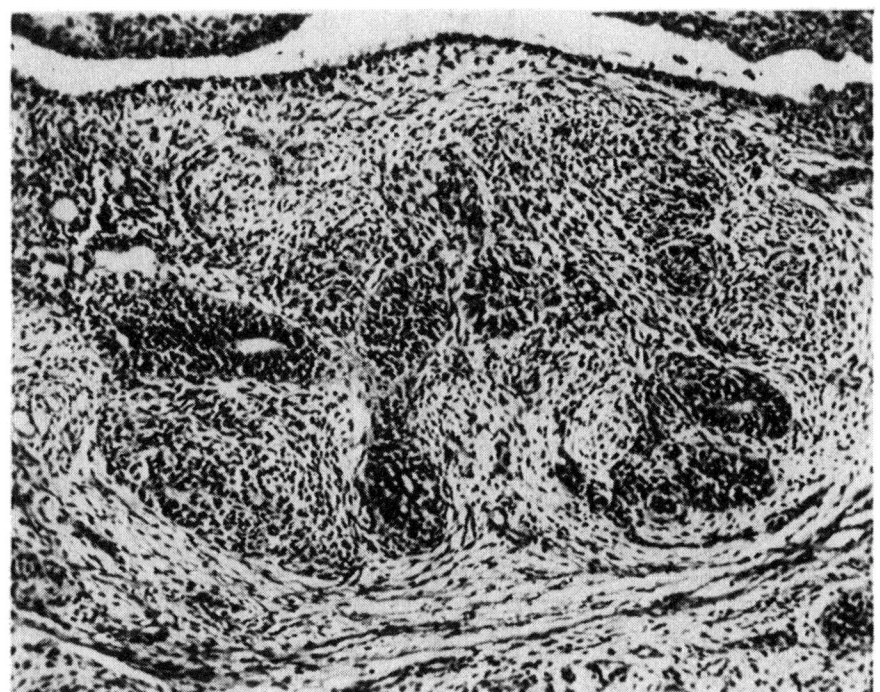

*Figure 8.* Immature Grade 2 teratoma containing primitive neuroepithelium that often produces rosettes. (From Kurman and Norris: Human Path 8:551, 1977.)

suggesting respiratory and gastrointestinal epithelium. The tissue elements in an immature teratoma may show varying degrees of immaturity, but the most primitive areas have a propensity to metastasize and, consequently, play the most important role in grading.

*2.4.5. Behavior and treatment.* Approximately 70% of tumors are Stage Ia. Bilateral involvement (Stage Ib or Ic) does not occur in the absence of diffuse peritoneal spread [39–41] (Table 4). About 5% of contralateral ovaries contain a benign cystic teratoma. Early spread occurs by direct extension to the adjacent pelvic tissues and by peritoneal implantation. Lymphatic invasion and extra-abdominal spread are rare.

For Stage I disease prognosis is related to the histologic grade of the tumor (Table 8). In view of the rarity or nonexistence of bilateral (Stage Ib) ovarian disease (Table 4), Stage I disease is best treated by unilateral salpingo oophorectomy. A biopsy of the opposite ovary should be examined by frozen section to rule out an occult metastasis from an unsuspected mixed malignant germ cell tumor that contains dysgerminoma in addition to teratoma. Patients with Grade 2 and 3, Stage I neoplasms require adjuvant chemotherapy because survival decreases to 60% and 25% respectively

*Table 8.* Immature teratoma–Stage I. Survival by grade and treatment.

A. Operation alone: patients surviving with no evidence of disease

| Author | Grade I patients surviving | Duration (months) | Grade II patients surviving | Duration (months) | Grade III patients surviving | Duration (months) |
|---|---|---|---|---|---|---|
| Norris et al. [40] | 14/14 | (20–156) | 11/20 | (6–396) | 2/6 | (206–210) |
| Nogales et al. [39] | 4/4 | (34–84) | 4/5 | (20–60) | 0/2 | (–) |
| Total | 18/18 (100%) | | 15/25 (60%) | | 2/8 (25%) | |

B. Operation and combination chemotherapy[a]: patients surviving with no evidence of disease

| Author | Grade I patients surviving | Duration (months) | Grade II patients surviving | Duration (months) | Grade III patients surviving | Duration (months) |
|---|---|---|---|---|---|---|
| Slayton et al. [32] | 2/2 | (10–30) | 2/2 | (15–35) | 3/3 | (8–37) |
| Curry et al. [127] | 2/2 | (21–73) | (–) | | 1/1 | (54) |
| Creasman et al. [22] | (–) | | 1/1 | (18) | 1/1 | (15) |
| Total | 4/4 (100%) | | 3/3 (100%) | | 5/5 (100%) | |

[a] 7 patients treated with MAC: methotrexate, actinomycin D, cytoxan.
5 patients treated with VAC: vincristine, actinomycin D, cytoxan.

(Table 8). Tumor rupture in Stage I was related to recurrence in 4 of 5 patients in the report of Norris *et al.* [40]. This outcome was worse than in the group without rupture and therefore suggests that this is an adverse prognostic feature and therefore merits adjuvant chemotherapy.

Once metastasis has occurred (Stage II and Stage III disease) the grade of the *metastasis* is the major prognostic determinant. Patients with Stage II and III disease require maximal surgical excision of all resectable disease for histologic grading and therapy. Those with Grade 0 metastases (Figure 7) all survive after surgery and need no further treatment provided the primary tumor is no worse than Grade 1. Prior to the use of recent combination chemotherapy, Norris and associates [40] showed that with Grade 1 or 2 metastases there is 40 to 50% survival and no patient with Grade 3 metastases survived. Recently there have been reports of patients with Stage II and III disease and histologic Grades 2 and 3 who were long-term (3–6 year) survivors following chemotherapy with vincristine, actinomycin-D and cyclophosphamide (VAC) (Table 9). Pathologic examination of residual disease at 'second look' operation following multiple courses of chemotherapy in 5 cases revealed Grade 0 (mature teratoma) exclusively [42, 43]. It appears, therefore, that the chemotherapy may eradicate the immature tissue leaving mature tissue which may either remain static or in some cases continue to grow superficially without causing symptoms.

*2.5. Mature teratoma*

Tumors in this group are composed entirely of mature tissue elements and may be either solid or cystic. The vast majority (99%) are cystic and are referred to as benign cystic teratomas (dermoid).

*2.5.1. Mature solid teratoma.* The mature solid teratoma occurs in the same age group as the immature teratoma and since most solid teratomas do contain immature tissue the tumor must be thoroughly sampled before it can be concluded with certainty that a solid teratoma is totally mature (Grade 0) and therefore benign.

*2.5.2. Gross features.* These tumors are usually large and have no specific features. Hemorrhage and necrosis are usually absent.

*2.5.3. Microscopic features.* The tumor is composed of mature tissue elements derived from all three germ layers and is therefore identical to the more common benign cystic teratoma.

*2.5.4. Behavior and treatment.* The tumors are invariably unilateral and consequently unilateral salpingo oophorectomy is adequate treatment. Oc-

Table 9. Immature teratoma–Stage I, II and III. Patients surviving[a] after operation and combination chemotherapy[b].

| Author | Stage I patients surviving | Duration (months) | Stage II patients surviving | Duration (months) | Stage III patients surviving | Duration (months) |
|---|---|---|---|---|---|---|
| Curry et al. [127] | 3/3 | (21–73) | 1/1 | (43) | 2/3 | (16–43) |
| Slayton et al. [32] | 7/7 | ( 8–37) | (–) | | 0/3 | (–) |
| Cangir et al. [8] | 5/5 | (24–55) | 1/1 | (80) | 1/1 | (78) |
| Creasman et al. [22] | 2/2 | (15–18) | (–) | | (–) | |
| Total | 17/17 (100%) | | 2/2 (100%) | | 3/7 (43%) | |

[a] No evidence of disease includes several patients with grade 0 implants at second look laparatomy.
[b] 20 patients treated with VAC: vincristine, actinomycin D, cytoxan.
 6 patients treated with MAC: methotrexate, actinomycin D, cytoxan.

casionally such a tumor may be associated with peritoneal implants, but if in fact the primary tumor is completely mature the implants will also be composed of mature (Grade 0) glial tissue. Implants should be surgically removed but adjuvant chemotherapy is not necessary.

*2.6. Mature cystic teratoma; benign cystic teratoma (dermoid)*

This teratoma, composed entirely of mature elements, is the most common tumor of the ovary, accounting for approximately one-fifth of all ovarian neoplasms [44–46]. Benign cystic teratomas are found in all ages, but 80% occur in patients between the ages of 20 and 30 years. Ten percent occur after the menopause.

*2.6.1. Histogenesis.* Teratomas of the ovary are sex chromatin-positive, 46XX. Recently Lindner and co-workers [47], using chromosome banding and electrophoretic techniques, demonstrated that homologous chromosomes in cells of benign cystic teratomas of the ovary of women have identical centromeric markers and are homozygous at some, but not all, genetic loci for which the host cells are heterozygous. For this to occur, the teratoma has to arise from a single germ cell after the first meiotic division, which occurs after crossing over and exchange of genetic material between homologous chromosomes.

*2.6.2. Clinical features.* Most of these tumors do not cause symptoms; they are discovered by a routine pelvic examination or as an incidental finding during X-ray examination of the abdomen or at the time of laporotomy. When symptoms do occur they usually are abdominal pain or swelling. Pain is often due to torsion, one of the most common complications that occurs in 9–16% of cases [44, 45]. Since slightly more teratomas occur in the right ovary, acute symptoms may mimic acute appendicitis. Other complications include rupture of the tumor into the bladder [44–46], rectum [44], uterus or peritoneal cavity. Teratomatous tissue may be found in endometrial curettings. Implantation of benign cystic teratoma has occurred from rupture and spillage of the cyst contents, but it is rare [44]. Other rare complications include infection of the tumor by Salmonella organisms, idiopathic autoimmune hemolytic anemia [44, 45] and virilization in pregnant patients [48]. In pregnant women, androgens are probably secreted by adjoining luteinized stromal cells, present in all recorded instances of virilization. Elevated levels of hCG may be responsible for the induction of stromal luteinization, since virilization in association with tumors that normally do not have a functional effect occurs relatively more often in pregnancy. Virilization with elevated serum levels of androgens and estrogens has been observed in a 73-year old woman [49]. Ten percent of benign cystic teratomas occur during pregnancy but decreased fertility has also been observed in patients with these neoplasms [50]. There is no apparent explanation for this finding.

*2.6.3. Gross features.* The gross appearance of a cystic teratoma with its smooth external surface and cystic interior containing sebaceous material, hair, bone, and cartilage, is characteristic. The average size of benign cystic teratomas is smaller than that of most other ovarian neoplasms, possibly because they are often incidental findings. In one study, 80% of these tumors were less than 10 cm in diameter [44].

*2.6.4. Microscopic features.* Microscopic examination reveals squamous epithelium in nearly all. Mesodermal differentiation, usually into fat and cartilage, occurs in at least 73%, and endodermal differentiation in the form of bronchial and gastrointestinal epithelium is present in 32% [44, 45, 51]. No doubt these figures would be higher if the neoplasms were sampled more thoroughly. The greatest variety of tissues is almost always located in a knobby solid nodule located at one margin of the cyst referred to as the dermoid (Rokitansky's) protuberance. The cyst wall is usually composed of stratified squamous epithelium often containing abundant sweat glands, sebaceous glands, and hair. Occasionally columnar cells having the appearance of gastrointestinal or bronchial epithelium are present in that location. Extrusion of sebaceous material into the cyst wall may lead to a foreign body giant cell reaction. A wide variety of tissues have been described in these tumors including glia, retina, choroid plexus, ganglia, bone, cartilage, smooth muscle, fibrous and adipose tissue, salivary glands and thyroid tissue. Rarely, lactating breast tissue [52] and even pituitary tissue have been reported [53].

*2.6.5. Behavior and treatment.* Benign cystic teratomas are bilateral in 10–15% of patients and treatment consists of cystectomy with conservation of residual ovarian tissue. In an unpublished study by Woodruff it was found that in 240 patients who underwent unilateral removal of a cystic teratoma with a normal appearing unbisected opposite ovary, 7 (3%) required subsequent laparatomy to remove a dermoid developing in the residual ovary [54]. In view of the reported decreased fertility in patients with dermoids it therefore does not seem necessary to bisect a normal appearing ovary searching for an occult benign cystic teratoma.

*2.7. Malignant transformation in benign cystic teratoma*

Between 1% and 2% of benign cystic teratomas undergo malignant transformation [45, 51, 55, 56]. Usually this event occurs in postmenopausal women. This malignant neoplasm arises within the mature element of a mature teratoma and is therefore distinct from immature teratoma which invariably occurs in children and young women and behaves in a malignant fashion because of immature tissue.

*2.7.1. Clinical features.* The presentation in the early stages of disease does not differ from that of a benign cystic teratoma except that ascites is occasionally present. In two-thirds of patients, however, invasion or metastasis has occurred before diagnosis [56] and in these women symptoms are those of epithelial cancers of equivalent stage.

*2.7.2. Gross pathology.* The gross specimen resembles a cystic teratoma that is larger than usual with a mass invading part of the wall, often with necrosis.

*2.7.3. Microscopic features.* Almost any component of a teratoma may undergo malignant change; in up to 80% of malignancies squamous cell carcinoma arises from the epidermal component [56]. The only other malignancies occurring with any frequency are carcinoids, struma ovarii and adenocarcinomas. There have been rare reports of leiomyosarcoma [55], osteosarcoma, bronchogenic carcinoma, chondrosarcoma [57], basal cell carcinoma, sebaceous tumors, nevi [58], melanoma [59] and melanotic 'retinal anlage tumor' [60]. A pseudosarcomatous change in stroma underlying areas of squamous carcinoma may also occur [61].

*2.7.4. Behavior and treatment.* Since the malignant component of these tumors is usually a squamous carcinoma, spread occurs by direct extension [55–57]. Although there are no reports of bilateral malignant transformation, these neoplasms almost always occur after the menopause, so total abdominal hysterectomy and bilateral salpingo oophorectomy is the treatment of choice. The prognosis depends on the type and stage of the malignancy. In patients with unruptured Stage I squamous cell carcinoma the five-year survival rate may be as high as 65% but it drops markedly with metastasis or rupture [56]. Few patients with adenocarcinoma or sarcoma have survived [51, 56, 57].

*2.8. Monodermal and highly specialized teratomas*

Tumors in this group constitute a rare variant of teratoma and account for perhaps 3% of all ovarian teratomas. They are characterized by highly specialized tissue derived from a single germ cell layer in contrast to teratomas containing elements of all the germ layers. The following subgroups are listed in order of decreasing frequency.

*2.8.1. Struma ovarii.* Thyroid tissue occurs in 5-15% of teratomas [44, 45, 51, 62, 63]. The term struma ovarii, however, is reserved for neoplasms in which thyroid tissue represents more than half of the tumor. At least 17% of struma ovarii are composed of thyroid tissue entirely. Since less than a quarter of teratomas containing thyroid tissue qualify as struma ovarii, struma represents only about 2% of all teratomas [45, 51]. It is found most frequently in the fifth decade although it has occurred in adolescence and elderly women [45, 51].

*2.8.2. Clinical features.* Most patients are asymptomatic but 5% display evidence of hyperthyroidism. Since 16% of these symptomatic patients have enlarged thyroid glands as well [51], it is not certain whether the hyperthyroidism is caused by the struma or by the enlarged thyroid gland. In at least 17 cases there has been good evidence that the ovarian thyroid tissue contributed to thyrotoxicosis [62-64]. Radioactive iodine uptake has, therefore, been advocated as an aid in diagnosis of tumor.

*2.8.3. Gross features.* The neoplasm is usually less than 10 cm in diameter. The exterior is smooth and the cut surface varies in appearance depending on the amount of thyroid tissue. The thyroid component is solid, homogeneous, brown and glistening depending on how much colloid is present.

*2.8.4. Microscopic features.* The tumor is similar to mature thyroid tissue and contains acini lined by a single layer of cuboidal epithelium with colloid in the lumens. On occasion the histologic appearance may suggest a nodular goiter, fetal adenoma, and even Hashimoto's thyroiditis.

*2.8.5. Behavior and treatment.* Most cases of struma ovarii are unilateral and benign so that unilateral salpingo oophorectomy will be sufficient therapy. The contralateral ovary contains a benign cystic teratoma in 5-15% of cases. Ascites has been reported in as many as 17% of cases, and may be accompanied by a pleural effusion. These effusions do not indicate a malignant course [65].

Malignant struma ovarii is exceedingly rare. In 5-10% of cases a diagnosis of carcinoma has been made [61-64] but metastases occurred in the minority [64, 65]. The frequency of malignancy has been exaggerated because the criteria for carcinoma in struma ovarii are not the same as those of primary follicular carcinoma of the thyroid gland. Thyroid tissue within a teratoma is not encapsulated, thereby giving the false impression of invasion; papillary processes within a struma do not signify malignancy.

The diagnosis of malignant struma ovarii should only be made when there are cytologic features of malignancy. Metastatic spread is usually over peritoneal surfaces but very infrequently peritoneal implants of benign thyroid tissue termed 'strumosis' occur with struma ovarii and should not be confused with malignancy.

*2.8.6. Carcinoid.* Carcinoid tumor is found in less than one percent of ovarian teratomas [66] and usually occurs in adults from the third to the ninth decade. Two distinctive histologic patterns have been described: the insular or midgut, and the trabecular variety [67] resembling foregut and hindgut carcinoid.

*2.8.7. Clinical features.* The carcinoid syndrome occurs only with the insular pattern and is present in just one-third of these patients [66]. Abnormal serum levels of 5-hydroxyindole acetic acid do not appear until tumors are 3 to 4 cm in diameter. Since blood from the ovary drains into the vena cava, bypassing the portal circulation, an ovarian carcinoid can produce the carcinoid syndrome without metastatic disease in the liver. Thus far no primary ovarian carcinoids associated with the carcinoid syndrome have had metastasis at the time of discovery.

*2.8.8. Gross features.* A carcinoid usually appears as a tan to yellow nodule or thickening in the wall of a benign cystic teratoma, or as a minor constituent of a mature solid teratoma [67, 68]. In about one-fourth of the cases, carcinoid is the sole component.

*2.8.9. Microscopic features.* Insular carcinoid is composed of clusters or 'islands' of uniform cells forming small acini. In some tumors there may be an accompanying dense fibrous stroma. In the trabecular carcinoid, the cells form ribbons of anastomosing trabecular columns. Argentaffin granules, reddish brown to orange by hematoxylin and eosin staining, can be identified with ferric ferricyanide or silver reactions in about 80% of cases. Ultrastructurally, the neurosecretory granules are larger and more pleomorphic in the insular pattern, whereas the granules are more uniform and round in trabecular carcinoids [69].

*2.8.10. Behavior and treatment.* There have been no bilateral primary carcinoids reported, although a benign cystic teratoma is sometimes present in the contralateral ovary [66, 67]. Primary carcinoids seldom metastasize. The patients have all been cured following the removal of the tumor except in two instances when death occurred 5 and 6 years following primary treatment. One patient developed progressive tricuspid insufficiency three years after a carcinoid was successfully removed and the carcinoid syndrome alleviated [66]. Primary ovarian carcinoid can be treated by unilateral salpingo oophorectomy in a young woman, in view of the benign behavior and unilaterality but in older age groups total abdominal hysterectomy and bilateral salpingo oophorectomy are warranted.

## 2.9. Strumal carcinoid

Thyroid tissue may be intermixed with a trabecular carcinoid or insular carcinoid and Scully [65] has proposed the term 'strumal carcinoid' for this unusual neoplasm. Strumal carcinoid has not been associated with the carcinoid syndrome or hyperthyroidism although one patient had virilization [70] apparently caused by luteinized ovarian stromal cells.

Although this neoplasm is being tentatively considered in the group of teratomas with monodermal differentiation, considerable controversy still exists over its precise origin. Strumal carcinoid shares some morphologic features with medullary carcinoma of the thyroid, a tumor thought to arise from parafollicular C-cells. Medullary thyroid carcinoma has been associated with carcinoid syndrome, and 5-hydroxytryptamine has been found in sheep parafollicular cells [71]. It has been postulated, therefore, that this neoplasm is derived from cells differentiating in the direction of both thyroid tissue and carcinoid [72]. This concept has been disputed by Ranchod and associates [68] who identified dense-core intracytoplasmic 'carcinoid' granules within both the carcinoid and strumal elements, leading them to the conclusion that the entire neoplasm was a carcinoid tumor (of pure neuroendocrine origin) that had differentiated into both strumal and carcinoid patterns. More recently both calcitonin and thyroglobulin have been identified immunohistochemically in the carcinoid and strumal tissues respectively [73]. Thus, the histogenesis of this neoplasm still remains a mystery; it may be an ovarian analogue of medullary carcinoma of the thyroid being derived from C-cells or it may be an ovarian carcinoid with C-cell differentiation.

## 2.10. Miscellaneous monodermal teratomas

There have been occasional reports of other tumors of presumed teratomatous origin that appear to represent unilateral development from one germ layer. These include a pure sebaceous gland tumor [74], epidermoid cyst [75], and an endodermal variant of a mature cystic teratoma composed of respiratory epithelium exclusively [76].

Although the majority of mucinous tumors of the ovary are considered to be of epithelial origin, the presence of Paneth and argentaffin cells in some of these tumors as well as their association with benign cystic teratoma in 5% of cases suggests that some may be monodermal teratomas.

## 2.11. Embryonal carcinoma

This tumor was included in the 1973 WHO classification [7] but has only recently been characterized as a separate clinico-pathologic entity by Kurman and Norris [77]. The tumor is analogous morphologically and immunohistochemically with embryonal carcinoma of the adult testis [12] but in the past was included with endodermal sinus tumor of the ovary; both terms were used interchangeably. Pure embryonal carcinoma in the ovary is rare, accounting for only 5% of malignant ovarian germ cell tumors in contrast to the testicular analogue that represents 35% of all testicular germ cell neoplasms.

*2.11.1. Histogenesis.* The histogenesis of embryonal carcinoma is closely related to that of endodermal sinus tumor, teratoma and choriocarcinoma, in that embryonal carcinoma is the neoplastic progenitor of all three of the other neoplasms. This view is supported by light microscopic and electron microscopic observations, animal transplantation experiments and most recently by studies of oncofetal antigens associated with these tumors. Thus, the light microscopic resemblances of embryonal carcinoma to endodermal sinus tumor and choriocarcinoma have been supported by ultrastructural studies that have shown a common origin of all germ cell tumors excepting germinomas [78-80] and their similarity to the embryonal carcinoma explants used in experimental induction of murine teratomas [81-83]. Current research in embryonic and fetal antigens has also provided further confirmation of a common histogenesis for these tumors [12]. The demonstration that the human fetal yolk sac synthesizes AFP [84, 85] supported Teilum's claim that the endodermal sinus tumor originates from the yolk sac [23]. Localization of hCG in syncytiotrophoblast in choriocarcinoma and the immature placenta further corroborated the trophoblastic nature of ovarian choriocarcinoma.

In its most primitive form embryonal carcinoma appears to be incapable of synthesizing either AFP or hCG since neither marker can be demonstrated in tissue sections of some embryonal carcinomas using immunocytochemical methods and 10% of patients with testicular embryonal carcinoma fail to show elevated serum marker levels [86-88]. In most instances, however, embryonal carcinoma shows either biochemical or morphologic evidence of differentiation along yolk sac or trophoblastic pathways. Based on immunoperoxidase studies it appears that biochemical differentiation precedes the more complex histologic differentiation [12]. This temporal relationship is manifested by localization of AFP in embryonal carcinoma cells showing no morphologic evidence of yolk sac differentiation. Early histologic differentiation into yolk sac is characterized by the formation of microcystic spaces lined by flattened embryonal carcinoma cells containing AFP (Figure 9) [12, 89, 90]. As these microcystic spaces become the dominant pattern in contrast to the solid masses of cells (Figure 10), the micro-

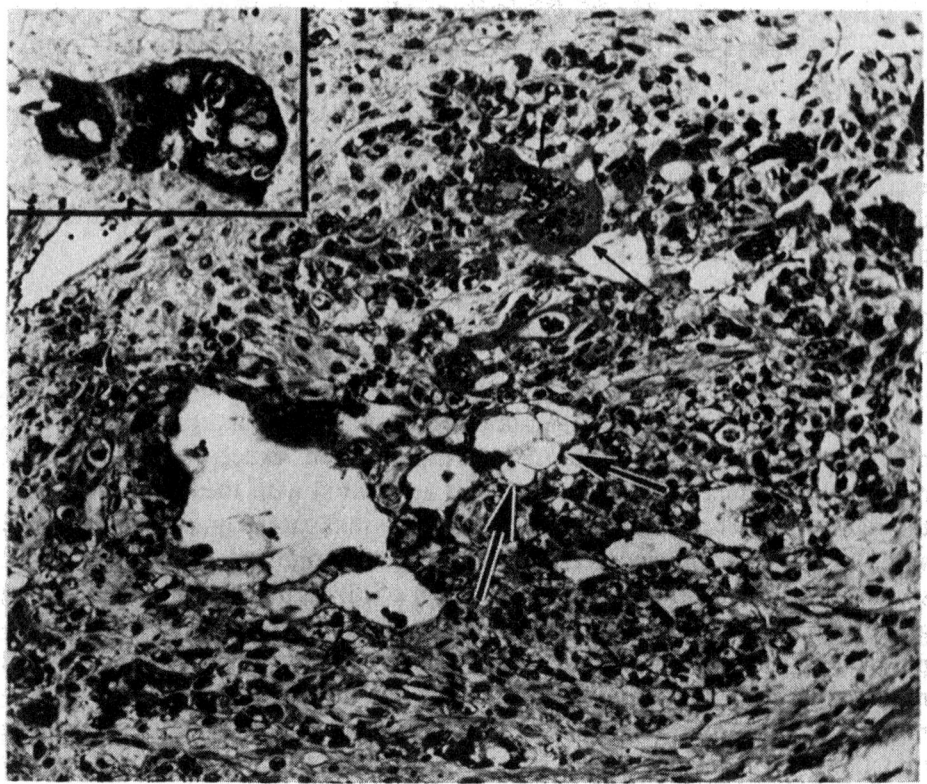

*Figure 9.* Early endodermal (yolk sac) differentiation within embryonal carcinoma manifested by focal microcystic formation (large arrows) and trophoblastic differentiation characterized by isolated syncytiotrophoblastic giant cells (small arrows). Insert – syncytiotrophoblastic cell containing hCG (dark intracytoplasmic reaction product) by immunoperoxidase.

cystic areas become the reticular pattern of endodermal sinus tumor (Figure 11) characterized by microcystic and macrocystic formation. These microcystic areas, reflect yolk sac differentiation, and occur more commonly in embryonal carcinoma than was previously suspected [91–93].

Differentiation of embryonal carcinoma along trophoblastic lines is manifested by the localization of hCG but not AFP within isolated syncytiotrophoblastic giant cells (Figure 9) and in the syncytiotrophoblast of bona fide choriocarcinoma [12]. Immunoperoxidase studies have also shown that syncytiotrophoblast contains pregnancy-specific beta globulin and human placental lactogen [90], further functional evidence of trophoblastic differentiation.

A tendency of embryonal carcinoma to differentiate towards teratomatous cell lines is manifested morphologically by the close association with cartilage and squamous epithelium [77]. Functional evidence of teratoma-

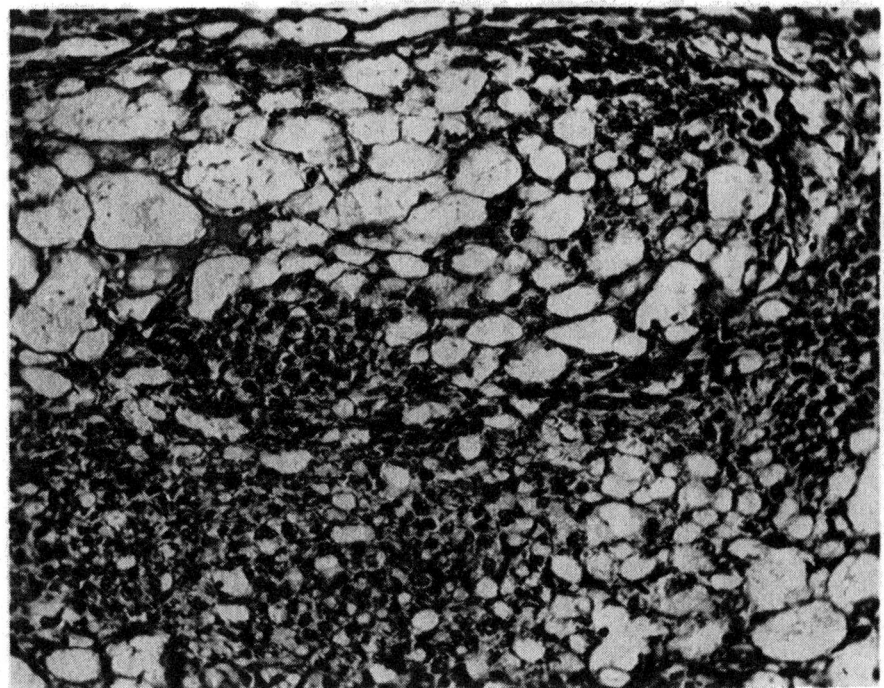

*Figure 10.* More extensive microcystic areas developing within solid masses of embryonal carcinoma cells.

tous differentiation in embryonal carcinoma is based on the presence of markers such as AFP, alpha-1 antitrypsin and CEA in both embryonal carcinoma and components of teratoma [90]. Embryonal carcinoma therefore appears to be comprised of a heterogeneous population of cells reflecting a dynamic process of differentiation along separate pathways.

*2.11.2. Clinical features.* The age range is 4 to 28 years with a median of 15 years. Nearly half of the patients are prepubertal [77]. Three-quarters of the patients have an abdominal or pelvic mass and half have abdominal pain. Symptoms tend to be of short duration (mean of 3 weeks) and occasionally mimic acute appendicitis or a ruptured ectopic pregnancy, especially when a positive pregnancy test is obtained.

Unlike patients with endodermal sinus tumors, most patients with embryonal carcinoma have manifestations of elevated hormone levels. Signs of precocious puberty are present in almost half of the prepubertal girls [77]. Amenorrhea or vaginal bleeding are found in one-third of the women in the reproductive age group. Mild hirsutism and virilization may result from stromal lutenization. Pregnancy tests have proved positive in all the patients tested including the children with precocious puberty.

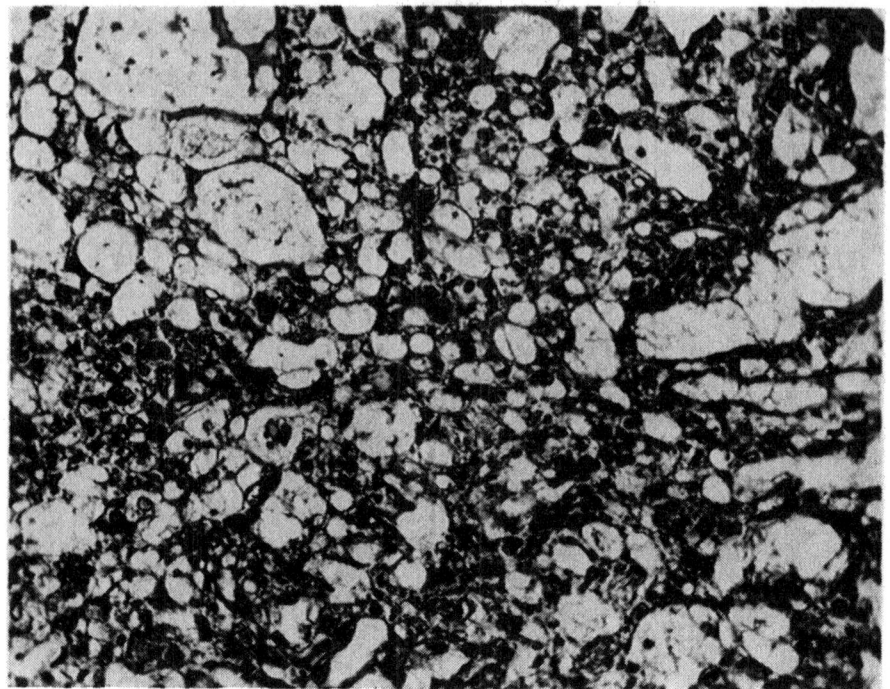

*Figure 11.* Extensive microcystic pattern within embryonal carcinoma. This represents a clearcut area of endodermal sinus tumor characterized by a microcystic or reticular pattern.

*2.11.3. Gross features.* Typically the tumor is large (median size 17 cm) encapsulated, and soft with a nondescript appearance. The cut surface is solid, gray-yellow and variegated with extensive hemorrhage and necrosis. Cysts are common.

*2.11.4. Microscopic features.* Pure embryonal carcinoma is composed of solid sheets of large primitive pleomorphic cells with amphophilic vaculated cytoplasm and vesicular nuclei with one or more nucleoli (Figure 12). These cells may form gland-like spaces and papillary processes but they lack the reticular, polyvesicular vitelline and festoon pattern of endodermal sinus tumor. A second cell type frequently present in embryonal carcinoma is a large multinucleated giant cell found at the periphery of the tumor or among solid masses of embryonal carcinoma cells or scattered haphazardly in the stroma. These syncytiotrophoblastic giant cells have eosinophilic or amphophilic cytoplasm and large vacuoles (Figures 9 and 13). Their nuclei are large, hyperchromatic and flattened into bizarre shapes. The supporting stroma of the tumor is variable, either myxoid and edematous or cellular with primitive spindle-shaped mesenchymal cells.

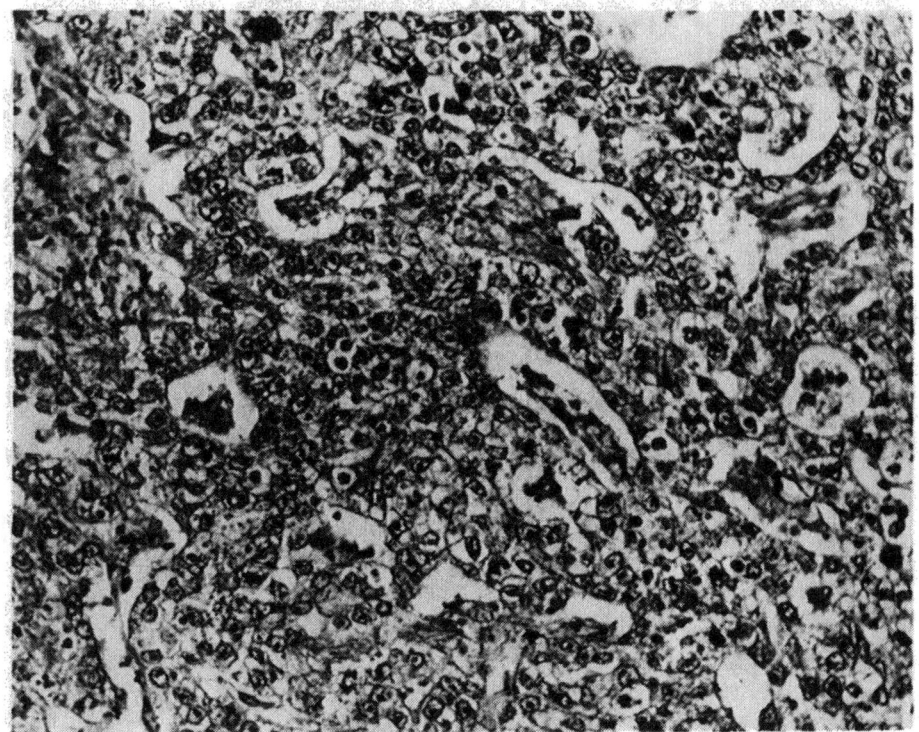

*Figure 12.* Sheets of embryonal carcinoma cells often forming clefts. These cells may contain AFP. (From Kurman and Norris: Cancer 38:2420, 1976.)

*2.11.5. Behavior and treatment.* The number of cases is too small for firm conclusions to be made about prognosis and treatment. Furthermore, few patients have had the benefit of combination chemotherapy.

The five-year actuarial survival before combination chemotherapy was 50 percent for Stage I disease and 39 percent for all stages combined (Table 3). Patients who developed recurrence after treatment die within two years from widespread intra-abdominal metastases, pulmonary metastases occurring late in the course of disease.

At initial laporotomy, 60% of tumors are localized to one ovary (Stage I) (Table 4). The remainder are divided equally between Stage II and III disease. Therapy is therefore the same as that for immature teratoma and endodermal sinus tumor and consists of complete excision of all resectable disease. Since metastasis to the opposite ovary without visible disease elsewhere is nonexistent (Table 4), unilateral salpingo oophorectomy for Stage I tumors should be performed. The opposite ovary, however, should be examined by frozen section since embryonal carcinoma may be admixed with dysgerminoma. In the series reported by Kurman and Norris [77], two

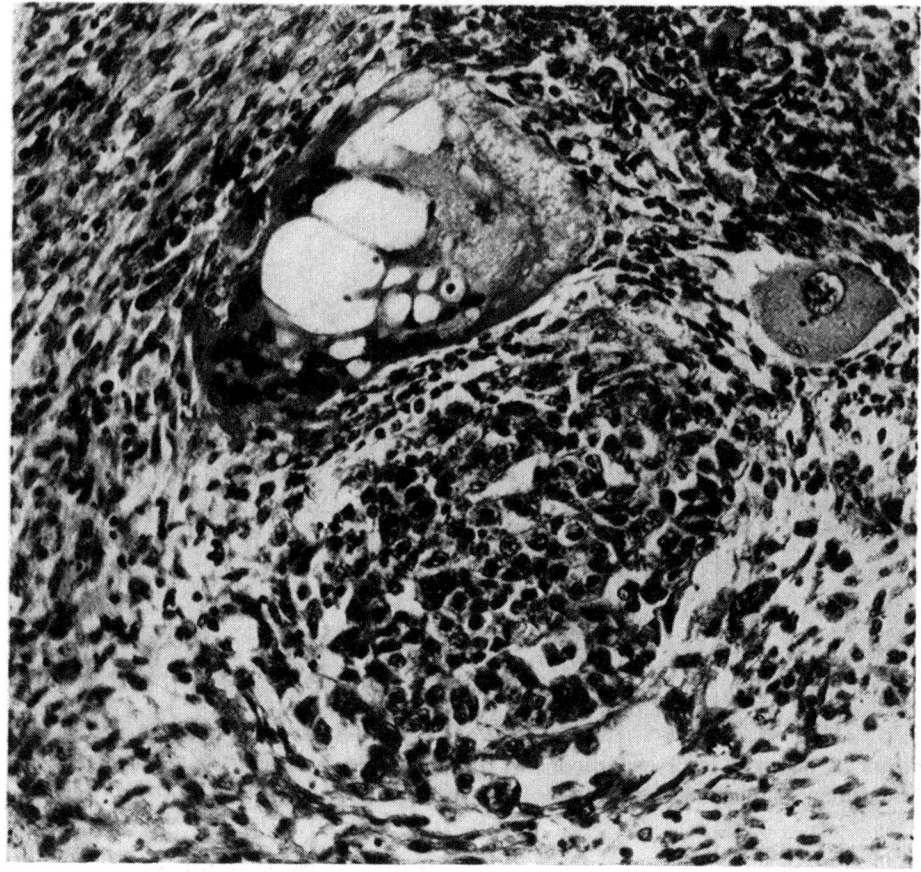

*Figure 13.* Syncytiotrophoblastic giant cells adjoining a nest of embryonal carcinoma cells. (From Kurman and Norris: Obstet Gynecol 48:579, 1976.)

of six patients undergoing biopsy of the contralateral ovary harbored microscopic foci of pure dysgerminoma when the main tumor contained foci of dysgerminoma along with embryonal carcinoma.

Since 50% of Stage I patients die if treated surgically only, adjuvant chemotherapy must be given postoperatively. Radiation is ineffective. The prognosis for embryonal carcinoma has improved with the use of multiple agent adjuvant chemotherapy [32].

### 2.12. Choriocarcinoma

Ovarian choriocarcinoma may be pure or, more commonly, part of a mixed germ cell tumor. The distinction is important because a pure tumor is more likely to be gestational than germ cell in origin. Gestational choriocarcinoma in the ovary is more likely a metastasis from a uterine or tubal primary malignancy than a primary choriocarcinoma from an ovarian pregnancy. Most nongestational choriocarcinomas in the ovary are mixed with teratoma, endodermal sinus tumor, embryonal carcinoma or dysgerminoma and are appropriately placed in the mixed malignant germ cell category. Only one-half of 40 examples of choriocarcinoma cited in the literature, were pure [51]. Among 5,000 ovarian tumors accessioned at the AFIP there were only two examples of pure nongestational ovarian choriocarcinoma.

*2.12.1. Histogenesis.* See embryonal carcinoma.

*2.12.2. Clinical features.* In a review of published cases of both mixed and pure choriocarcinoma, the age range was 7 months to 35 years with a mean of about 13 years [51]. An unequivocal derivation from germ cells of an ovarian choriocarcinoma can only be established in a prepubertal child. Half of the patients present with abdominal enlargement and pain. Only half of the premenarchal girls have signs of precocious puberty.

*2.12.3. Gross features.* Choriocarcinoma is soft and characteristically hemorrhagic. The purer tumors are associated with the more extensive hemorrhage. Other gross characteristics depend on the proportions of other germ cell elements.

*2.12.4. Microscopic features.* Choriocarcinoma is composed of two populations of cells, cytotrophoblast and syncytiotrophoblast, arranged in a characteristic biphasic plexiform pattern. The syncytiotrophoblast, which secretes hCG usually caps islands of cytotrophoblast (Figures 14 and 15). Both elements must be present in order to distinguish choriocarcinoma from embryonal carcinoma. Viable tumor is typically scanty, since most of the tissue is hemorrhagic and necrotic. The presence of large masses and aggregates of cells should suggest a poorly-differentiated carcinoma because choriocarcinoma does not contain a supporting stroma and is always intimately associated with areas of hemorrhage.

*2.12.5. Behavior and therapy.* In older reports, nongestational choriocarcinoma of the ovary has not proved as amenable to methotrexate as gestational choriocarcinoma of the uterus, but this is because some cases either represented misdiagnosed embryonal carcinoma or were poorly sampled and probably contained other malignant germ cell elements such as endodermal sinus tumor or teratoma that require other chemotherapeutic agents.

Radiation is of no value. Modern treatment depends on surgical excision and a choice of combination chemotherapy based upon the histologic composition of the neoplasm [94].

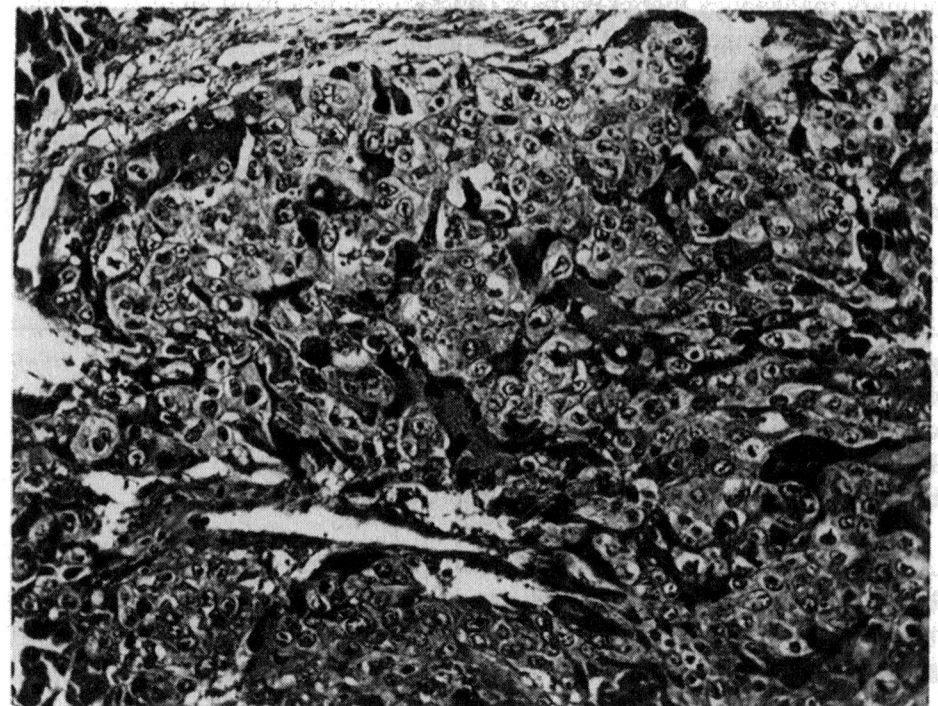
*Figure 14.* Choriocarcinoma of the ovary characterized by an intimate mixture of syncytio- and cytotrophoblast growing in a plexiform pattern.

## 2.13. Malignant mixed germ cell tumors

Germ cell tumors that contain more than one malignant germ cell component are referred to as malignant mixed germ cell tumors [95]. They represent 8% of malignant ovarian germ cell tumors in the AFIP files compared to 40% of testicular germ cell tumors.

*2.13.1. Clinical features.* The age of the patients ranges from 5 to 30 years with a median of 16 years. Forty percent are prepubertal and one-third of these children have precocious puberty. Pregnancy tests are positive in 38% of nonpregnant patients [95]. The majority present with nonspecific signs of an abdominopelvic mass; 50% have lower abdominal pain. The mean duration of symptoms is 4 weeks.

*2.13.2. Gross features.* These tumors tend to be large with a mean diameter of 15 cm. The outer surface is smooth and the appearance of the cut surface depends on the type and quantity of the components of the neoplasm. Solid fleshy areas correspond to dysgerminoma, mucoid cystic areas to teratoma

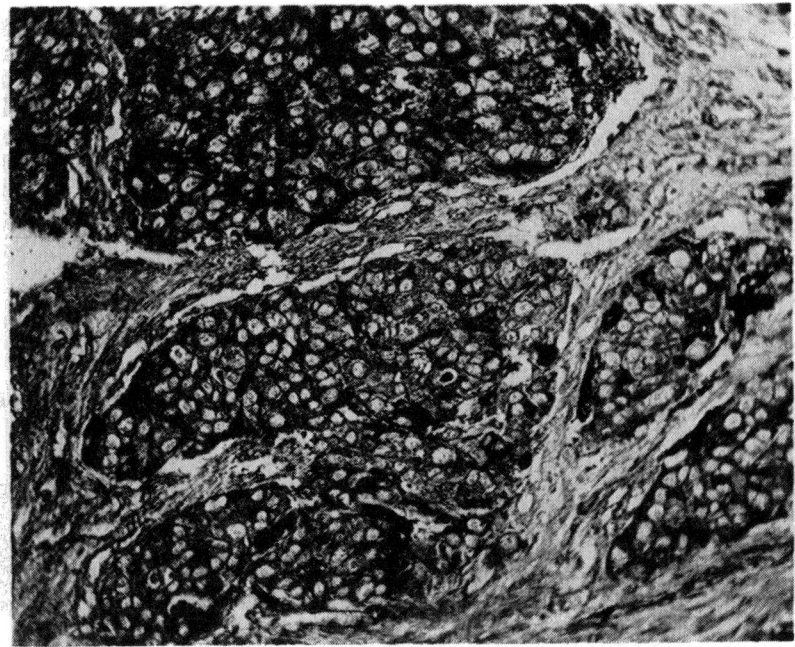

*Figure 15.* Choriocarcinoma showing localization of hCG (dark black intracytoplasmic reaction product) in syncytiotrophoblast by immunoperoxidase.

or endodermal sinus tumor and hemorrhagic necrotic areas to choriocarcinoma or endodermal sinus tumor.

Careful microscopic sampling of the gross specimen is essential. Quantitation of the various components is critical to an assessment of the behavior of the tumor.

*2.13.3. Microscopic features.* By definition at least two malignant components are present. The most common component is dysgerminoma, found in 80% of tumors followed by endodermal sinus tumor in 70%, immature teratoma in 53%, choriocarcinoma in 20%, and embryonal carcinoma in 13% [95]. In two-thirds of the tumors only two malignant components are present. The most frequently encountered mixture is dysgerminoma and endodermal sinus tumor which represents one-third of the cases (Figure 16).

*2.13.4. Behavior and treatment.* Two-thirds of patients at laparotomy have Stage I disease, with no microscopic involvement of the opposite ovary (Table 4) and these patients have an actuarial survival of 50%. Survival according to stage after combination chemotherapy is shown in Table 10. Disease tends to involve the pelvic and abdominal viscera. Metastasis to the

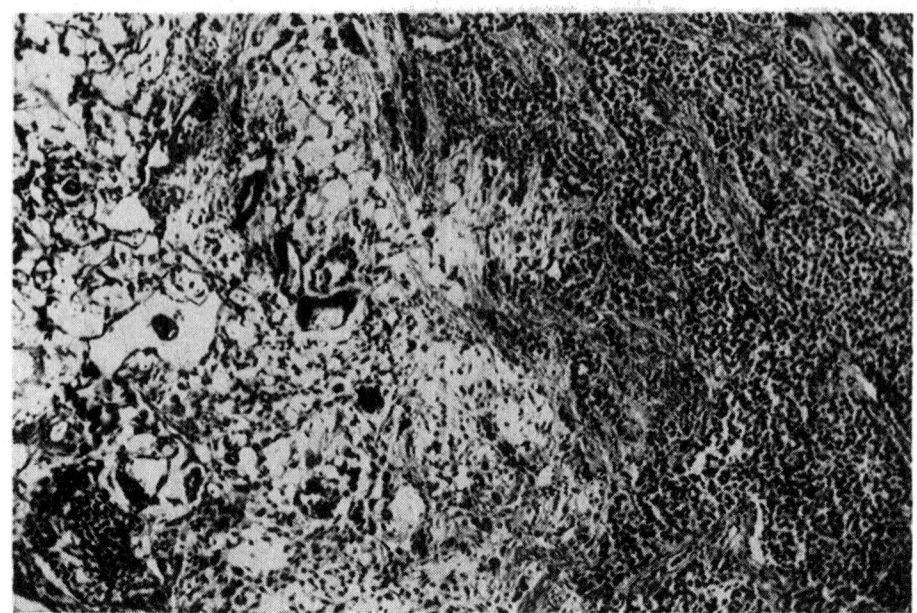

*Figure 16.* Mixed malignant germ cell tumor composed of 95% dysgerminoma (right) and 5% endodermal sinus tumor (left). The patient was treated by surgery and radiotherapy and is alive 4 years later without evidence of disease. (From Kurman and Norris: Path Ann 13:291, 1978.)

lungs is infrequent and late. The prognosis for patients with Stage I mixed germ cell tumors can be determined if the neoplasm is adequately sampled (1 block of tissue for every centimeter of maximum tumor diameter). The two most important factors in predicting the outcome for patients with Stage I tumors are the size and the histologic composition of the neoplasm.

*Table 10.* Mixed germ cell tumors-stage and survival after operation and combination chemotherapy[a].

| Stage | Surviving patients | Percent | Survival duration (months) |
| --- | --- | --- | --- |
| I | 10/10 | 100 | 18–114 |
| II | 4/4 | 100 | 19–154 |
| III | 3/5 | 60 | 41–120 |
| IV | 0/3 | 0 | – |

[a] 11 patients treated with vincristine, actinomycin D, cytoxan.
  9 patients treated with methotrexate, actinomycin D, cytoxan.
  2 patients treated with actinomycin D, 5-FU and cytoxan.
  6 patients also had radiation therapy: 4 Stage I, 1 Stage II and 1 Stage III.
From Cangir *et al.* [8], Slayton *et al.* [32],
    Creasman *et al.* [22], and Kurman and Norris [95].

Those that are larger than 10 cm and are more than one-third endodermal sinus tumor, choriocarcinoma, or Grade 3 teratoma have a poor prognosis and consequently require adjuvant chemotherapy. In contrast patients with tumors (1) smaller than 10 cm, or (2) less than one-third endodermal sinus tumor, choriocarcinoma, or Grade 3 teratoma, or (3) composed exclusively of combinations of dysgerminoma, embryonal carcinoma, or Grade 1 or 2 teratoma have a much more favorable outlook [95]. Thus a Stage I mixed tumor containing only small foci of highly malignant elements can be considered pure as far as adjuvant treatment is concerned. Surgical treatment of Stage I tumors in young women can be unilateral salpingo oophorectomy, as only 1 of 30 patients in the AFIP series [95] had bilateral neoplasms. The contralateral ovary should be biopsied if unilateral oophorectomy is contemplated because mixed germ cell tumors containing dysgerminoma may have occult metastasis of dysgerminoma in a visibly normal ovary.

## 2.14. Polyembryoma

This tumor pattern is rare and best classified as a malignant mixed germ cell tumor with embryoid formation, rather than as a separate entity. Peyron's [96] description of a testicular teratoma of this type has been followed by other reports of ovarian polyembryomas associated with dysgerminoma, endodermal sinus tumor, embryonal carcinoma, and teratoma. This tumor has never been reported as a pure neoplasm. Embryoids are microscopic structures resembling the embryonic disc, yolk sac and amniotic cavity (Figure 17). Embryoid bodies are described as complete, imperfect or

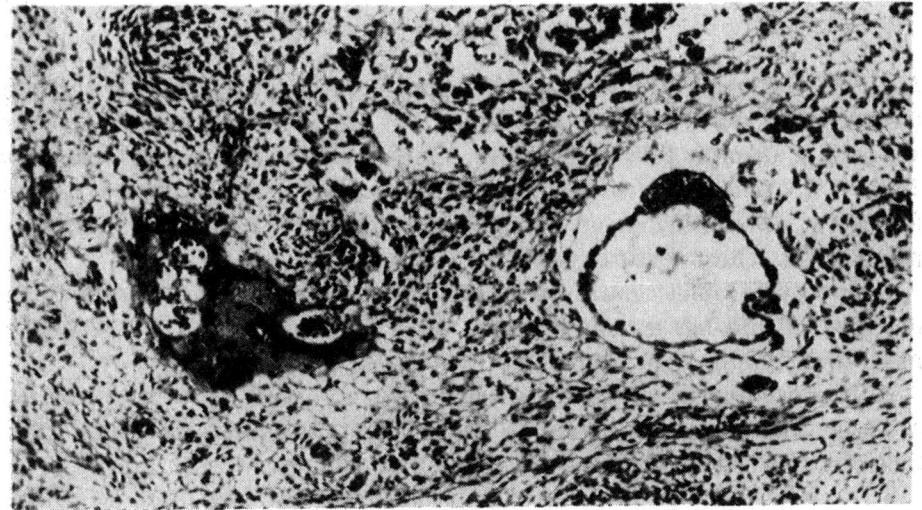

*Figure 17.* Malignant mixed germ cell tumor with embryoid formation (right). A syncytiotrophoblastic giant cell is on the left. (From Kurman and Norris: Obstet Gynecol 48:579, 1976.)

amorphous depending on the degree of organization [97]. Embryoids have been observed in transplanted embryonal carcinoma after its germ cells were no longer identifiable, suggesting that embryoids are a stage in the differentiation of embryonal carcinoma form primitive multipotential cells [78, 98].

## 3. MIXED GERM CELL AND STROMAL TUMORS

This category includes tumors that contain large numbers of germ cells resembling dysgerminoma and gonadal stromal cells. The most common tumor is the gonadoblastoma. Talerman has described another type of mixed germ cell and sex cord stromal tumor with distinctive clinical and pathologic features that justify separation from gonadoblastoma but that tumor is extremely rare [99-101].

### 3.1. Gonadoblastoma

Gonadoblastoma is generally regarded as a neoplasm although there is considerable evidence to indicate that it represents a maldeveloped gonad in a genetically abnormal individual. It is referred to as a neoplasm in this section since this view currently prevails. Gonadoblastoma is the most common neoplasm of abnormal gonads from which it arises almost exclusively. Twenty-two percent arise in a streak gonad, and 18% in a cryptorchid testis. The majority, however, originate in an abnormal gonad of indeterminate type [102].

*3.1.1. Histogenesis.* The gonadoblastoma is generally regarded as a benign germ cell neoplasm with a propensity for the development of a superimposed malignant germ cell tumor. On the other hand, gonadoblastoma displays a number of features which suggest that it may represent a malformation developing in an abnormal gonad and therefore qualifies as a hamartoma. These features include the following:

1. The gonadoblastoma is frequently small, sometimes a few millimeters in diameter and has a striking resemblence to 'ring tubules' thought to be malformed seminiferous tubules present in cryptorchid testes [51].

2. Microscopically, the gonadoblastoma is composed of several different cell types arranged in an organized fashion more suggestive of a hamartoma than the haphazard cellular arrangement of a tumor.

3. Leydig cells are preent in gonadoblastoma but they become evident only when the child reaches puberty in the same manner that Leydig cells appear in the normal testis.

4. Although Sertoli cells in addition to germ cells are an integral part of

the gonadoblastoma, only the germ cells have the capacity for metastasis. Such selective metastatic behavior would be unusual for a neoplasm.

5. When it can be positively identified, the underlying gonadal tissue is almost always a testis and patients almost invariably have a Y chromosome although there have been rare reports of gonadoblastoma in women with XX karyotypes and normal ovaries [103]. Thus, rather than being an *in situ* malignancy, the gonadoblastoma may be a malformation arising in a 'cryptorchid testis'. Such gonads have a high likelihood of malignant transformation as evidenced by the increased incidence of malignant germ cell tumors arising in intra-abdominal testes of both normal males and individuals with testicular feminization. In both groups of these patients as in that group with gonadoblastoma, the malignant germ cell tumor is almost always a seminoma (dysgerminoma).

*3.1.2. Clinical features.* Patients with gonadoblastomas range in age from 1 to 40 years and typically have some type of congenitally abnormal gonad associated with sexual maldevelopment. The gonadal abnormality is characterized by either bilateral streak gonads or a unilateral streak and a contralateral testis. Patients with the former condition fall into the category of either pure gonadal dysgenesis or Turner's syndrome whereas those with the latter are considered to have mixed gonadal dysgenesis. Those with pure gonadal dysgenesis have a 46XX karyotype and are sexually immature but grow to a normal height while patients with Turner's syndrome have a 46XO karyotype, are also sexually immature but are less than 5 feet in height and have one or more congenital anomalies, i.e., webbed neck, shield-shaped chest, coarctation of the aorta, etc. Patients with mixed gonadal dysgenesis generally have a 45X/46XY karyotype and are phenotypic females with varying degrees of masculinization. The development of a gonadoblastoma in individuals with maldeveloped gonads has been shown to depend on the presence of a Y chromosome. Thus, although 80% of patients with gonadoblastoma are phenotypic females, 90% have a Y chromosome [102]. An abnormal ring type of Y chromosome has also been reported [104]. Reports of gonadoblastoma occurring in normal women with 46XX karyotype [103, 105, 106] who have become pregnant and had normal offspring are rare as are gonadoblastomas occurring in true hermaphrodites [107, 108]. Some of these patients may be hidden mosaics and in some patients the gonadoblastoma may have arisen as a hamartomatous malformation in a polyovular follicle [101].

*3.1.3. Gross features.* Gonadoblastomas vary from a few millimeters in diameter to a large solid mass, which may be soft, firm, or gritty, depending on the degree of calcification and the extent of the germinomatous component. Dystrophic calcification is common and may be recognized in abdominal roentgenograms prior to surgery.

*3.1.4. Microscopic features.* Gonadoblastoma is composed of a mixture of germ cells resembling primordial germ cells or dysgerminoma cells in association with cells that have the same ultrastructure as luteinized ovarian stromal cells or testicular Leydig cells, but do not contain crystals of Reinke. In two-thirds of tumors, cells identical to luteinized stromal cells are present [102]. The cells are probably Sertoli cells that surround the germs cells and tend to be oriented around spaces, creating a microfollicular pattern (Figure 18). In some neoplasms these structures are aligned along the periphery of solid nests of germ cells and some may surround individual germ cells. Approximately half of gonadoblastomas are overgrown by germinoma. Rarely, they are associated with endodermal sinus tumor, embryonal carcinoma or choriocarcinoma [109].

*3.1.5. Behavior and treatment.* Gonadoblastomas can synthesize both androgens and estrogens [110]. Steroid production appears to be independent of the presence of Leydig cells or luteinized stromal cells since in some

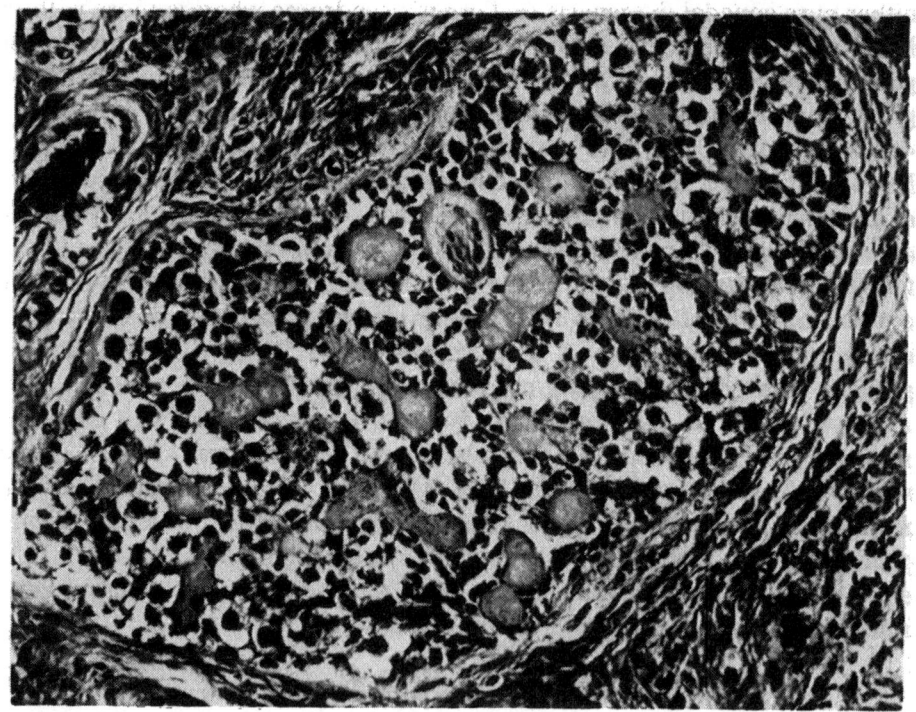

*Figure 18.* Gonadoblastoma. Germ cells and Sertoli-like cells surround round hyaline bodies creating a microfollicular pattern. (Courtesy of Dr. Henry J. Norris, AFIP, Washington, D.C.)

instances the tumor may elaborate androgens in the absence of these cells when examined by light microscopy [15]. Any patient with gonadal dysgenesis and a Y chromosome runs a high risk of developing a germ cell tumor, particularly gonadoblastoma. In Scully's review [102], at least 90% of gonadoblastomas arose in these patients.

A review of several studies shows that the median incidence of malignant germ cell tumors in patients with gonadal dysgenesis and a Y chromosome is 25% [108].

Total abdominal hysterectomy and bilateral salpingo oophorectomy is indicated in patients with gonadoblastoma because most tumors arise in patients with gonadal dysgenesis and the contralateral ovary is usually abnormal. The gonadoblastoma tends to be overgrown by malignant elements and a third of tumors are bilateral though frequently evident only on microscopic examination.

Thorough sampling of all these tumors is important. Pure gonadoblastoma does not metastasize but half contain germinoma. Surprisingly, metastases from germinoma arising in gonadoblastoma are uncommon even when the tumor is large and bilateral. In contrast, other combinations consisting of endodermal sinus tumor, embryonal carcinoma, or choriocarcinoma have been fatal within $1\frac{1}{2}$ years [109]. Further treatment is therefore determined by the histologic nature of the other malignant germ cell elements.

### 3.2. Mixed germ cell–sex cord stromal tumor

Talerman [99, 100, 111] has described a tumor containing a mixture of germ cells and gonadal stromal cells that is distinct from gonadoblastoma. In contrast to gonadoblastoma, mixed germ cell stromal tumors have a trabecular or a tubular pattern rather than a circumferential nesting arrangement. These tumors arise in normal gonads, and are not associated with other malignant germ cell neoplasms. They are extremely rare, and only a handful of cases have been reported. They have ocurred in both normal phenotypic males and females.

#### 3.2.1. Clinical features. 
The patients have been children who have been presented with an abdominal tumor. One child had precocious puberty. The patients have otherwise been phenotypically normal with no abnormalities of the external or internal genitalia.

#### 3.2.2. Gross features. 
The tumors have been large ranging from 7 to 18 cm and have had no distinctive appearance.

#### 3.2.3. Microscopic features. 
The tumor has two histologic patterns which may merge. In one a trabecular pattern is present composed of long ramify-

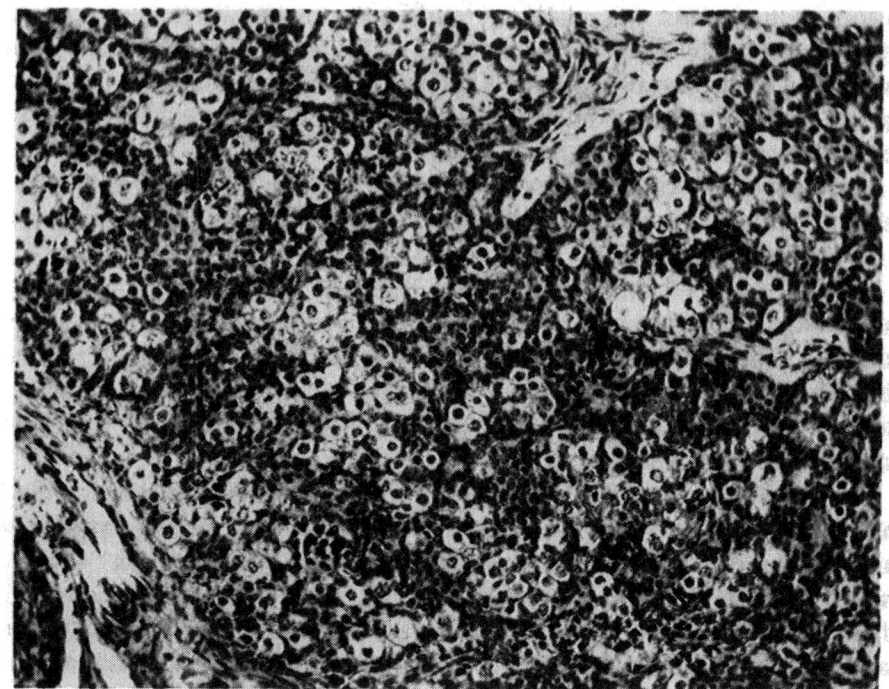

*Figure 19.* Mixed germ cell-stromal tumor. Germ cells are admixed with uncommitted gonadal stromal cells.

ing columns of stromal cells (granulosa or Sertoli cells) containing variable numbers of larger round cells having the appearance of primitive germ cells. The other pattern is tubular in which there is no lumen. The tubules are composed of sex cord stromal and admixed germ cells (Figure 19). Leydig cells may be present but eosinophilic hyaline bodies and the calcification as found in gonadoblastoma are absent.

*3.2.4. Behavior and treatment.* The tumor has always been confined to one ovary and has behaved in a benign fashion. Biopsies of the contralateral ovary have contained normal ovarian tissue. The neoplasm has never been observed in an extragonadal site, nor have chromosomal abnormalities been identified. In view of its unilaterality and benign behavior, conservative treatment consisting of unilateral salpingo oophorectomy is the treatment of choice.

4. MANAGEMENT USING TUMOR MARKERS

There has been dramatic improvement during the past few years in the results of therapy for germ cell tumors. These results can be attributed mainly to the use of effective combination chemotherapy, but tumor markers have played an important role in this achievement. By providing functional correlates of the traditional morphologic classification of germ cell tumors, the immunohistochemical data have provided a classification that accurately reflects the natural history, prognosis and response of these tumors to therapy [12] (Table 11).

Although a number of oncofetal and placental proteins have been identified in germ cell tumors, systematic correlation of serologic marker levels and histopathologic localization in tissue sections has been performed only with AFP and hCG [12, 112-118] (see also Chapter 2, Sections 3 and 4).

These studies have shown that the serum levels of AFP and hCG are an accurate reflection of the histologic composition of the tumor. The present management of germ cell tumors is therefore based on the measurement of both these markers in the serum using radioimmunoassay techniques and in

Table 11. Histogenetic and immunohistologic classification of germ cell tumors.

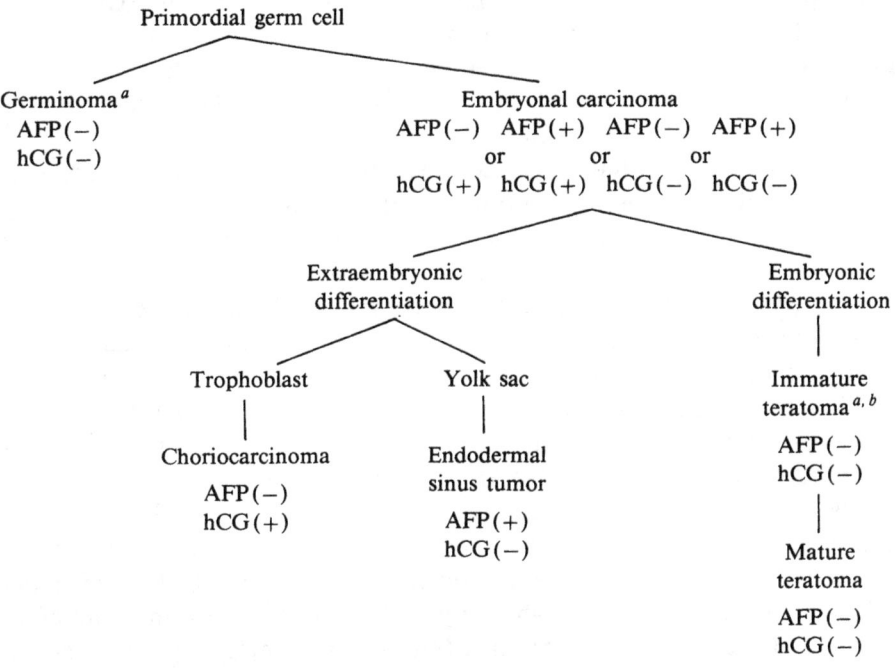

[a] Syncytiotrophoblastic giant cells may occasionally be associated with these neoplasms in which case hCG will be present.
[b] AFP is occasionally localized within this tumor and may be associated with elevated serum levels.

tissue sections using immunocytochemical methods, usually immunoperoxidase. Approximately 65% of all ovarian germ cell tumors excluding dysgerminomas, gonadoblastomas and teratomas can be expected to have an associated elevation of serum levels of either one or both markers (Table 11).

Elevation of either AFP or hCG levels in the serum of a child or young woman with an adnexal mass strongly suggests the presence of a malignant germ cell tumor. Normal serum levels, however, do not exclude a germ cell tumor since dysgerminoma and immature teratoma are generally not associated with the production of AFP or hCG. In contrast, endodermal sinus tumor is invariably associated with high circulating levels of AFP and choriocarcinoma with high levels of hCG. Embryonal carcinoma may be associated with elevated levels of both markers, AFP alone, hCG alone or may have no marker elevation, depending on the degree and direction of differentiation along yolk sac (AFP production) or trophoblastic (hCG production) pathways (see histogenesis of embryonal carcinoma) (Table 11). The pattern of tumor marker production by mixed germ cell tumors containing two or more pure cell types depends on the various histologic components that comprise the tumor. Thus, a mixed germ cell tumor composed exclusively of dysgerminoma and teratoma would not be expected to show a serum elevation of either marker, whereas a mixed germ cell tumor composed of dysgerminoma, endodermal sinus tumor and choriocarcinoma is likely to have elevations of both AFP and hCG levels.

Although valuable in diagnosis, the most effective use of these markers is in monitoring the response of the tumor to therapy and in detection of early recurrence at a time when the tumor burden is small (markers often become detectable months before other clinical signs) and can be most effectively eradicated by chemotherapy. Several groups of investigators have confirmed that the activity of disease can be accurately monitored after initial therapy with the use of serial determinations of serum AFP and hCG values [112–118]. Marker levels should be determined before and after each therapeutic intervention, and at 1 to 3 month intervals while the patient remains at high risk of recurrence (usually 2 years). In monitoring serum markers it must be remembered that the time required for an elevated serum level to return to normal depends on the serum half-life of the individual marker and the actual serum marker level before treatment. The half-life of hCG is 18 hours and that of AFP is 3–5 days. High preoperative levels of AFP may therefore take several weeks to return to normal. In following tumor response, a single elevated postoperative level is of little value. Serial determinations must be performed and can themselves be used to calculate the acutal rate of decline compared with the expected regression rate. It has been shown that persistent tumor can be identified if the rate of fall of the marker is slower than expected [113]. If the marker levels plateau or rise, persistent or recurrent disease is invariably present. No false-positive values have been reported when reliable assays are used [118]. In contrast, negative serum tumor marker levels do not necessarily assure the absence of active disease. In addition to true remission, serum marker levels may be negative if the tumor has differentiated into mature tissue which does not produce a marker, i.e., mature teratoma or if the tumor has reverted to a completely undifferentiated state, i.e., undifferentiated embryonal carcinoma incapable of marker synthesis. The marker patterns reflect the response of heterogeneous populations of cells to chemotherapy; each marker is synthesized by a different cell type [12]. Chemotherapy may interfere with marker production without destroying the cells or may selectively destroy marker producing or nonmarker producing cells. The patterns of serum marker levels following surgery have been referred to as concordant if AFP and hCG rise and fall in a parallel fashion or discordant if they do not [119].

As a result of refinements in immunocytochemical methods and the increased use of serologic assays, greater attention is being focused on these immunologic techniques for diagnosis and management. Thus, tumor markers provide a functional tool to assess the presence and extent of these neoplasms quite distinct from the traditional anatomic studies (roentegenograms, scintigrams) used to follow the course of most tumors. A comparable situation exists in the management of patients with gestational trophoblastic disease where it has been shown that the serum level of hCG and its regression pattern in response to chemotherapy is even more important in management than the histologic grading system [120-123]. Currently, AFP and hCG are the primary tumor markers in the diagnosis and management of germ cell tumors. As greater clinical experience is gained with other markers such as pregnancy-specific beta globulin, human placental lactogen, alpha-1 antitrypsin, CEA and ferritin, tumors may be further classified by qualitative and quantitative patterns of a panel of multiple tumor markers. In the future, the pathologist may report that a tumor displays a particular pattern of tumor markers determined by immunocytochemistry and thereby indicate to the clinician which markers may be useful to monitor the effect of therapy. This information may complement the morphologic diagnosis and prove to be more relevant to the management of the patient.

REFERENCES

1. Abell MR, Johnson VJ, Holtz F: Ovarian neoplasms in childhood and adolescence I. — Tumors of germ cell origin. Am J Obstet Gynecol 92:1059, 1965.
2. Norris HJ, Jensen RD: Relative frequency of ovarian neoplasms in children and adolescents. Cancer 30:713, 1972.
3. Ashley DJB: Origin of teratomas. Cancer 32:390, 1973.

4. Witschi E: Migration of the germ cell of human embryos from the yolk sac to the primitive gonadal folds. Contrib Embryol Carnegie Instit 32:67, 1948.
5. Friedman NB: The comparative morphogenesis of extragenital and gonadal teratoid tumors. Cancer 4:265, 1951.
6. Asadourian LA, Taylor HB: Dysgerminoma. An analysis of 105 cases. Obstet Gynecol 33:370, 1969.
7. Serov SF, Scully RE, Sobin LH: International histological classification of tumours, No. 9. Histological typing of ovarian tumours. Geneva: WHO, 1973.
8. Cangir A, Smith J, Van Eys J: Improved prognosis in children with ovarian cancers following modified VAC (vincristine sulfate, dactinomysin and cyclophosphamide) chemotherapy. Cancer 42:1234, 1978.
9. Gallion H, van Nagell JR, Powell DF, Donaldson ES, Hanson M: Therapy of endodermal sinus tumor of the ovary. Am J Obstet Gynecol 135:447, 1979.
10. Higuchi K, Kato T: Dysgerminoma of the ovary. J Jpn Obstet Gynecol Soc 5:206, 1958.
11. Krepart G, Smith JP, Rutledge F, Delclos L: The treatment for dysgerminoma of the ovary. Cancer 41:986, 1978.
12. Kurman RJ, Scardino PT, McIntire KR, Waldmann TA, Javadpour N, Norris HJ: Malignant germ cell tumors of the ovary and testis. An immunohistologic study of 69 cases. Ann Clin Lab Sci 9:462, 1979.
13. Meyer R: The pathology of some special ovarian tumors and their relation to sex characteristics. Am J Obstet Gynecol 22:697, 1931.
14. Manuel M, Katayama KP, Jones HW Jr: The age of occurrence of gonadal tumors in intersex patients with a Y chromosome. Am J Obstet Gynecol 124:293, 1976.
15. Hou-Jensen K, Kempson RL: The ultrastructure of gonadoblastoma and dysgerminoma. Human Pathol 5:79, 1974.
16. Day S, Silverberg SG, Schatski PF: Ultrastructure of an ovarian dysgerminoma. Report of a case featuring neurosecretory-type granules in stromal cells. Am J Clin Pathol 58:458, 1972.
17. Ueda G, Hamanaka N, Hayadawa K, Tanizawa O, Ichii H, Nakagawa H, Mineda H, Furuyama J, Matsumoto K, Mori M: Clinical, histochemical and biochemical studies of an ovarian dysgerminoma with trophoblasts and Leydig cells. Am J Obstet Gynecol 114:748, 1972.
18. Freel JH, Cassir JF, Pierce VK, Woodruff J, Lewis JL: Dysgerminoma of the ovary. Cancer 43:798, 1979.
19. Kurman RJ, Norris HJ: Malignant germ cell tumors of the ovary. Human Path 8:551-564, 1977.
20. Burkons DM, Hart WR: Ovarian germinomas (dysgerminomas). Obstet Gynecol 51:221, 1978.
21. Cohen SM, Goldsmith MA: Prolonged chemotherapeutic remission of metastatic ovarian dysgerminoma. Report of a case. Gynecol Oncol 5:299, 1977.
22. Creasman WT, Fetter BF, Hammond CB, Parker RT: Germ cell malignancies of the ovary. Obstet Gynecol 53:226, 1979.
23. Teilum G: Endodermal sinus tumors of the ovary and testis. Comparative morphogenesis of the so-called mesonephroma ovarii (Schiller) and extraembryonic (yolk sac-allantoic) structures of the rat's placenta. Cancer 12:1092, 1959.
24. Scully RE, Barlow JF: 'Mesonephroma' of the ovary. Tumor of mullerian nature related to the endometrioid carcinoma. Cancer 20:1405, 1967.
25. Kurman RJ, Norris HJ: Endodermal sinus tumor of the ovary. A clinical and pathologic analysis of 71 cases. Cancer 38:2420, 1976.

26. Teilum G: The concept of endodermal sinus (yolk sac) tumor. Scand J Immunol 8:(Supp 8) 75, 1978.
27. Nogales FF, Matilla A, Nogales-Ortiz F, Galera-Davidson HL: Yolk sac tumors with pure and mixed polyvesicular vitelline patterns. Human Path 9:553–566, 1978.
28. Ito T, Shirai T, Naka A, Matsumoto S: Yolk sac tumor and alphafetoprotein. Clinicopathological study of four cases. Gann 65:215, 1974.
29. Palmer PE, Safaii H, Wolfe HJ: Alphal-antitrypsin and alphafetoprotein. Protein markers in endodermal sinus (yolk sac) tumors. Am J Clin Pathol 65:575, 1976.
30. Schabel FM Jr: Concepts for treatment of micrometastasis. Cancer 35:15–24, 1975.
31. DeVita VT: Cell kinetics and the chemotherapy of cancer. Cancer Chemother Rep 2:23–33, 1971.
32. Slayton RE, Hreshchyshyn MD, Silverberg SG, Shingleton HM, Park RC, DiSaia PJ, Blessing JA: Treatment of malignant ovarian germ cell tumors. Cancer 42:390, 1978.
33. Smith JP, Rutledge F, Sutow WW: Malignant gynecologic tumors in children. Current approaches to treatment. Am J Obstet Gynecol 166:261, 1973.
34. Einhorn LH, Donohue J: Cis-diaminodichloroplatinum, vinblastine and bleomycin combination chemotherapy in disseminated testicular cancer. Ann Int Med 87:293, 1977.
35. Julian CG, Barnett JM, Richardson RL, Greco FA: Bleomycin, vinblastine and Cis-platinum in the treatment of advanced endodermal sinus tumor. Obstet Gynecol 56:396, 1980.
36. Lockey JL, Baker JJ, Price NA, Winokur SH: Cis-platinum, vinblastine and bleomycin for endodermal sinus tumor of the ovary. Ann Int Med 94:56, 1981.
37. Jacobs AJ, Harris M, Deppe G, DasGupta I, Cohen CJ: Treatment of recurrent and resistant germ cell tumors with Cis-platinum, vinblastine and bleomycin. Obstet Gynecol 59:129–132, 1982.
38. Forney JP: Pregnancy following removal and chemotherapy of endodermal sinus tumor. Obstet Gynecol 52:360–362, 1978.
39. Nogales FF, Favara BE, Major FJ, Silverberg SG: Immature teratoma of the ovary with a neural component ('solid teratoma'). Hum Pathol 7:625, 1976.
40. Norris HJ, Zirkin HJ, Benson WL: Immature (malignant) teratoma of the ovary. A clinical and pathologic study of 58 cases. Cancer 37:2359, 1976.
41. Robboy SJ, Scully RE: Ovarian teratoma with glial implants on the peritoneum. An analysis of 12 cases. Hum Pathol 1:643, 1970.
42. DiSaia PJ, Saltz A, Kagan AR, Morrow CP: Chemotherapeutic retroconversion of immature teratoma of the ovary. Obstet Gynecol 49:346, 1977.
43. Piver MS, Sinks L, Barlow JJ, Tsukada Y: Five year remissions of metastatic solid teratoma of the ovary. Cancer 38:987, 1976.
44. Caruso PA, Marsh MR, Minkowitz S, et al.: An intense clinico pathologic study of 305 teratomas of the ovary. Cancer 27:343, 1971.
45. Matz MH: Benign cystic teratomas of the ovary. Obstet Gynecol Surv 16:591, 1961.
46. Pantojo E, Noy MA, Axtmayer RW, et al.: Ovarian dermoids and their complications. Comprehensive historical review. Obstet Gynecol Surv 30:1, 1975.
47. Lindner D, McCan BK, Hecht F: Parthenogenic origin of teratomas. N Engl J Med 292:63, 1975.
48. Ober WB: Solid ovarian teratoma with struma ovarii theca lutein reaction and endometrial hyperplasis. J Obstet Gynaecol Br Commonw 67:451, 1960.
49. Robboy SJ, Scully RE, Norris HJ: Carcinoid metastatic to the ovary-clinocopathologic analysis of 35 cases. Cancer 33:798, 1974.
50. Blackwell WJ, Dockerty MB, Masson JC, Mussey RD: Dermoid cysts of the ovary; clinical and pathological significance. Am J Obstet Gynecol 51:151, 1976.

51. Fox H, Langley FA: Tumors of the Ovary. London: W. Heinemann Medical Books, 1976.
52. Oi RH, Dubbs M: Lactating breast tissue in benign cystic teratoma. Am J Obstet Gynecol 130:729, 1978.
53. McKeel DW, Askin FB: Ectopic hypophyseal hormonal cells in benign cystic teratoma of the ovary. Arch Pathol Lab Med 102:122, 1978.
54. Woodruff JD: Cited by Jones HJ in Obstet Gynecol Surv 26:547, 1971.
55. Kelley RR, Scully RE: Cancer developing in dermoid cysts of the ovary. Cancer 14:989, 1961.
56. Peterson WF: Malignant degeneration of benign cystic teratomas of the ovary: a collective review of the literature. Obstet Gynecol Surv 12:793, 1957.
57. Climie ARW, Heath LP: Malignant degeneration of benign cystic teratomas of the ovary. Cancer 22:824, 1968.
58. Herman WJ Jr, Humes JJ: A compound nevus in a benign cystic teratoma of the ovary. Am J Clin Pathol 66:54, 1976.
59. Leo S, Rorat E, Parekh M: Primary malignant melanoma in a dermoid cyst of the ovary. Obstet Gynecol 41:205, 1973.
60. Hameed K, Burslem MRG: A melanotic ovarian neoplasm resembling the retinal 'anlage tumor'. Cancer 25:564, 1970.
61. Czernobilsky B, Rotenstreich L, Lancet M: Ovarian dermoid with squamous carcinoma – pseudosarcoma. Arch Pathol 93:141, 1972.
62. Bortolozzi G: Lo struma ovarico. Ann Obstet Gynec 89:310, 1967.
63. Emge LA: Functional and growth characteristics of struma ovarii. Am J Obstet Gynecol 40:738, 1940.
64. Yannopoulos D, Yannopoulos K, Ossowski R: Malignant struma ovarii. Pathol Annu 11:403, 1976.
65. Scully RE: Recent progress in ovarian cancer. Hum Pathol 1:73, 1970.
66. Robboy SJ, Norris HJ, Scully RE: Insular carcinoid primary in the ovary. A clinicopathologic analysis of 48 cases. Cancer 36:404, 1975.
67. Robboy SJ, Scully RE, Norris HJ: Primary trabecular carcinoid of the ovary. Obstet Gynecol 49:202, 1977.
68. Ranchod M, Kempson RL, Dorgeloh JR: Strumal carcinoid of the ovary. Cancer 37:1913, 1976.
69. Serratani FT, Robboy SJ: Ultrastructure of primary and metastatic carcinoids: Analysis of 11 cases. Cancer 36:157, 1975.
70. Dikman SH, Toker C: Strumal carcinoid of the ovary with masculinization. Cancer 27:925, 1971.
71. Gonzalez-Licea A, Hartmann WH, Yardley JH: Medullary carcinoma of the thyroid. Ultrastructural evidence of its origin from the parafollicular cell and its possible relationship to carcinoid tumors. Am J Clin Path 49:512, 1968.
72. Robboy SJ, Scully RE: Strumal carcinoid tumor of the ovary. An analysis of 50 cases of a distinctive tumor composed of thyroid tissue and carcinoid. Cancer 46:2019, 1980.
73. Greco MA, LiVolsi VA, Pertschuk LP, Bigelow B: Strumal carcinoid of the ovary. An analysis of its components. Cancer 43:1389, 1979.
74. Straus AF, Gates HS: Giant sebaceous gland tumor of the ovary. Am J Clin Path 41:78, 1964.
75. Nogales FF, Silverberg SG: Epidermoid cysts of the ovary: A report of five cases with histogenetic considerations and ultrastructural findings. Am J Obstet Gynecol 124:523, 1976.
76. Clement PB, Dimmick JE: Endodermal variant of mature cystic teratoma. Cancer 43:383, 1979.

77. Kurman RJ, Norris HJ: Embryonal carcinoma of the ovary. A clinicopathologic entity distinct from endodermal sinus tumor resembling embryonal carcinoma of the adult testis. Cancer 38:2420, 1976.
78. Pierce GB, Dixon FJ: Testicular teratomas. I. Demonstration of teratogenesis by metamorphosis of multipotential cells. Cancer 12:573, 1959.
79. Pierce GJ Jr: Ultrastructure of human testicular tumors. Cancer 19:1963, 1966.
80. Pierce GB Jr, Stevens LC, Nakane PK: Ultrastructural analysis of the early development of teratocarcinomas. J Natl Cancer Inst 39:755, 1967.
81. Stevens LC, Hummel KP: A description of spontaneous congenital testicular teratomas in strain 129 mice. J Natl Cancer Inst 18:719, 1957.
82. Stevens LC Jr: The biology of teratomas including evidence indicating their origin from primordial germ cells. Ann Biol 11:585, 1962.
83. Stevens LC: Experimental production of testicular teratomas in mice. Proc Natl Acad Sci USA 5:661, 1964.
84. Gitlin D, Petricelli A: Synthesis of serum albumin, prealbumin, alphafeto-protein, alpha-1-antitrypsin and transferrin by the human yolk sac. Nature 228:995, 1970.
85. Gitlin D: Normal biology of alphafeto-protein. Ann NY Acad Sci 259:7, 1975.
86. Waldman TA, McIntyre KR: The use of radioimmunoassay for alphafeto-protein in the diagnosis of malignancy. Cancer 34:1510, 1974.
87. Grigor KM, Detre SI, Kohn J, Neville AM: Serum alphafeto-protein levels in 153 male patients with germ cell tumors. Brit J Cancer 35:52, 1977.
88. Kohn J, Orr AH, Mcelwain TJ, Bentall M, Peckham MJ: Serum alphafeto-protein in patients with testicular tumors. Lancet 2:433, 1976.
89. Beilby JOW, Horne CHW, Milne GD, Parkinson C: Alphafeto-protein, alpha-1 antitrypsin and transferrin in gonadal yolk-sac tumors. J Clin Pathol 32:455, 1979.
90. Jacobsen GK, Jacobsen M, Clausen PP: Distribution of tumor associated antigens in the various histologic components of germ cell tumors of the testis. Am J Surg Path 5:257, 1981.
91. Neville AM, Grigor K, Heyderman E: Clinicopathologic role of tumor index substances in paediatric neoplasia. In: Recent Advances in Histopathology, Anthony PP, Woolf N (eds). Edinburgh, London, New York: Churchill Livingstone, 1978, pp 13–44.
92. Parkinson C, Beilby JOW: Features of prognostic significance in testicular germ cell tumors. J Clin Pathol 30:113, 1977.
93. Talerman A: The incidence of yolk sac (endodermal sinus tumor) elements in germ cell tumors of the testis in adults. Cancer 36:211, 1975.
94. Gerbie MV, Brewer JI, Tamini H: Primary choriocarcinoma of the ovary. Obstet Gynecol 46:720, 1975.
95. Kurman RJ, Norris HJ: Malignant mixed germ cell tumors of the ovary. A clinical and pathological analysis of 30 cases. Obstet Gynecol 48:579, 1976.
96. Peyron A: Faits nouveaux relatifs à l'origine et à l'histogenèse, 1939.
97. Marin-Padilla M: Origin, nature and significance of the 'embryoids' of human teratomas. Virchows Arch (Pathol Anat) 340:105, 1965.
98. Stevens LC Jr: Embryonic potency of embryoid bodies derived from a transplantable testicular teratoma of the mouse. Dev Biol 2:285, 1960.
99. Talerman A: A distinctive gonadal neoplasm related to gonadoblastoma. Cancer 30:1219, 1972.
100. Talerman A: A mixed germ cell–sex cord stroma tumor of the ovary in a normal female infant. Obstet Gynecol 40:473, 1972.
101. Hughesdon PE, Kumarasamy T: Mixed germ cell tumors (gonadoblastomas) in normal and dysgenetic gonads. Virchows Arch (Pathol Anat) 349:258, 1970.
102. Scully RE: Gonadoblastoma, a review of 74 cases. Cancer 25:1340, 1970.

103. Bergher de Bacalao E, Dominguez I: Unilateral gonadoblastoma in a pregnant woman. Am J Obstet Gynecol 105:1279, 1969.
104. Khudr G, Benirschke K: Y ring chromosome associated with gonadoblastoma *in situ*. Obstet Gynecol 41:879, 1973.
105. McDonough PG, Rogers Byrd J, Freedman MA: Gonadal dysgenesis with ovarian function. Clinical and cytogenetic findings in six patients. Obstet Gynecol 37:868, 1971.
106. Salet J, de Gennes JL, de Grouchy J, Musset R, Pelissier I, Yaneva H, Sebaoun M, Netter A: A propos d'un cas de gonadoblastome 46XX. Ann Endocrinol 31:927, 1970.
107. McDonough PG, Rogers Byrd J, Tho, PT, Otken L: Gonadoblastoma in a true hermaphrodite with a 46XX karyotype. Obstet Gynecol 47:355, 1976.
108. Schellhas HF: Malignant potential of the dysgenetic gonad – I. Obstet Gynecol 44:302, 1974.
109. Talerman A: Gonadoblastoma associated with embryonal carcinoma. Obstet Gynecol 43:138, 1974.
110. McDonough PG, Ellegood JO, Byrd JR, Mahesh VB: Ovarian and peripheral venous steroids in XY gonadal dysgenesis and gonadoblastoma. Obstet Gynecol 47:351, 1976.
111. Talerman A, Van der Harten JJ: A mixed germ cell–sex cord stroma tumor of the ovary associated with isosexual precocious puberty in a normal girl. Cancer 40:889, 1977.
112. Perlin E, Engeler JE Jr, Edson M, *et al.*: The value of serial measurement of both human chorionic gonadotropin and alphafeto-protein for monitoring germinal cell tumors. Cancer 37:215, 1976.
113. Thompson DK, Haddow JE: Serial monitoring of serum alphafeto-protein and chorionic gonadotropin in males with germ cell tumors. Cancer 43:1820, 1979.
114. Javadpour N, McIntire KR, Waldmann TA, Bergman S, Anderson T: The role of the radioimmunoassay of serum alphafeto-protein and human chorionic gonadotropin in the intensive chemotherapy and surgery of metastatic testicular tumors. J Urol 119:759, 1978.
115. Scardino PT, Skinner DG: Germ-cell tumors of the testis: Improved results in a prospective study using combined modality therapy and biochemical tumor markers. Surgery 86:86, 1979.
116. Sell A, Sogaard H, Norgard-Pederson B: Serum alphafeto-protein as a marker for the effect of post-operative radiation and/or chemotherapy in eight cases of ovarian endodermal sinus tumor. Int J Cancer 18:574, 1976.
117. Skinner DG, Scardino PT: Relevance of biochemical tumor markers and lymphadenectomy in management of non-seminamatous testis tumors. Current perspective. J Urol 123:378, 1980.
118. Scardino PT, Cox HD, Waldmann TA, *et al.*: The value of serum tumor markers in the staging and prognosis of germ cell tumors of the testis. J Urol 118:994, 1977.
119. Braunstein GD, McIntire KR, Waldmann TA: Discordance of human chorionic gonadotropin and alphafeto-protein in testicular teratocarcinomas. Cancer 31:1065, 1973.
120. Elston CW, Bagshawe KD: The value of histological grading in the management of hydatidiform mole. J Obstet Gynecol Br Cmwlth 79:717, 1972.
121. Bagshawe KD: Risk and prognostic factors in trophoblastic neoplasia. Cancer 38:1373, 1976.
122. Curry SL, Hammond CB, Tyrey L, Creasman WT, Parker RT: Hydatidiform mole. Diagnosis, management and long-term follow-up of 347 patients. Obstet Gynecol 45:1, 1975.
123. Morrow CP, Kletzky OA, DiSaia PJ, Townsend DE, Mishell DR, Nakamura RM: Clinical and laboratory correlates of molar pregnancy and trophoblastic disease. Am J Obstet Gynecol 128:424, 1977.
124. Alfridi MA, Vontagma V, Tsukada Y, Piver MS: Dysgerminoma of the ovary: Radiation therapy for recurrence and metastases. Am J Obstet Gynecol 126:190, 1976.

125. Jimerson GK, Woodruff JD: Ovarian extraembryonic teratoma I. Endodermal sinus tumor. Am J Obstet Gynecol 127:73, 1977.
126. Smith JP: The treatment of embryonal carcinoma of the ovary. In: Diagnosis and Treatment of Ovarian Neoplastic Alterations. H Dewatteville (ed) American Elsevier Publishing Co., New York, 1975, pp 214–216.
127. Curry SL, Smith JP, Gallagher HS: Malignant teratoma of the ovary: prognostic factors and treatment. Am J Obstet Gynecol 131:845, 1978.
128. Malkasian GD, Webb MJ, Jorgensen EO: Observations on chemotherapy of granulosa cell carcinomas and malignant ovarian teratomas. Obstet Gynecol 44:885, 1974.
129. Boyes DA, Pankratz E, Galliford BW, White GW, Fairey RN: Experience with dysgerminomas at the Cancer Control Agency of British Columbia. Gynecol Oncol 6:123, 1978

# 5. Treatment of Advanced Trophoblastic Disease

RICHARD H.J. BEGENT and KENNETH D. BAGSHAWE

## 1. INTRODUCTION

Knowledge of the diverse behaviour of trophoblastic tumours has increased greatly over the 25 years since the introduction of methotrexate [1] and methods of treatment have developed accordingly. The best possible management of the individual patient now involves complex considerations leading to treatment chosen according to the particular characteristics of the patient and her tumour. This has been achieved by sustained work in a limited number of specialized centres but in spite of the advances some of these young women still die. Many of the deaths can be attributed to inappropriate treatment started in centres lacking experience in this group of diseases. There remains a strong case for the continued referral of patients to units where experience has accumulated and where old lessons do not have to be re-learned.

For the present purpose we have chosen to define advanced trophoblastic disease as those invasive moles and choriocarcinomas which require cytotoxic chemotherapy. Since this definition includes patients with localized lesions which respond readily to treatment, as well as advanced metastatic disease, our justification for this rests on the more or less continuous nature of the clinical spectrum, presented by trophoblastic tumours. We exclude from the definition hydatidiform mole.

There is usually little difficulty in distinguishing invasive mole from choriocarcinoma by histological examination of the excised uterus but the distinction may not be possible clinically and hysterectomy may be both disadvantageous and unnecessary. Moreover, within the generality of early post-mole tumours is a small minority which do not respond fully to treatment which eradicates the majority and it is necessary to identify this important, potentially resistant minority at the earliest possible stage.

*Griffiths, C. T. and Fuller, A. F. (eds.), Gynecologic Oncology.*
© *1983, Martinus Nijhoff Publishers, Boston. ISBN 0-89838-555-5.*
*Printed in The Netherlands.*

## 2. INDICATIONS FOR TREATMENT WITH CYTOTOXIC DRUGS

One of the curious facets of gestational trophoblastic tumours is their genetic derivation. They arise from complete moles which are now known to be 'androgenic' in that the complete nuclear genetic content is of male parent origin although they are usually female (46XX) in constitution [2]. They may arise also from partial moles which are usually triploid and they may arise from apparently normal conceptions, 46XX or 46XY. Choriocarcinomas arising from these diverse sources appear to behave similarly although further study may reveal differences.

Trophoblastic activity or persistence is most reliably monitored by HCG values in serum or urine. The main problem in deciding whether or not to treat a patient with evidence of trophoblastic activity which is not associated with a normally progressing pregnancy, arises from differences in the natural history of the trophoblast or hydatidiform mole and non-mole pregnancy. After a term pregnancy, trophoblastic activity generally becomes undetectable within 3-4 weeks of delivery and HCG production, if not normal by this time has to be assumed to be due to choriocarcinoma until proved otherwise. After first trimester non-mole abortion trophoblastic activity may be detectable for somewhat longer but rarely more than 7 weeks post-evacuation and similar considerations to those after term pregnancy generally apply.

However, 'trophoblastic pseudotumours' first described by Kurman *et al.* [3] have added somewhat to the complexity of the scene. They have been described as an exaggerated placental site reaction, a histological picture which has previously been described by some authors as 'syncytial endometritis'. This is important since these lesions are essentially cytotrophoblastic and indeed distinguished by their lack of syncytial formation. Cytotrophoblastic tumours would perhaps be a more appropriate description and they seem to occur predominantly though not exclusively after non-mole pregnancies. These lesions seem not to metastasize readily but the spectrum of behaviour is wide and deep pelvic invasion has occurred in one patient in our series after hysterectomy. Others have proved resistant to chemotherapy. We have also seen one case associated with nephrotic syndrome and know of another similar case where the nephrotic syndrome responded only to hysterectomy.

After a partial mole or a complete mole is evacuated, HCG levels sometimes fall as quickly as after normal pregnancy but in many patients the process may be slow and it may take six months or more before HCG becomes undetectable by sensitive radioimmunoassay. During this time it is clear that trophoblast persists either in the uterus or elsewhere. If hysterectomy is performed invasive mole is usually found but this is scant justification for the operation unless the patient has completed childbearing. There is strong evidence that most invasive moles die out spontaneously but because they may cause uterine or intraperitoneal haemorrhage and may prove difficult to distinguish from choriocarcinoma a proportion of them require treatment with drugs. Only about 3% of moles give rise to choriocarcinoma but the percentage of mole patients treated with cytotoxic drugs ranges from about 6% to 25% or more. These differences arise from different policies and in comparing the results of different methods of treatment this must be borne in mind. Whereas for the patient with choriocarcinoma cytotoxic drugs are potentially life saving, for invasive mole they are, for the most part, preserving fertility.

In the USA it has been common policy to treat 20% or more of mole patients with cytotoxics on the basis of any level of HCG activity detectable 6 weeks' post evacuation [4, 5]. In addition at least one group gives chemotherapy before evacuating the mole on the basis of an assessment of the probability that the mole is aggressive. The rationale for these policies is the proposition that early treatment is more likely to be effective than late treatment. In Europe, on the other hand, the overriding consideration has been the wish to avoid using potentially mutagenic cytotoxic drugs in women of childbearing age except where absolutely necessary and on this basis 10% or less are treated with drugs.

At Charing Cross Hospital approximately 400 patients are registered each year for supervision of their follow-up and the following indications for treatment after hydatidiform mole are applied:

1. Histological evidence of choriocarcinoma or evidence of a trophoblastic tumour after non-mole pregnancy.
2. Opacities on chest radiograph or CT scan with constant or increasing HCG values; if HCG values are falling the patient remains under observation.
3. Persistent uterine or vaginal haemorrhage necessitating repeated transfusion.
4. Metastases at any site other than vagina or lung.
5. Very high HCG values (e.g. > 20,000 IU/L) persisting 4 weeks' post evacuation and after careful curettage. (These patients have a high risk of uterine perforation by invasive mole or less commonly by choriocarcinoma.)
6. HCG values progressively increasing for more than 4 weeks at any time after evacuation of mole.
7. Any level of HCG activity persisting 4-6 months after evacuation of mole.

## 3. PREVENTIVE MEASURES

It is proper to consider whether advanced trophoblastic disease can be prevented. The incidence of mole increases to high levels in mothers over 45 years of age but although much has been learned in recent years about the genetics of hydatidiform mole we are unable to prevent moles or to prevent choriocarcinoma after term pregnancy. Nevertheless the high proportion of trophoblastic tumours that follow hydatidiform mole has imposed the obligation to see how problems might best be reduced. We have already referred to the different solutions proposed in different centres. Some others have taken the view that 'prophylactic therapy' meaning cytotoxic therapy before or soon after the evacuation of mole is likely to be highly effective. An absence of proof that prophylactic therapy eliminates the need for later chemotherapy has however tended to reinforce the case for selection.

In the UK gynaecologists register patients with hydatidiform mole at one of three centres from which a systematic monitoring of human chorionic gonadotrophin (HCG) is undertaken on specimens posted by the patient to the laboratory. This has nearly eliminated follow-up failures and has facilitated the selection of patients for treatment at a stage when eradication can be confidently anticipated. A further benefit of such a registration scheme has been the ability to collect data which could not be obtained at a single centre.

### 3.1. Method of evacuation of the uterus

Analysis of the patients registered at Charing Cross Hospital [6] showed that vacuum extraction, curettage and spontaneous evacuation carried the smallest risk of sequelae requiring chemotherapy, whereas medical induction with oxytocin or prostaglandins, hysterotomy and hysterectomy carried a 2 to 3-fold greater risk. Vacuum extraction appeared to be the safest technique with respect to late sequelae and may have the added advantage that a large hydatidiform mole can usually be evacuated with little blood loss [7]. The greater risk of sequelae associated with uterine evacuation induced by oxytocin or prostaglandins may be attributed to deportation of trophoblast induced by uterine contractions. For the same reason the administration of these drugs during evacuation is not recommended. However, the use of ergometrine to control bleeding after evacuation of mole is sometimes unavoidable.

Hysterotomy seems to incur surprisingly increased risks of malignant sequelae and hysterectomy for mole *in situ* or soon after evacuation of mole by other means, is no guarantee that all trophoblastic elements have been removed. One such patient in our series had a hysterectomy for a mole at the age of 17, only to present at 34 with advanced choriocarcinoma. If hysterectomy is indicated for a woman who has completed her childbearing, it may be better deferred until the mole has fully regressed, or if performed while still active, follow-up by sensitive assay remains essential and pregnancy test follow-up is inadequate.

The available data relating to methods of evacuation are unfortunately limited in value by the absence of information on pre-evacuation uterine size. It is possible that large moles are associated with a poor prognosis and that uterine size influenced the choice of method of evacuation in favour of hysterectomy or hysterotomy. Nevertheless vacuum extraction appears to be the method of choice in many circumstances.

*3.2. Oestrogens and progestogens*

The first suggestion that oestrogens and progestogens might adversely affect the prognosis of gestational trophoblastic tumours came in the 1960s [8]. Patients who took oral contraceptives immediately after completing treatment for choriocarcinoma appeared to have a higher relapse rate. At about the same time attempts to use oestrogen or progestogen to stimulate trophoblastic mitosis and render the cells more amenable to cytotoxic kill sometimes seemed to achieve the former effect but not the latter. Further, as might have been expected, an increasing proportion of patients with post-mole trophoblastic neoplasia reported taking oral contraceptives soon after evacuation of mole. Since 1972 all patients followed up after mole evacuation were asked to record whether or not they were taking oral contraceptives and the first 600 cases have been analyzed [9]. This showed that patients taking oral contraceptives between the time of evacuation and the first normal urinary HCG value had approximately twice the risk of requiring treatment as those who did not. Oral contraceptives taken after normal gonadotrophin values were obtained had no discernible effects. The relationship of oral contraception to causation has also been raised by Baltazar [10]. The dangers of oral contraceptives have recently been challenged [11] but the data from London and Boston are not comparable [12]. Ideally, a prospective randomized controlled clinical trial is required to resolve this question but the emotional, ethical and organizational problems which it would present have so far inhibited such a course.

4. CLINICAL FEATURES

*4.1. Invasive mole*

Since choriocarcinoma has been demonstrated to arise in only about 3% of mole patients in properly documented series and since in our centre we treat up to 10% of mole patients with drugs we must conclude that 7 out of 10 of our treated patients have invasive mole. In a series treating 20% of mole patients we must assume that 17 out of 20 have invasive mole and thus comparisons between series may be invalid.

It is worth emphasizing the temporal relationship between hydatidiform mole, invasive mole and choriocarcinoma with a generalization. Most trophoblastic lesions in the early months after evacuation are invasive moles but a trophoblastic tumour present six or more months after evacuation of a mole is most likely a choriocarcinoma.

Curettage sometimes helps to distinguish invasive mole from choriocarcinoma but it cannot be relied upon to do so. The finding of villi, whether macroscopic or microscopic, confirms that the lesion is invasive mole but finding trophoblast without villi is not proof that it is choriocarcinoma. The indications for treatment (see above) are designed to avoid the necessity for making the distinction at the clinical level.

The careful use of frequent HCG assays and the indications for treatment outlined above, help to anticipate the problems which in earlier times resulted from invasive mole so that hysterectomy or ligation of vaginal metastases are now rarely needed. Symptoms may still occur in the form of persistent slight blood loss or pain from theca lutein cysts but the majority of patients undergoing treatment for persisting trophoblastic lesions after hydatidiform mole have few symptoms. If theca lutein cysts cause pain and anxiety at a time when HCG levels are falling aspiration of the cyst fluid is probably the only surgical procedure required.

*4.2. Choriocarcinoma*

*Choriocarcinoma* is much more diverse than invasive mole in its clinical features and time of presentation. Patients may be seen in the early weeks after the antecedent pregnancy or symptoms may be delayed for months or even years. The longest interval in our series was 17 years after hysterectomy for hydatidiform mole but several other patients had latent periods of 10 years or more.

While gynaecological manifestations, usually uterine bleeding, are the most common forms of presentation, non-gynaecological manifestations of choriocarcinoma may produce the presenting features in as many as a third of the patients [13]. The most common forms of presentation are pulmonary metastases producing haemoptysis, dyspnoea, pleuritic pain or coughing. Pulmonary hypertension may be produced by growth of choriocarcinoma within the pulmonary artery.

Metastases in the central nervous system (Figure 1) are associated with surrounding oedema and may produce focal neurological signs. Intracerebral or subarachnoid haemorrhage may be the presenting event and chorio-

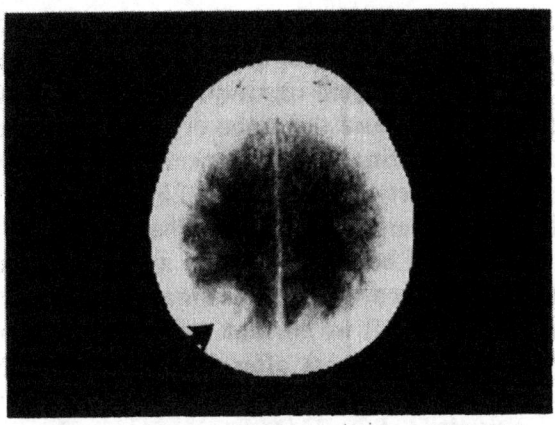

*Figure 1.* Computerized axial tomography (CT) of the brain of a patient with drug-resistant choriocarcinoma. A deposit is seen in the occipital lobe (arrowed).

carcinoma should always be remembered as a possible cause in women who have had a pregnancy. The spinal cord and cauda equina may rarely be the site of metastases.

The small or large bowel may be involved and severe gastrointestinal bleeding may occur in either case. Deposits in the liver, spleen and kidneys may produce intraperitoneal haemorrhage but lymph node and bone involvement are very rare. Deposits in the skin are also unusual as presenting features and are more often seen in patients with late drug-resistant disease.

## 5. DIAGNOSTIC METHODS

### 5.1. Biochemical markers

Normal trophoblast is remarkable for its repertoire of synthesizing activity which includes a range of steroid hormones and glycoproteins and for the way in which this repertoire changes during the normal gestational period. In the context of malignant trophoblast these are important because of the utility in monitoring the course of the disease. It is interesting that substances most useful for malignant trophoblast are the products most evident during early placental development, when trophoblastic invasion is active. In essence, human chorionic gonadotrophin (HCG) remains the principal marker although placental glycoprotein ($SP_1$) may give additional information in a small minority of cases [14].

*5.1.1. Human chorionic gonadotrophin.* In the presence of clinically evident disease, pregnancy tests are generally positive. They are not necessarily unreliable but a negative result does not exclude a trophoblastic tumour. Whenever this diagnosis is suspected, quantitative measurement by a sensitive radioimmunoassay or enzyme immunoassay is essential. Although trophoblastic tumours may produce the alpha or beta sub-unit of HCG there is little to be gained by measuring these independently of intact HCG. Only a few antisera discriminate between HCG and LH and assays are now usually performed with antisera raised against the beta sub-unit of HCG. Such assays provide an index of both intact HCG and its free beta sub-unit.

A good assay will indicate a value of less than 2 milli International Units per ml (5 mIU/ml ≃ 1.0 ng/ml) in normal serum. Assays on urine are still useful in the follow-up of patients after hydatidiform mole although the 'background noise' on urine assays tends to be higher than on serum so that values up to the equivalent of 30 IU/24 hours may not be significant. (Urine estimations should be based on timed collections; the preferred preservative for immunoassay is merthiolate ≡ THIOMERSAL 100 mg per 24-hour collection.) These sensitive assays can be performed using 2–3-hour incubation times although for most purposes an overnight incubation giving a result within 24 hours of the specimen being received in the laboratory is satisfactory. Using double antibody or solid phase particulate methods these assays have been automated and performed on a large scale [15, 16]. The use of RIA with extracted urine provides a very sensitive method for the detection of HCG but is laborious and difficult to justify as a routine procedure at present.

*5.1.2. Interpretation of HCG values.* Any excess of HCG not accounted for by pregnancy or recent uterine evacuation is likely to be due to tumour activity, either in a gestational trophoblastic neoplasm, a malignant teratoma or other malignancy. In many thousands of samples analyzed in our laboratory only one exception to this has been found; this young woman with elevated levels of HCG, $SP_1$ and alpha foeto-protein has not been found to have tumour in ovaries or uterus but the possibility of a teratoma elsewhere cannot be excluded nor has it become apparent during more than 4 years' observation.

Malignant teratomas, usually in the ovary or the mid-line, commonly produce HCG though the site of origin, histology and common finding of AFP production usually allow discrimination from gestational trophoblastic tumours. HCG production can be ectopic, that is by non-trophoblastic tumour. It has been reported that about 12–14% of tumours of various histological type produce detectable serum levels of HCG, but in our experience and that of others the figure is lower and only occasional tumours are associated with serum concentrations > 100 IU/L. Nevertheless HCG production cannot be equated with trophoblastic tumours exclusively.

In general, in a young woman with a recent pregnancy, the presence of HCG in the body fluids is strongly suggestive of a trophoblastic tumour when a new pregnancy has been excluded.

The broad quantitative relationship between HCG concentration in excretion rate and viable tumour mass is of course of particular value in monitoring the course of the disease (Figures 7-11). Rises and falls in these values provide a much more sensitive guide to the course of the disease than changes in radiographs and other physical diagnostic methods since the former relate to viable cell mass.

Allowance must be made however for the half-life of HCG, of the order of 30-48 hours, so that clearance takes a finite time. Cessation of HCG production is not accompanied by an instantaneous fall in serum and urine values. Also, it has to be recognized that the use of cytotoxic agents is often associated with an initial increase in serum and urine values for HCG and a significant fall may not be evident for 2 weeks after the start of an effective cytotoxic regimen.

Immunofluorescent and peroxidase methods for localizing HCG in sections of trophoblastic tumours suggest that synthesis is more active in the syncytium than in cytotrophoblast. Although the production of HCG by different tumours proceeds at different rates we have no evidence that gestational choriocarcinomas ever fail to synthesize HCG and failure to find HCG in the presence of clinically detectable masses results either from incorrect histological diagnosis or inadequate methodology for HCG assay.

*5.1.3. Frequency of estimation.* In patients undergoing treatment twice weekly assays probably provide all the information that is required. After completion of treatment assays should be performed every 1-2 weeks for 3 months and then progressively less frequently, until after 3 years 6 monthly assays are adequate. Relapses have occurred up to 8 years after terminating treatment.

*5.1.4. Brain metastases.* Although computerized axial tomography has made a substantial advance in the localization of brain metastases and should eventually become a routine investigation for patients with choriocarcinoma (see below), the most sensitive method for the detection of brain metastases remains a disturbance in the ratio of HCG in serum and spinal fluid (CSF). The CSF concentration is normally less than 1:60 of that in serum [17]. However, where serum concentrations are falling rapidly, slow equilibrium between CSF and serum may produce temporary disturbance. The CSF/serum ratio is sometimes normal when a small trophoblastic embolus or growth has produced either a cerebral haemorrhage or a cerebral infarction.

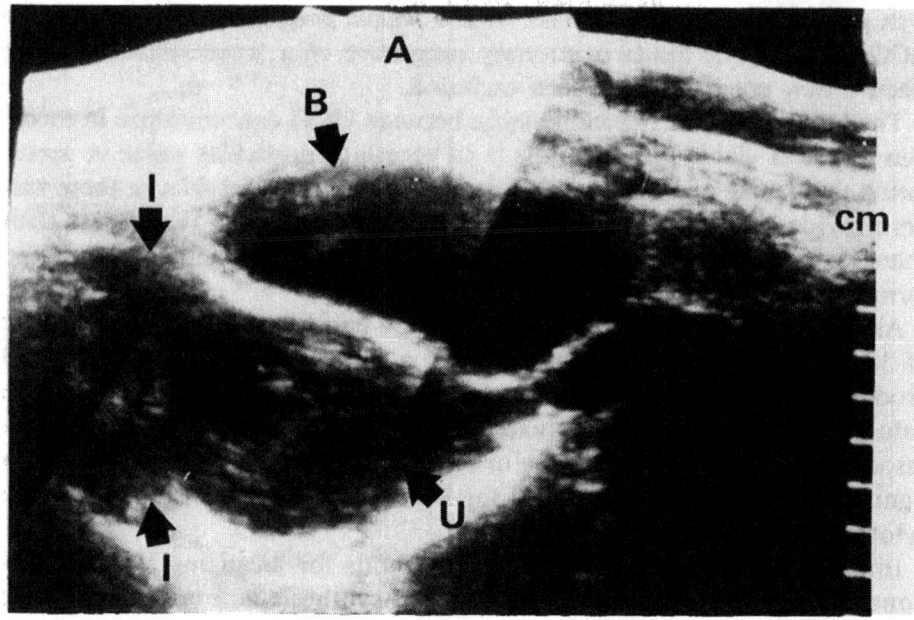

*Figure 2.* Ultrasound image of the pelvis in a patient with invasive mole. Transverse section showing anterior abdominal wall (A), bladder (B), uterus (U) and infiltration of mole into the parametrium (I).

## 5.2. Ultrasound

Grey scale ultrasound has proved the best method of discrimination between hydatidiform mole and normal pregnancy and is of use not only in the initial diagnosis of hydatidiform mole but also before the institution of chemotherapy in making sure that the rising HCG is the result of a trophoblastic tumour rather than a normal pregnancy. In some patients with invasive mole it is capable of demonstrating infiltration through the uterine wall (Figure 2) and of discriminating between this and corpus lutein cyst of the ovary (Figure 3). Ultrasound has been used to monitor the progress of the disease [18] but it is undoubtedly less sensitive than monitoring HCG, even where disease is confined to the uterus, and it should not be used as a substitute.

## 5.3. Pelvic arteriography

This investigation has taught us much about the vascular structure of trophoblastic tumours. The vascular connections of vaginal metastases were previously unsuspected and the extraordinary dilatation of ovarian arteries and veins, long reported by surgeons and sometimes resulting in surgical disasters, was revealed to all by this technique. It is probably no longer necessary to perform this investigation as a routine and it is important to

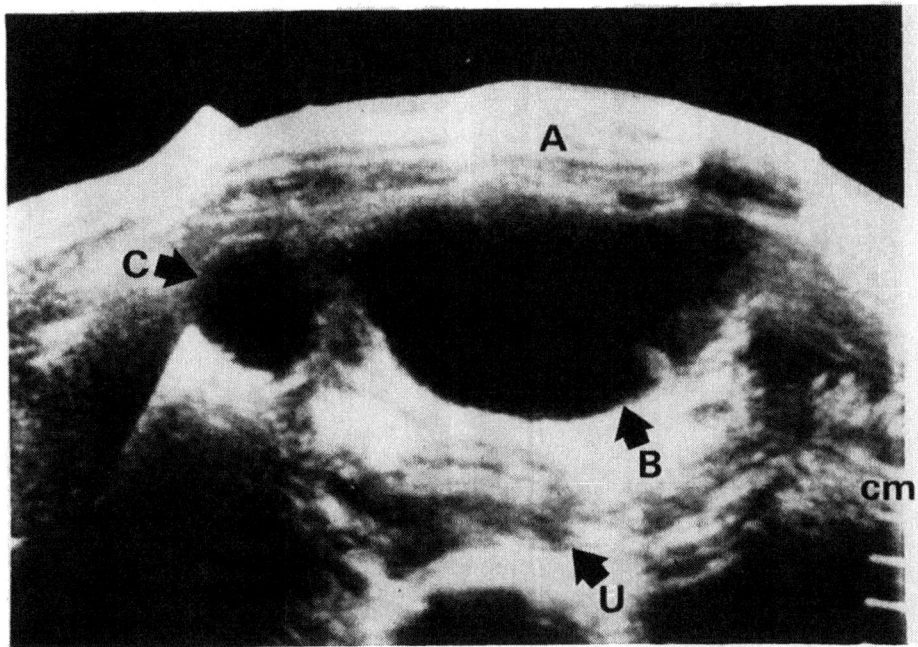

*Figure 3.* Ultrasound of the pelvis in a patient with persistently raised concentrations of HCG 4 months after evacuation of a hydatidiform mole. Transverse section showing anterior abdominal wall (A), bladder (B), uterus (U) and an ovarian cyst (C).

note that the atypical circulation sometimes persists after eradication of the tumour. Nevertheless where hysterectomy is contemplated arteriography is worthwhile, since an extensive extrauterine circulation should be a deterent unless hysterectomy is being undertaken as a last resort in drug-resistant disease.

### 5.4. Radiography of the lungs

Chest radiography is an essential investigation in all patients, some deposits only being seen on a lateral film. Pulmonary metastases may be discrete and multiple (Figure 4), solitary (Figure 5) or of miliary pattern. Opacities are sometimes present when HCG has returned to normal but when excised these have usually proved to contain only necrotic tissue. If not removed, these opacities slowly become smaller and usually disappear after months or occasionally 1-2 years. Whole lung tomography is of some value when trying to determine whether pulmonary metastases are resectable but has now been surpassed in sensitivity by computerized tomography (Figure 4).

When considering the cardiorespiratory system it is important to look for evidence of pulmonary hypertension induced by growth of choriocarcinoma in the pulmonary artery and also to perform electrocardiography for evi-

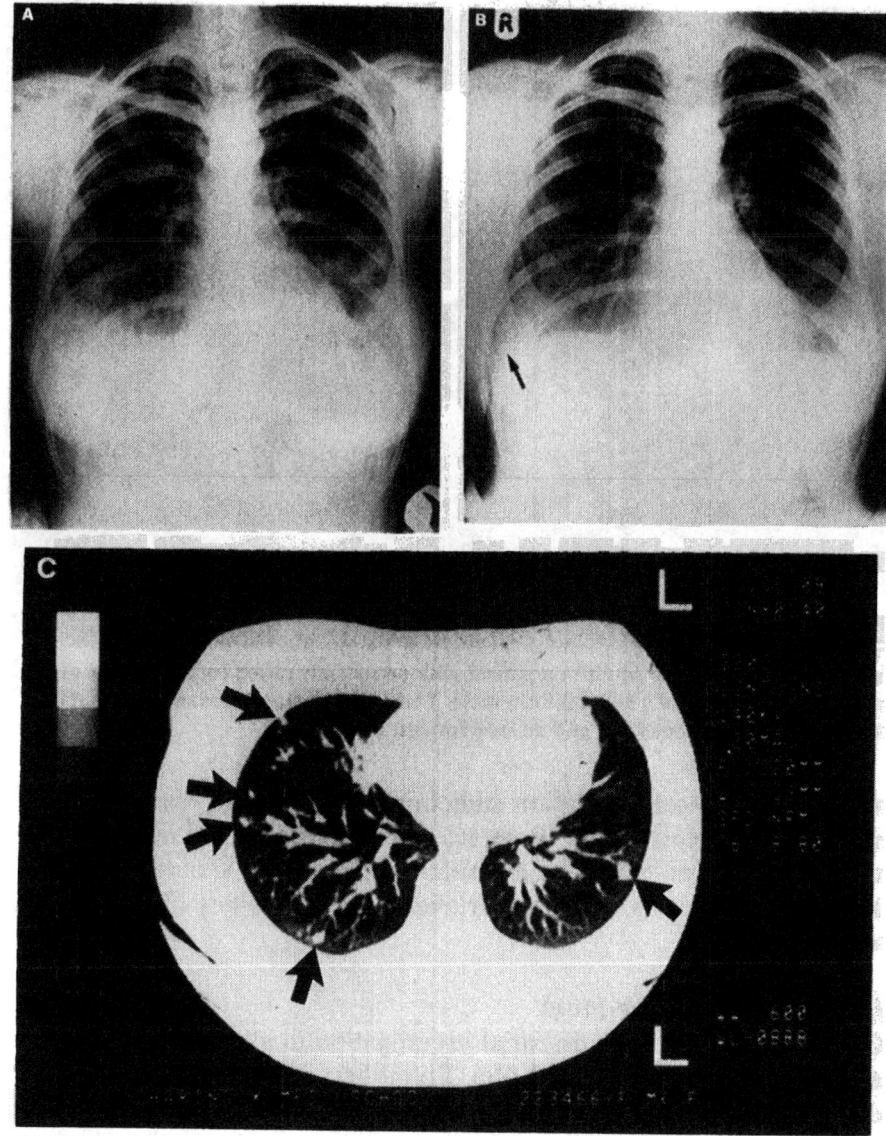

*Figure 4.* (A) Posteroanterior radiograph of the chest in a patient with choriocarcinoma showing multiple small metastases. (B) After chemotherapy for 4 months only one deposit is clearly identified (arrowed). CT at this time (C) showed that multiple lung deposits were still present (arrowed).

dence of right ventricular hypertrophy or strain induced by the same pathology.

## 5.5. *Investigation of the central nervous system*

Measurement of the ratio of HCG in CSF, to that in serum (see above)

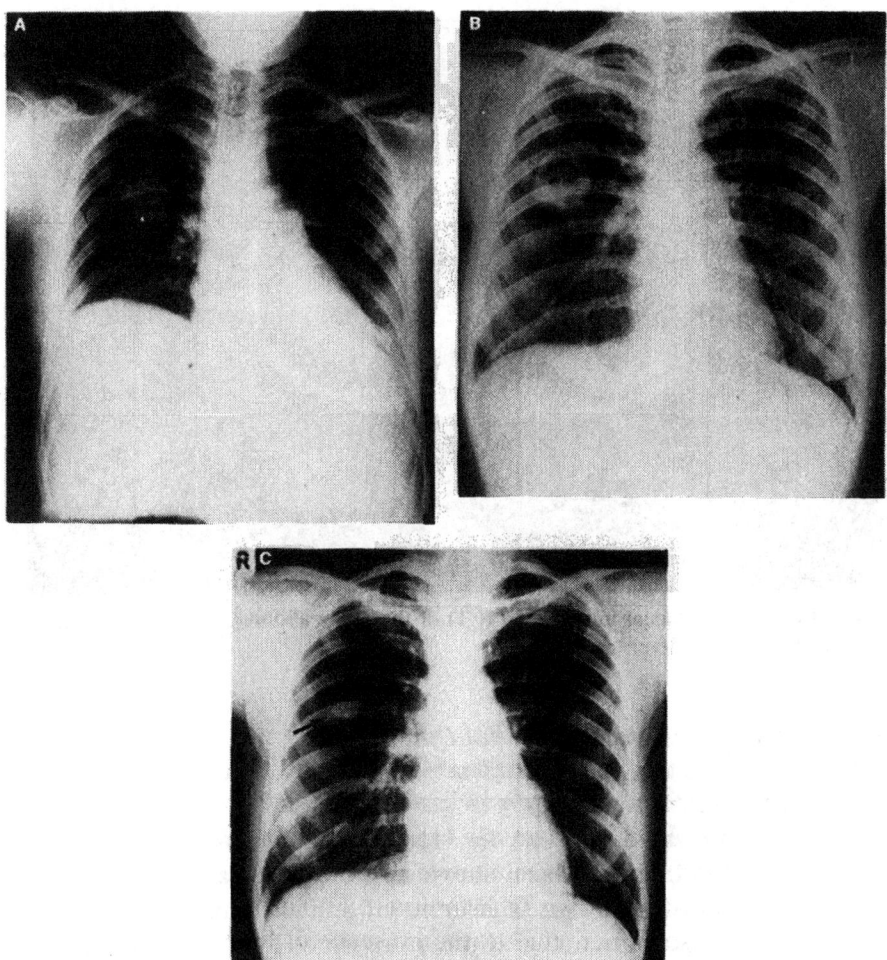

*Figure 5.* Plain radiographs of the chest of patient with choriocarcinoma. (A) A solitary metastasis present before treatment. (B) Cavitation occurring in association with a response to treatment after 5 weeks. (C) A residual opacity after 18 weeks chemotherapy. This was subsequently excised and found to contain only necrotic tissue.

has proved adequate as a screening test in those patients where there is no particular reason to suspect brain metastases. If there is reason for doubt, computerized tomography of the brain should also be performed (Figure 1). The method is clearly superior to isotope scans which may be useful if CT is not available. In some patients with involvement of the spinal cord or cauda equina, myelography is capable of demonstrating the lesions but the need for urgent therapy may be an overriding consideration where clinical signs are clear.

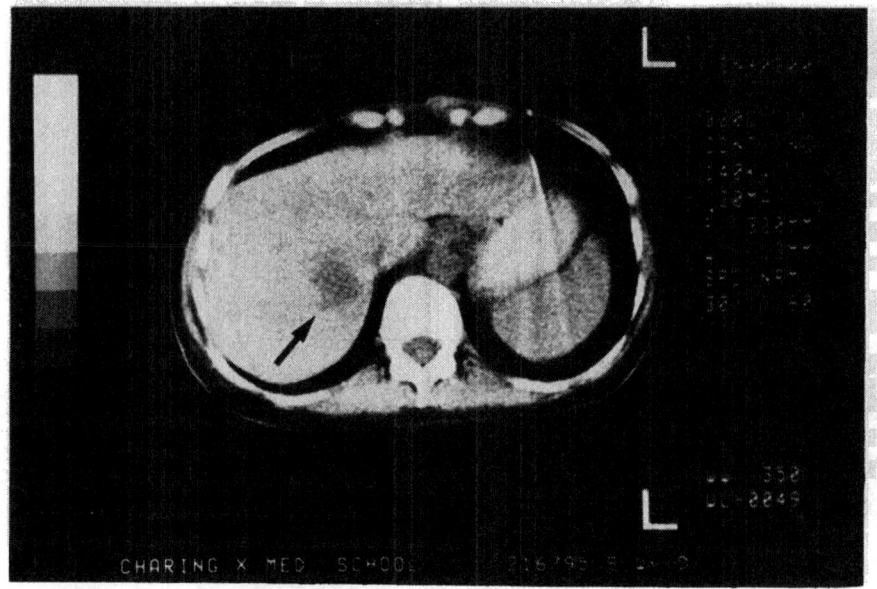

*Figure 6.* Computerized axial tomography (CT) of the upper abdomen showing a metastasis of choriocarcinoma in the liver (arrowed).

## 5.6. *Investigation of gastrointestinal tract*

Liver metastases may be demonstrable by colloid isotope liver scan, ultrasound, computerized tomography (Figure 6) or selective arteriography. The choice of method will depend on the expertise within a particular institution and no one method has yet been shown to be superior although arteriography may be the most sensitive. Measurement of plasma bilirubin and hepatic enzymes may also give a clue to the presence of liver deposits but elevation of these parameters may also be caused by nonspecific factors such as hepatitis. One patient in our series who had antibodies to hepatitis B antigen became positive for hepatitis B antigen after chemotherapy and developed fulminating hepatitis. It is therefore wise to look for the presence of both hepatitis B antigen and antibody before starting treatment.

## 5.7. *Other biochemical investigations*

The toxicity of those cytotoxic drugs excreted by the kidney will be greatly magnified in the presence of impairment of glomerular filtration rate and both plasma urea and creatinine clearance or other measurement of glomerular filtration rate must be determined before starting treatment. Choriocarcinoma may be present with features of thyrotoxicosis apparently caused by the similarity of the alpha sub-unit of HCG and that of thyroid stimulating hormone [19]. Whilst this syndrome usually resolves with chemotherapy of the trophoblastic tumour, it is helpful to define this problem by measurement of T3 and T4 before treatment.

*5.8. Radioimmunolocalization (see Chapter 2, Section 3)*

In this method radiolabelled antibodies directed against HCG are injected intravenously. They become specifically concentrated in HCG-producing tumours which can then be localized by external scintigraphy. The method requires elaborate purification of antibody and the use of a subtraction technique in order to allow for the substantial fraction of radiolabelled antibody which persists in the normal tissues and circulation. Nevertheless deposits of choriocarcinoma have been localized in this way with a sensitivity comparable to that of CT scanning. The method has the theoretical advantages that a deposit at any previously unknown site in the body may be identified and that viable tumour may be discriminated from deposits of necrotic tissue [20, 21]. Subsequently antibodies directed against HCG have been shown to be retained specifically in xenografts of human choriocarcinoma in nude mice [22].

It is likely that the method of RIL will improve during the next few years as a result of the use of antibodies labelled with isotopes more suitable for imaging with current gamma cameras, by use of 3-dimensional imaging methods, by improved methods of removal of background radioactivity and possibly by use of monoclonal antibodies.

## 6. RISK AND PROGNOSIS

Prognosis of malignant tumours is usually determined by the natural history of a particular histological type and by the stage of disease. Given that it is usually desirable for a patient to retain her uterus, histology at the time treatment is indicated is often not available. In patients with progressing trophoblastic tumours the early occurrence of haematogenous spread and rapid rate of growth of choriocarcinoma means that disease progression to death is usually only a matter of weeks unless therapy is successful. Early micrometastatic spread casts surgery in the adjuvant role and chemotherapy is the principle method of treatment.

A number of factors have been shown to affect the risk of a tumour becoming drug-resistant. These appears to operate additionally to each other. Analysis of the 317 patients treated at Charing Cross Hospital up to 1973 has identified these factors and given an indication of the weight to be attached to each [23]. An analysis confined to patients with metastases was also performed by Hammond *et al.* [24].

The interval between the end of the antecedent pregnancy and the start of chemotherapy was one of the two most powerful effects. This was not simply a measure of tumour burden although that also proved to be a powerful effect as judged by HCG values at the start of treatment. The combined effect of tumour age and HCG values were illustrated by zero fatality rate in 72 patients whose initial HCG excretion rates were below 10,000 IU/day when treated within 7 months of the antecedant pregnancy, whereas the fatality rate was 50% in 84 patients where the interval was greater than 7 months and HCG excretion rate greater than 100,000 IU/day. Metastases in the brain, gastrointestinal tract, liver or kidneys were unfavourable as were very large metastases at any site or very numerous metastases of moderate size.

The patient's blood group was found to have an effect in that patients in group B and AB had the worst survival rate whereas those with group B or AB consorts had a better prognosis. Parity appeared to have a complex effect with survival rates falling as parity increased up to four but it improved with those with more than four pregnancies. Survival was also somewhat improved in the younger age group but this effect was not statistically significant. Term antecedent pregnancies were less favourable than abortion or mole and as might be expected previous chemotherapy had an adverse effect. Lymphocytic infiltration of the tumour [25] was associated with a relatively good prognosis but this was only applicable where suitable material was available for histological examination. Immunological unreactivity as judged by tests of humoral and cell mediated immunity carried an adverse effect.

On the basis of these factors it was possible to construct a basis for a more precise staging system than is currently available for other cancers. The system has been described as 'prognostic scoring'.

*6.1. Prognostic score*

On the basis of the magnitude of the various factors discussed in the previous section a scoring system was devised (Table 1). A group (low score) could be defined with 100% survival and at the other extreme a group with no survivors. The system has now been in use for six years and patients are ascribed to a low, medium or high risk group, according to their cumulative score. Various attempts have been made to simplify the system and it has proved acceptable to omit data for lymphocytic infiltration and immune status, patients being accorded a score of 10 for each of these factors and the same numerical limits for each risk group being retained. Other attempts at simplification have so far proved less successful in predicting the patients who show drug-resistance or relapse after treatment.

Table 1

| Risk factors | Score | | | |
|---|---|---|---|---|
| | 0 | 10 | 20 | 40 |
| Age | <39 | >39 | | |
| Parity | 1, 2, 4 | 3 or 4 | | |
| Antecedent pregnancy (AP) | Mole | Abortion | Term | |
| Interval (AP-chemotherapy) in months | <4 | 4 to 7 | 7 to 12 | >12 |
| HCG (plasma IU/L or urine IU/day) | $10^3$–$10^4$ | <$10^3$ | $10^4$–$10^5$ | >$10^5$ |
| ABO ♀ × ♂ | A×A ×B ×AB | O×O A×O | B× AB× | |
| No. of metastases | Nil | 1–4 | 4–8 | >8 |
| Site of metastases | Not detected Lungs Vagina | Spleen Kidney | GI tract Liver | Brain |
| Largest tumour mass | <3 cm | 3–5 cm | >5 cm | |
| Lymphocytic infiltration | Marked | Moderate Unknown | Slight | |
| Immune status | Reactive | Unknown | Unreactive | |
| Previous chemotherapy | Nil | | Single drug | Two drugs or more |

Scores for individual risk factors are added and risk group determined by the total score as follows:
Low risk 50 or less    Medium risk 55–95    High risk >100

## 7. TREATMENT

The aim of treatment is eradication of the tumour and cytotoxic chemotherapy is the method of choice for this purpose. Having defined the relatively small group of patients who require this treatment, the success of therapy can best be determined by twice weekly measurement of HCG during treatment. In this way it is possible to follow the response of the tumour to chemotherapy and to detect drug resistance at an early stage (Figures 7–11). The number of courses of treatment is determined individually. HCG values below the limit of detection by a serum radioimmunoassay (less than 2 IU/L) mean that there are fewer than $10^4$–$10^5$ tumour cells. If treatment of choriocarcinoma is discontinued at this point relapse is likely. In some cases one can extrapolate the rate of fall of HCG down to the theoretical zero cell level to determine the minimum duration of treatment. In general the worse the prognostic factors the longer treatment needs to be continued after attaining undetectable HCG levels. Low risk cases generally need 2 or 3 courses lasting for 6 weeks, whereas patients at highest risk may need 4 months' treatment after reaching sustained normal HCG values. There is often a delay of up to 2 weeks after starting treatment before HCG values are seen to decrease. The net change in HCG values between the beginning of one course of treatment and the start of the next is a measure of response and can be given a numerical value. In the early stages of treatment HCG values should fall to less than 1/10 of their pre-treatment values with each course. A fall in HCG values to only half the pre-treatment value indicates only a poor response.

*7.1. Choice of drugs*

The activity of drugs available up to 1977 has been reviewed by Bagshawe [26]. Combination therapy with methotrexate and 6-mercaptopurine as introduced in 1958 proved unnecessarily toxic for early post-mole cases. Non-toxic regimens such as methotrexate with folinic acid can eradicate tumour in most patients treated after hydatidiform mole and some after non-molar pregnancies. Between 1962–1969 almost all patients in our series began treatment in this way and those developing resistance went on to other more toxic drug schedules. There is a theoretical risk in this approach that resistance to all the available agents will be induced without achieving the optimal anti-tumour effect. The alternative is to use intensive and often toxic combination chemotherapy from the outset in patients with a poor prognosis. The latter policy has been followed consistently since 1973, with a reduction in the number of high risk patients dying from drug resistance. While it seems likely that the use of combination therapy from the outset is preferable this has not been submitted to a prospective controlled trial.

The current policy therefore is to divide patients into three groups: low risk, scoring less than 60 (Table 1); medium risk, scoring 60–90 and high risk, 100 or above.

*7.2. Low risk patients*

The combination of intramuscular methotrexate with folinic acid shown in Table 2 is used for low risk patients. Most patients have no toxicity but oral ulceration and methotrexate-induced pleurisy [27] is seen in a small proportion. Myelosuppression is rare and alopecia does not occur. This regimen has been compared with weekly methotrexate infusions at a dose of 300 mg/m$^2$. The low dose or prolonged regimen shown in Table 2 was superior [28]. Evidence of drug resistance is seen in approximately 20% and such patients are then transferred to the medium risk regimen (Table 3)

*Table 2.* Low-risk patients

| | |
|---|---|
| Day 1 | MTX 50 mg i.m. at noon |
| Day 2 | FA 6 mg i.m. at 6.00 p.m. |
| Day 3 | MTX 50 mg i.m. at noon |
| Day 4 | FA 6 mg i.m. at 6.00 p.m. |
| Day 5 | MTX 50 mg i.m. at noon |
| Day 6 | FA 6 mg i.m. at 6.00 p.m. |
| Day 7 | MTX 50 mg i.m. at noon |
| Day 8 | FA 6 mg i.m. at 6.00 p.m. |

Courses are usually repeated after an interval of 7 days.

*Table 3.* 'Medium-risk' regimen.

**Course A**

| Day | | |
|---|---|---|
| 1. | Hydroxyurea | 500 mg p.o. 12 hourly for 2 doses |
| 2. | Methotrexate (MTX) | 50 mg i.m. at noon |
| 3. | Folinic acid (FA) | 6 mg i.m. at 6.00 p.m. |
| | 6-mercaptopurine (6-MP) | 75 mg p.o. |
| 4. | MTX | 50 mg i.m. at noon |
| 5. | FA | 6 mg i.m. at 6.00 p.m. |
| | 6-MP | 75 mg p.o. |
| 6. | MTX | 50 mg i.m. at noon |
| 7. | FA | 6 mg i.m. at 6.00 p.m. |
| | 6-MP | 75 mg p.o. |
| 8. | MTX | 50 mg i.m. at noon |
| 9. | FA | 6 mg i.m. at 6.00 p.m. |
| | 6-MP | 75 mg p.o. |

**Course B**

| | |
|---|---|
| Actinomycin-D | 0.5 mg i.v. daily for 5 days |

**Course C**

| | |
|---|---|
| Days 1 and 3 | Vincristine 0.8 mg/m$^2$ i.v. |
| Days 1 and 3 | Cyclophosphamide 400 mg/m$^2$ i.v. |

Courses are given in the sequence ABAC with intervals usually of 7 days between each course.

except that the methotrexate-containing regimen is omitted. 128 patients in this group have been treated in this way between 1973 and 1980 and there has been one death due to malignant lymphoma which was present before treatment for the trophoblastic tumour. A typical response is shown in Figure 7 with another example in a patient showing resistance to methotrexate

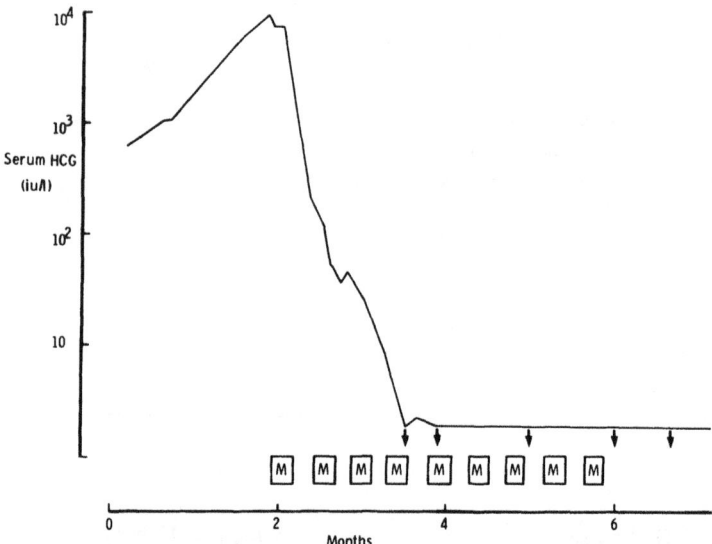

*Figure 7.* Chart of HCG values and chemotherapy in a patient after evacuation of hydatidiform mole. HCG values rose progressively so that chemotherapy was required 3 months after evacuation. The patient was in the 'low risk' group and was treated with courses of methotrexate and folinic acid (M) as shown in Table 2. In this patient treatment was continued until HCG had remained normal for 9 weeks.

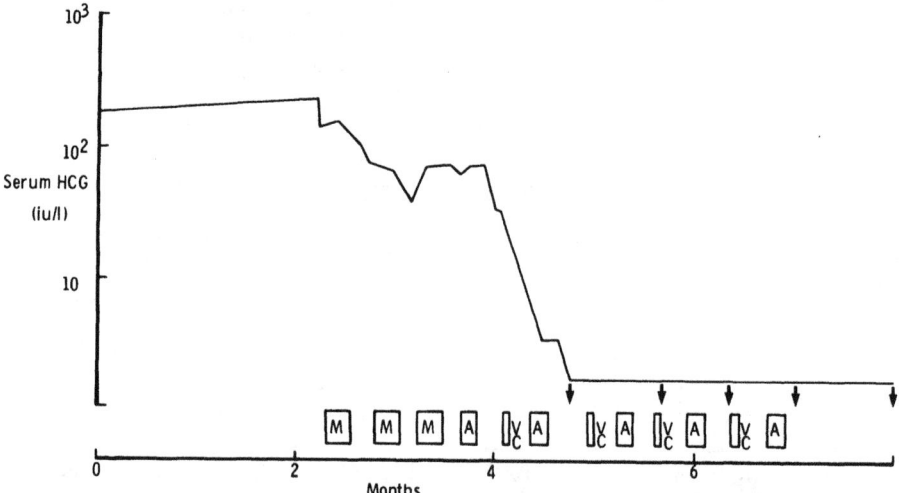

*Figure 8.* Chart showing HCG values and chemotherapy in a patient after evacuation of hydatidiform mole. HCG values were still raised six months after evacuation of a hydatidiform mole, indicating a risk of the development of choriocarcinoma. The patient fell into the low risk group and was treated initially with methotrexate and folinic acid (M) (Table 2). HCG values did not fall at a satisfactory rate, indicating drug resistance but complete remission was obtained when treatment was changed to courses of actinomycin-D (A) and vincristine (V) with cyclophosphamide (C).

but later responding to treatment with actinomycin-D, vincristine and cyclophosphamide, in Figure 8.

## 7.3. Medium risk patients

Patients in this group receive a series of regimens (Table 3), which introduce six different cytotoxic agents over a period of 6 weeks, after which the cycle is repeated. Some toxicity occurs in most patients. Alopecia is slight to moderate. Mucositis and vomiting may or may not develop and some degree of myelosuppression is common, though it is rarely necessary to extend the period between courses to more than 7 or 8 days. There have been 3 deaths all due to drug-resistance in 103 patients falling into this group between 1973 and 1980. In the early part of the study patients developing drug-resistance were transferred to the CHAMOCA regimen (Table 4) used for high risk patients but from 1977 the epipodophylotoxin derivative, VP.16-213 has been investigated in these patients and found to have activity [29]. Because of this success VP.16-213 has now been incorporated in the regimen for the medium risk patients, being given as the first treatment in a dose of 100 mg/m$^2$ as an i.v. infusion over approximately 20 minutes daily for 5 days. Vincristine and cyclophosphamide are then omitted from the treatment but methotrexate, 6-mercaptopurine and hydroxyurea and actinomycin-D are still used. An example of a patient treated this way is shown in Figure 9. The early fall of HCG induced by VP.16-213 is demonstrated.

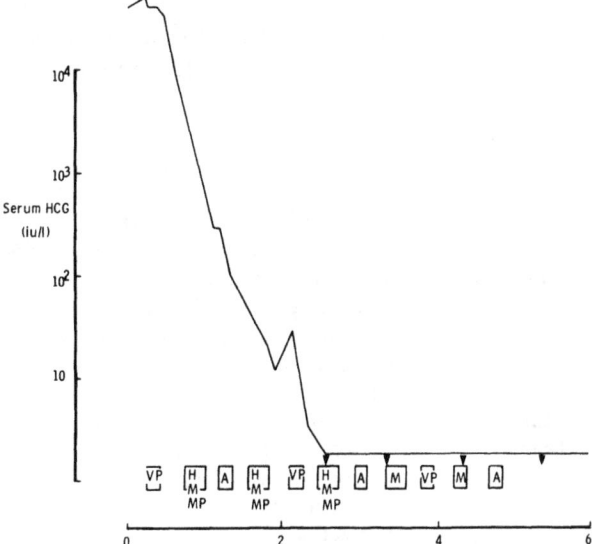

Figure 9. Chart showing HCG values and chemotherapy in a patient requiring treatment 4 months after evacuation of a hydatidiform mole. The patient fell into a 'middle risk' group and was treated successfully with courses of VP.16-213 (VP), hydroxyurea (H), methotrexate and folinic acid (M), 6-mercaptopurine (MP) and actinomycin (A).

## 7.4. High risk patients

Seventy-two of 303 patients treated at Charing Cross Hospital between 1973 and 1980 fell into this group. This exaggerates the true incidence of high risk patients in the UK since several were referred from abroad with advanced disease.

Chemotherapy has been based on the CHAMOCA regimen (Table 4). This produces alopecia in nearly all patients but mucositis and vomiting are variable and can be severe. A minimum interval of 10 days is required between courses of treatment although this is frequently more prolonged because of myelosuppression. Approximately 50% of patients attained complete remission with this regimen alone. However about 80% of patients finally achieved sustained complete remission. A number of factors in addition to the basic chemotherapy regimen must therefore be considered.

### 7.4.1. Initial extent of disease.
Metastases from choriocarcinoma may sometimes cause the patient to present with life-threatening complications such as haemorrhage from a cerebral metastasis (see below), rapidly progressive dyspnoea from extensive pulmonary deposits or tumour thrombus in pulmonary arteries. She may have a large hepatic or renal metastasis threatening intraperitoneal haemorrhage or diffuse gastrointestinal metastases causing massive gastrointestinal haemorrhage. The potential variety and complexity of these conditions makes generalization about management difficult and dangerous.

In a recent analysis of 72 patients in the high risk group treated at Charing Cross Hospital since 1973, metastatic disease outside the pelvis was present

Table 4. Chamoca.

| Day | Time | Treatment |
|---|---|---|
| Day 1 | | Hydroxyurea 1 gm q.d.s. for 24 hours |
| Day 2 | 10.00 a.m. | Vincristine 1.0 mgs/m$^2$ stat i.v. |
| | 3.00 p.m. | Methotrexate 100 mgs/m$^2$ stat i.v. |
| | | Methotrexate 200 mgs/m$^2$ 12-hour infusion i.v. |
| Day 3 | 3.00 p.m. | Folinic acid 15 mgs i.m. or p.o. |
| Day 4 | 8.00 a.m. | Folinic acid 15 mgs i.m. or p.o. |
| | 10.00 a.m. | Cyclophosphamide 600 mgs/m$^2$ i.v. |
| | | Actinomycin-D 0.5 mgs i.v. |
| | 8.00 p.m. | Folinic acid 15 mgs i.m. or p.o. |
| Day 5 | 8.00 a.m. | Folinic acid 15 mgs i.m. or p.o. |
| | 10.00 a.m. | Actinomycin-D 0.5 mgs i.v. |
| Day 6 | 10.00 a.m. | Actinomycin-D 0.5 mgs i.v. |
| Day 7 | | No treatment |
| Day 8 | | No treatment |
| Day 9 | | Adriamycin 30 mgs/m$^2$ i.v. [a] |
| | | Cyclophosphamide 400 mgs/m$^2$ i.v. |

[a] Check WBC and platelets before giving.

at the start of treatment in 64 (89%), lungs being the commonest site (79% of patients), followed by the brain (15%) and liver (8%) [30].

It may at first appear tempting to deal with such presentations by local surgery or radiotherapy. This is rarely wise because such action usually prohibits effective chemotherapy for up to three weeks, a course of action which courts disaster in a tumour which is almost always disseminated in this 'high risk' group. Also large masses of choriocarcinoma at whatever site are usually enmeshed in a network of large and delicate vessels so that surgery may be hazardous. The multiplicity of gastrointestinal lesions may also defeat surgical resection. Surgery does however have a place after the use of chemotherapy (see below). Chemotherapy therefore is almost invariably preferable as the initial treatment but is not without its problems. A rapid tumour response may often be associated with increasing oedema around the tumour or haemorrhage into it, thus discrete pulmonary metastases may become diffuse as a result of chemotherapy, the patient proceeding to respiratory failure. In these circumstances great care must be taken that fluid overloading does not occur. Even in the absence of fluid retention, diuretics may produce temporary improvement. In such conditions infection readily supervenes and should be treated without delay. Particular measures in relation to the initial treatment of central nervous system metastases are considered below. In spite of increasing experience in this area, between 5 and 10% 'high risk' patients in our series have died as a result of the initial extent of disease.

*7.4.2. Drug-resistance.* This leads to death in approximately 10% of patients with 'high risk' choriocarcinoma and attempts to improve the results are based on the use of new drugs, better use of surgery and special attention to the treatment of metastases in the central nervous system.

*7.5. New drugs*
*7.5.1. VP 16-213 (Etoposide).* This epipodophylotoxin derivative has been shown to be effective in choriocarcinoma resistant to other agents [29] and in the initial treatment of patients in the 'medium risk' group. Principal toxicities are myelosuppression and alopecia. Rarely, anaphylactic reactions have occurred. An example of the use of this drug is given in Figure 10, where it has been used in alternation with CHAMOCA. Toxicity is reduced in this way and it seems likely that the chances of tumour eradications are enhanced with this drug although this regimen has not been submitted to a controlled trial comparing it with CHAMOCA alone. The MECA regimen (Table 5) is presently being studied as the initial treatment for patients in the 'high risk' group. It is less toxic than CHAMOCA and has good antitumour effect. However, it is too early to know whether survival of patients

*Table 5.* 'MECA' pilot study for 'high risk' choriocarcinoma.

| Course 1 | |
|---|---|
| Day 1 | Actinomycin-D 0.5 mg i.v. stat |
| Day 1 | VP.16-213 100 mg/m$^2$ i.v. infusion over 30 minutes |
| Day 1 | Methotrexate 100 mg/m$^2$ i.v. stat |
| Day 1 | Methotrexate 200 mg/m$^2$ i.v. 12-hour infusion |
| Day 2 | Actinomycin-D 0.5 mg i.v. stat |
| Day 2 | VP.16-213 100 mg/m$^2$ i.v. infusion over 30 minutes |
| Day 2 | Folinic acid 15 mg p.o./i.m. b.d. for 4 doses starting 24 hours after the start of methotrexate |
| 5-day interval and if no mucositis | |

| Course 2 | |
|---|---|
| Day 1 | Vincristine 1.0 mg/m$^2$ i.v. stat |
| Day 2 | Cyclophosphamide 600 mg/m$^2$ i.v. infusion over 30 minutes |
| 6-day interval and if no mucositis | |

| Course 1 | |
|---|---|
| As above | |
| 5-day interval and if no mucositis | |

| Course 2 | |
|---|---|
| As above | |

Intervals between courses should not be increased unless WBC < 1,000 and platelets are < 50,000 or mucositis develops. If mucositis occurs, delay next course until it has healed.

treated in this way will be as good as that achieved when CHAMOCA is given as the initial treatment and VP.16-213 held in reserve for use if drug-resistance develops.

*7.5.2. Cis-platinum.* This agent has been studied both alone and in combination with vincristine and methotrexate [31]. The combination was found to be more effective. Vincristine was given in a dose of 1 mg/m$^2$ at 10.00 a.m. on Day 1 and methotrexate 100 mg/m$^2$ i.v. stat at 3.00 p.m. on the same day, followed by methotrexate 200 mg/m$^2$ over the next 12 hours by i.v. infusion. Folinic acid rescue was started in the dose of 15 mg i.m. 24 hours after the start of the methotrexate and continued 12 hourly for a further 3 doses. Cis-platinum was given in the dose of 120 mg/m$^2$ on the third day with intense hydration, based on the work of Hayes [32]. Mannitol was given in the dose of 10 g hourly for each of 6 hours. One litre of i.v. fluids (alternating normal saline with 5% dextrose, each containing 1 g of

KCl) was given hourly for 3 hours before the Cis-platinum, which was given as a short i.v. infusion. Intravenous fluids were continued at a rate of 1 litre hourly for a further 3 hours. Hydration was continued until all vomiting had stopped. When the drugs were used in this way two courses could usually be given without significant nephrotoxicity. Ototoxicity is usually measurable by audiogram after one course and 4 courses tend to produce measurable deterioration in glomerular filtration and socially noticeable high frequency hearing loss. Significant hypomagnesemia commonly occurs after repeated courses due to renal tubular losses. Unless anticipated this may be sufficiently severe to produce tetany. Platinum may also be given in a dose of 20 mg/m$^2$ daily, 3–5 days in succession. This may also be combined with vincristine and methotrexate or with VP.16-213, or with all four drugs used together.

Cis-platinum is probably best reserved for circumstances where there is clear-cut evidence of drug-resistance such as seen in the patient illustrated in Figure 10, where a complete response was achieved with the use of Cis-platinum when resistance to all other drugs was evident.

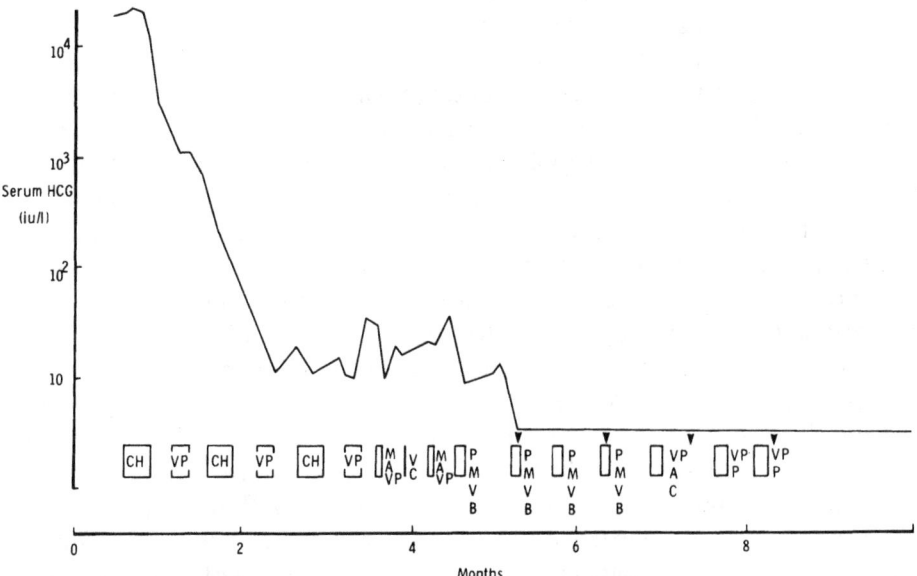

*Figure 10.* Chart showing HCG values and chemotherapy in a patient with choriocarcinoma 13 months after a normal pregnancy, who fell into the 'high risk' group. After a satisfactory initial response to CHAMOCA (CH) and VP.16-213 (VP), drug resistance becomes manifest. Different drug scheduling of methotrexate and folinic acid (M), actinomycin-D (A) and VP.16-213 failed to produce a response but complete remission was finally achieved with Cis-platinum in combination with vincristine (V), methotrexate and bleomycin (B). The patient remains disease-free one year after finishing treatment.

## 7.6. Surgery for drug-resistant disease

There is a small group of patients with drug-resistant disease in whom the tumour is restricted to a sufficiently small number of sites to be resectable. Accurate localization of these deposits is essential for success. Conventional radiographs, ultrasound, isotope scanning and computerized tomography should be used as appropriate. We have found the latter particularly useful in this context. It is sometimes difficult to tell whether deposits identified in this way contained viable or necrotic material. The new technique of radioimmunolocalization using radiolabelled antibody directed against HCG appears to have the potential to identify viable deposits of choriocarcinoma [20]. Three patients whose residual tumours appeared to be viable by this method have had successful resection of tumour which was in each case found to contain viable choriocarcinoma. All three subsequently achieved complete remission. The method is still in a state of development, however, and appears to have restricted application in the region of the uterus because of artefacts produced by free isotope in the bladder.

If tumour appears to be restricted to potentially resectable sites surgery should be considered. In the absence of known active tumour at other sites, hysterectomy should be performed and if HCG is not normal within 14 day or so, it has to be assumed that there is tumour elsewhere.

Thoracotomy may be successful in removing solitary or even multiple lesions. Solitary lesions within the abdomen can sometimes be excised successfully though it is wise to perform arteriography beforehand to determine the extent of the vascular supply. It is our practice to give methotrexate 50 mg intravenously at the time of operation to try and prevent metastases caused by manipulation of the tumour. The dose is reduced and folinic acid rescue given if renal function is impaired. Methotrexate is less likely to cause vomiting than some other cytotoxic agents but other drugs may be appropriate. Chemotherapy is restarted as soon as possible after surgery but rarely is this advisable before 10–14 days have passed, particularly when the intensive regimens described here are used. Ten to 14 days is usually also necessary between the preceding chemotherapy and surgery, thus four weeks or more usually passes when little or no systemic chemotherapy is given. If all the tumour is not completely excised there is a risk that the patient may have a larger tumour burden by the time she receives her next course of chemotherapy than she had before surgery. Experience with this approach has also been described by Hammond *et al.* [33] who advocate operation at the start of treatment, usually hysterectomy. Our experience leads us to avoid this approach in women wishing to have more children; primary hysterectomy can prove hazardous because of the profusion of delicate vessels within the pelvis.

In drug-resistant disease, however, the effects of surgery may be dramatic

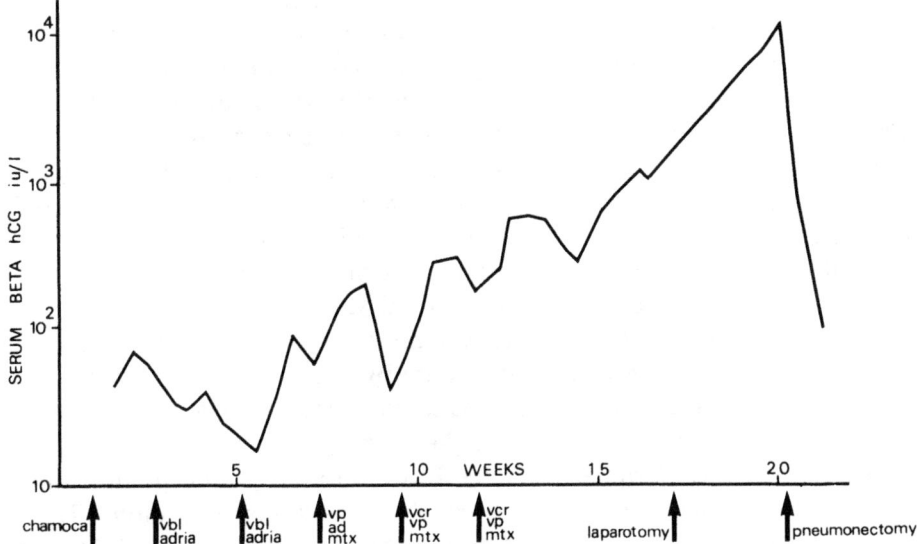

*Figure 11.* Chart showing HCG values and treatment in a patient with choriocarcinoma. The tumour had been extensively treated previously and was drug resistant as shown by rising HCG values in spite of treatment with CHAMOCA, vinblastine (VBL) adriamycin (Adria), VP.16-213 (VP), actinomycin-D (AD), vincristine (VCR), and methotrexate and folinic acid (MTX). A laparotomy was performed in search of resectable abdominal tumour but none was found. Finally radioimmunolocalization with antibody directed against HCG suggested the presence of viable tumour in the left lung. Pneumonectomy was performed with a dramatic response in HCG. The patient achieved a complete response with further chemotherapy and has been off treatment for 1 year.

and undoubtedly contribute to cure in selected patients. An example of this effect is given in Figure 11.

### 7.7. Radiotherapy

Radiotherapy is capable of producing responses in localized choriocarcinoma, but most of the patients reported here received chemotherapy in addition so that the tumour eradication with irradiation alone appears to be exceptional [34, 35]. In this respect it has less to offer than surgery while compromising the administration of cytotoxic chemotherapy to a similar degree.

### 7.8. Central nervous system metastases

CNS metastases of choriocarcinoma were associated with pulmonary deposits in 65 of 69 patients treated at Charing Cross Hospital; some were present on referral, others developed during chemotherapy [36]. For this reason, all patients with lung deposits or high risk choriocarcinoma are given prophylactic intrathecal methotrexate 12.5 mg with each course of chemotherapy which does not contain a moderately high dose ($0.3 \text{ g/m}^2$ or more) or systemic methotrexate. For this purpose, intrathecal or high dose systemic methotrexate should be given no less frequently than every two weeks. When these measures have been employed no patient has developed CNS metastases unless disease elsewhere had become drug-resistant and presumably reseeded the brain. By contrast brain metastases were the only site of progressive disease in 19 patients who did not receive CNS prophylaxis [36]. Thus, the disease outside the CNS was responding to systemic chemotherapy while that in the brain was progressing, presumably due to inadequate penetration of drugs into the CNS.

When CNS metastases are evident at the start of treatment the poor access of drugs into the CSF is overcome by use of high dose methotrexate together with intrathecal methotrexate in standard doses (12.5 mg). An intravenous infusion of $3 \text{ g/m}^2$ over 24 hours gives CSF methotrexate concentrations of $>10^{-6}$ molar at the end of the infusion and the data of Tattersall indicate that $1 \text{ g/m}^2$ also gives therapeutic concentrations [37]. Although lower doses sometimes produce responses, it is our policy to give methotrexate $1 \text{ g/m}^2$ as a 24-hour infusion with folinic acid (Leucovorin) 30 mg, 12-hourly for three days, starting 32 hours after the start of the infusion. It is essential to maintain urine flow above 2.5 l/day. The dose of intravenous methotrexate and folinic acid in the CHAMOCA and MECA regimens may be increased to these levels. Provided that there is no evidence of raised intracranial pressure, intrathecal methotrexate is given approximately once every two weeks either between courses of systemic chemotherapy or concurrent with those regimens which do not contain intravenous methotrexate. Intrathecal cytosine arabinoside and thiotepa have also been used, but there is insufficient data to assess their usefulness.

The greatest risk to patients presenting with CNS metastases is during the first month of treatment; eight of 33 patients in our series died during this time [36]. These patients all had severe neurological damage on presentation which can sometimes be ameliorated by dexamethazone. It is possible that high dose methotrexate at the onset may exacerbate oedema or cause cerebral haemorrhage as the tumour becomes necrotic. The alternative of using a lower dose, however, may predispose to drug-resistance. Apart from the eight patients dying in the first month another nine have died of drug-resistant disease during ensuing 43 months. Sixteen patients have been off treatment for a mean of 111 months. Since 1974 when treatment was based on the principles outlined above, only one of eight patients has died of drug-resistance. Mortality during the first month of treatment has remained at 25%.

The prognosis is grave for patients developing CNS metastases while on chemotherapy. The disease is usually drug-resistant from the outset and only three of 36 patients in our series [36] have survived, although two are still on treatment. The remaining patient is worthy of note in that a solitary metastasis was localized by CT and successfully resected.

## 8. IMMUNOTHERAPY

During the 1960s the expected expression of paternal histocompatibility antigens by choriocarcinoma led to attempts at immunotherapy by skin grafting from patients' consorts. The experiments proved unsuccessful, but the idea of directing therapy at an antigen which is relatively specific for choriocarcinoma has continued to stimulate interest. Early attempts at therapy with antiserum or purified antibody to HCG in our department have been hampered by difficulty in assessing results. The therapeutic antibody interferes with assays for HCG and it is difficult to tell whether any fall in HCG is due to clearance from the blood by antibody or a true anti-tumour effect. The demonstration by radioimmunolocalization that antibody to HCG can be concentrated in choriocarcinomatous tissue in patients [20] stimulates further interest in tissue culture experiments in which cytotoxicity of various compounds is enhanced when they are coupled with tumour-directed monoclonal antibodies [38]. Further exploration of radioimmunolocalization as a means of increasing the tissue concentration of cytotoxic agents is needed in experimental systems and later in patients.

## 9. CONCLUSION

The regular follow-up of HCG values in serum or urine after evacuation of hydatidiform mole permits early recognition of the need for chemotherapy at a time when prognosis is good and treatment relatively nontoxic. There is little doubt that this procedure has been a major contribution to survival after hydatidiform mole and has increased awareness of the possibility of early diagnosis of choriocarcinoma after non-molar pregnancies. The procedure has been shown to be cost-effective when performed in a centre using automated radioimmunoassay to handle large numbers of samples [39, 16]. Having recognized those patients for whom treatment is needed, the use of prognostic factors allows identification of groups in which relatively nontoxic chemotherapy will nearly always eradicate the disease.

The major outstanding problems are presented by the 'high risk' group. Disease can now be eradicated in the majority of these patients. In a recent series of 72 such patients treated in this unit 13 of 72 (18%) died [30]. Very advanced disease at the time of presentation is one of the most frequent causes of death that could sometimes be avoided by earlier recognition of the clinical and biochemical features of the disease. Thanks to new drugs and surgery in carefully selected patients, death from drug-resistance is becoming less frequent. This problem is not completely solved, however, and new therapeutic agents are needed for those young women who still die of drug-resistant choriocarcinoma.

ACKNOWLEDGEMENTS

We are grateful to the many gynaecologists who have referred patients, making this work possible and also to our colleagues in the Department of Medical Oncology at Charing Cross Hospital. We would also like to thank Dr J. E. Boultbee for his work on ultrasound and our many other colleagues at Charing Cross Hospital who have contributed to the studies.

The support of the Cancer Research Campaign and the Medical Research Council is gratefully acknowledged.

REFERENCES

1. Li MC, Hertz R, Spencer DB: The effect of methotrexate therapy upon choriocarcinoma and chorioadenoma. Proc Soc exp Biol (NY) 93:361–366, 1956.
2. Kajii T, Ohama K: Androgenetic origin of hydatidiform mole. Nature 268:633–634, 1977.
3. Kurman RJ, Scully RE, Norris HJ: Trophoblastic pseudotumor of the uterus. An exaggerated form of 'syncytial endometritis' simulating a malignant tumor. Cancer 38:1214–1226, 1976.
4. Goldstein DP: Prevention of gestational trophoblastic disease by use of actinomycin-D in molar pregnancies. J Obstet Gynecol 43:475–479, 1974.
5. Hatch KD, Shingleton HM, Austin JM, Boots LR, Younger JB, Soong SJ: Southern regional trophoblastic disease centre, 1972–1977. Southern Med J 71:1334–40, 1978.
6. Stone M, Bagshawe KD: An analysis of the influences of maternal age, gestational age, contraceptive method and mode of primary treatment of patients with hydatidiform moles on the incidence of subsequent chemotherapy. Brit J Obstet Gynaecol 86:782–792, 1979.
7. Brandes JM, Grunstein S, Peretz A: Suction evacuation of the uterine cavity in hydatidiform mole. Obstet Gynecol 28:689–691, 1966.
8. Bagshawe KD: Choriocarcinoma: The Clinical Biology of the Trophoblast and its Tumours, p 261. London: Arnold, 1969.
9. Stone M, Dent J, Kardana A, Bagshawe KD: Relationship of oral contraception to development of trophoblastic tumour after evacuation of a hydatidiform mole. Br J Obstet Gynaecol 83:913–916, 1976.
10. Baltazar JC: Epidemiological features of choriocarcinoma. Bull WHO 54:523–532, 1976.
11. Berkowitzrs, Marean AR, Goldstein DP, Bernstein MR: Oral contraceptives and post-molar trophoblastic tumours. Lancet ii:752, 1980.
12. Bagshawe KD, Stone M: Oral contraceptives and post-molar trophoblastic tumours. Lancet ii:1250, 1980.

13. McGrath IT, Golding PR, Bagshawe KD: Medical presentations of choriocarcinoma. Brit Med J 2:633-637, 1971.
14. Searle F, Leake BA, Bagshawe KD, Dent J: Serum-SP$_1$-pregnancy-specific-$\beta$-glycoprotein in choriocarcinoma and other neoplastic disease. Lancet i:579-581, 1978.
15. Kardana A, Bagshawe KD: A rapid, sensitive and specific radioimmunoassay for human chorionic gonadotrophin. J Immunol Methods 9:297-305, 1976.
16. Bagshawe KD: Computer controlled automated radioimmunoassay. Lab Practice (September):573-575, 1975.
17. Bagshawe KD, Harland S: Immunodiagnosis and monitoring of gonadotrophin-producing metastases in the central nervous system. Cancer 38:112-118, 1976.
18. Requard CK, Mettler FA: The use of ultrasound in the evaluation of trophoblastic disease and its response to therapy. Radiology 135:419-422, 1980.
19. Cave WT, Durn JT: Choriocarcinoma with hyperthyroidism: probable identity of the thyrotropin with human chorionic gonadotrophon. Ann Int Med 85:60-63, 1976.
20. Begent RHJ, Searle F, Stanway G, Jewkes RF, Jones BE, Vernon P, Bagshawe KD: Radioimmunolocalization of tumours by external scintigraphy after administration of $^{131}$I antibody to human chorionic gonadotrophin. J Roy Soc Med 23:624-630, 1980.
21. Goldenberg DM, Kim EE, Deland FM, van Nagell JR, Javadpour N: Clinical radioimmunodetection of cancer with radiolabelled antibodies to human chorionic gonadotrophin. Science 208:1284-1286, 1980.
22. Searle F, Boden J, Lewis JCM, Bagshawe KD: A human choriocarcinoma xenograft in nude mice; a model for study of antibody localization. Brit J Cancer 44:137-144, 1981.
23. Bagshawe KD: Risk and prognostic factors in trophoblastic neoplasia. Cancer 38:1373-1385, 1976.
24. Hammond CB, Borchert LG, Tyrey L, Creasman WT, Parker RT: Treatment of metastatic trophoblastic disease: good and poor prognosis. Am J Obstet Gynecol 115:451-457, 1973.
25. Elston CW, Bagshawe KD: Cellular reaction in trophoblastic tumours. Br J Cancer 28:245-256, 1973.
26. Bagshawe KD: Treatment of trophoblastic tumours. Recent Results in Cancer Research 62:192-199, 1977.
27. Walden PAM, Mitchell-Heggs PF, Coppin C, Dent J, Bagshawe KD: Pleurisy and methotrexate treatment. Brit Med J 2:867, 1980.
28. Bagshawe KD, Newlands ES: High dose methotrexate in patients with trophoblastic tumours. In: High Dose Methotrexate, Pharmacology, Toxicology and Chemotherapy. Pereti P (ed), Firenze, Italy: Editrice Ginntina, 1978, pp 281-288.
29. Newlands ES, Bagshawe KD: Anti-tumour activity of the epipodophyllin derivative VP. 16-213 (Etoposide: NSC - 141540) in gestational choriocarcinoma. Europ J Cancer 16:401-405, 1980.
30. Begent RHJ, Bagshawe KD: The management of high risk choriocarcinoma. Seminars in Oncology, 9:198-203, 1982.
31. Newlands ES, Bagshawe KD: Activity of high dose Cis-platinum (NCI 119875) in combination with vincristine and methotrexate in drug-resistant choriocarcinoma. A report of 17 cases. Brit J Cancer 40:943-945, 1979.
32. Hayes DM, Cvitkovic E, Golbey RB, Scheiner E, Helson L, Krakoff RH: High dose Cis-platinum diammine dichloride. Amelioration of renal toxicity by mannitol diuresis. Cancer 39:1372-1381, 1977.
33. Hammond CB, Weed JC, Curie JL: The role of operation in the current therapy of gestational trophoblastic disease. Am J Obstet Gynecol 136:844-858, 1980.

34. Weed JC, Hammond CB: Cerebral metastatic choriocarcinoma: Intensive therapy and prognosis. Obstet Gynecol 55:89–94, 1980.
35. Brace KC: The role of irradiation in the treatment of metastatic trophoblastic disease. Radiology 91:540–544, 1968.
36. Athanassiou A, Begent RHJ, Newlands ES, Parker D, Rustin GJS, Bagshawe KD: Central nervous system metastases of chorio carcinoma: 23 years experience at Charing Cross Hospital. Cancer (in Press).
37. Tattersall MHN, Parker LM, Pittman SW, Frei E: Clinical pharmacology of high dose methotrexate. Cancer Chemother Rep 6:25–29, 1975.
38. Gregoriadis G: Targeting of drugs: Implications in medicine. Lancet ii:241–246, 1981.
39. Bagshawe KD: Choriocarcinoma: Can we afford to cure cancer? Ann Roy Coll Surg of England 60:34–41, 1978.

# 6. The Immunobiology of Ovarian Carcinoma

ROBERT C. BAST Jr. and ROBERT C. KNAPP

1. INTRODUCTION

Knowledge of the immunobiology of ovarian carcinoma may aid in the detection, staging, and treatment of this malignancy. In all probability, the immune response to ovarian carcinoma is affected by many of the same factors which influence immunological resistance to tumors that arise from other organs. In addition, several facets of ovarian tumor immunology almost certainly reflect the unique biology of epithelial neoplasms that develop at this particular site.

*1.1. Principles of tumor immunology*

A central concept of tumor immunology is that many, if not all, neoplasms bear distinctive antigens which are not associated with normal tissues and which permit the host to recognize tumor tissue as foreign. Tumor-associated antigens can be detected at the cell surface, in the cytoplasm, or within the nucleus. Antigens associated with the cell surface membrane are most accessible for interaction with antibodies or specifically sensitized lymphocytes. Different antigens may or may not remain localized on or within tumor cells. Substantial quantities of tumor-associated antigens can be released into cyst fluid, ascites, lymph or blood. Release of antigens can occur through tumor necrosis, blebbing of cytoplasmic vesicles or shedding of antigen from the cell surface membrane at a molecular level [1]. Shed antigens might provide appropriate markers for diagnosing or monitoring occult tumor that cannot be readily detected by noninvasive techniques. Not all antigens are shed readily. Some remain closely associated with the tumor cell surface. Antigens that remain associated with the cell surface membrane should be appropriate targets for immunodetection or immunotherapy *in situ* using antibodies of appropriate specificity.

Not all cells within a tumor may display a particular antigen. Expression

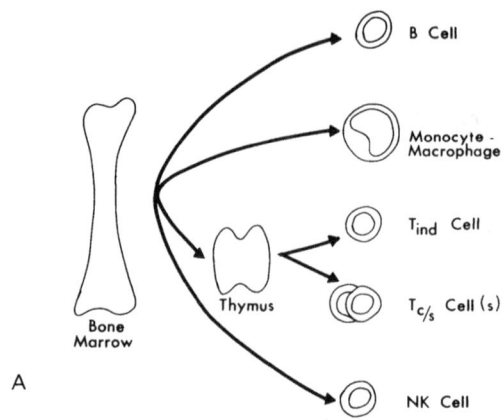

*Figure 1.* A. Bone marrow provides the ultimate source of several cell types which participate in immunologically-mediated tumor cell killing. B cells, monocytes, and natural killer (NK) cells are derived directly from bone marrow. T cells differentiate under the influence of the thymus into subsets that mediate induction ($T_{ind}$) or cytotoxicity and suppression ($T_{c/s}$). B. $T_{ind}$ cells stimulate the proliferation and/or differentiation of B cells, monocytes, and $T_{c/s}$ cells. A protion of $T_{c/s}$ cells can, in turn, suppress the activity of $T_{ind}$ cells. C. Monocytes can also facilitate the proliferation and differentiation of B cells and T cells. Plasma cells are derived from B cells and produce specific immunoglobulins of different subclasses. IgG and IgM immunoglobulins mediate antibody-dependent tumor cell lysis in the presence of complement components. IgG also mediates tumor cell lysis in the presence of cellular effectors. $T_{c/s}$ cells produce specific tumor cell lysis in the absence of antibody. Activated macrophages participate in delayed hypersensitivity, destruction of intracellular pathogens, and lysis of tumor cells independent of specific tumor-associated antigens. In addition, activated macrophages can suppress the proliferation and differentiation of T cells and B cells. Natural killer cells lyse tumor cells bearing antigens to which the host has not been intentionally exposed. (Reproduced by permission of Lea and Febiger. From: Cancer Medicine, 2nd ed, Holland JF, Frei E III (eds).

of antigens can also vary quantitatively with phases of the cell cycle [2]. Binding of antibody to certain tumor-associated antigens can result in their redistribution or complete disappearance from the tumor cell surface, i.e., antigenic modulation [3, 4]. Not all tumor-associated antigens modulate, but loss of antigens from the tumor cell surface may provide one mechanism by which some tumors evade host defense. Growth of clones which lack antigen may not be detected by immunodiagnostic tests and antigenic loss or modulation may limit the efficacy of serotherapy.

Immunological resistance to tumor growth must ultimately be mediated by lymphocytes, macrophages, antibodies and/or complement (Figure 1). Over the last two decades immunologists have demonstrated that small lymphocytes can be separated into T cells and B cells based upon distinctive cell surface phenotypes [5]. B cells bear cell surface immunoglobulin and are the precursors for antibody forming cells (Table 1). T cells form 'rosettes'

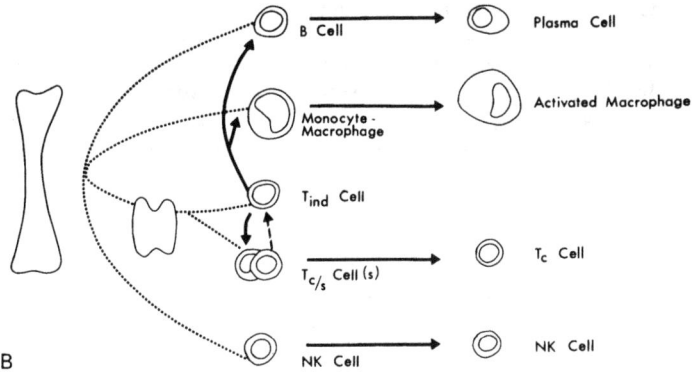

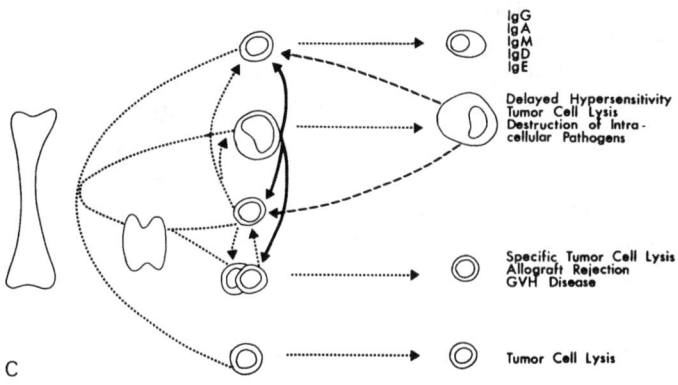

with sheep erythrocytes and bear antigens that are acquired in the thymus (Table 1). After stimulation with antigen, T cells proliferate, differentiate and release mediators. Stimulated T cells contribute to cell-mediated reactions including delayed cutaneous reactivity, allograft rejection and graft *versus* host disease. In addition to their effector function, T cells regulate the activities of macrophages, B cells and other T cells. Among the T cells, distinct subsets either promote or suppress the cellular and humoral response to different antigens [6]. Inducer or 'helper' T cells permit rapid amplification of the immune response by attracting, arresting and activating macrophages or by stimulating the proliferation and differentiation of other T cells and B cells. Suppressor T cells limit the superfluous production of antibody or the excessive proliferation of lymphocytes following exposure to new antigens. In addition suppressor cells may prevent immunological destruction of normal host tissue. Several tumor-associated antigens studied

Table 1. Characteristics of lymphocytes and monocytes.

|  | Bear thymic antigens | Synthesize surface $I_g$ | Bear specific receptors | Adhere to surfaces | Phagocytize particles |
|---|---|---|---|---|---|
| T cells | + | − | + | − | − |
| B cells | − | + | + | +/− | − |
| Null cells | − | − | − | − | − |
| Monocytes | − | − | − | + | + |

to date resemble normal determinants found in embryonic or adult tissue [7]. Consequently, the immune response to tumor-associated antigens may be actively suppressed to avoid destruction of subtly 'altered self'.

At least five mechanisms have been proposed for the immunological destruction of tumor cells: T cell mediated cytotoxicity, antibody-dependent complement-mediated cytotoxicity, antibody-dependent cell-mediated cytotoxicity, natural killing and macrophage-mediated cytotoxicity. Only T cells and B cells bear receptors with specificity for different antigens (Table 1). Specific elimination of tumor cells can be mediated by those clones of T lymphocytes which bear receptors for unique antigens associated with the tumor cell surface (Figure 2). Direct contact between specifically programmed T lymphocytes and tumor cells produces membrane damage and

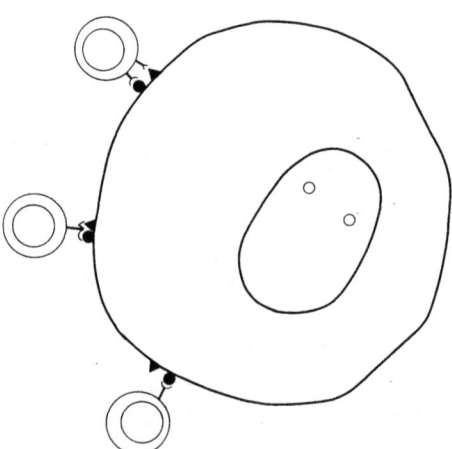

Figure 2. Tumor cells can be lysed by specifically sensitized T cells that bear receptors for tumor-associated antigens (●) and, in some cases, for cell surface antigens encoded by the major histocompatibility complex (▲). Recognition of both structures may be required for effective T cell-mediated cytotoxicity.

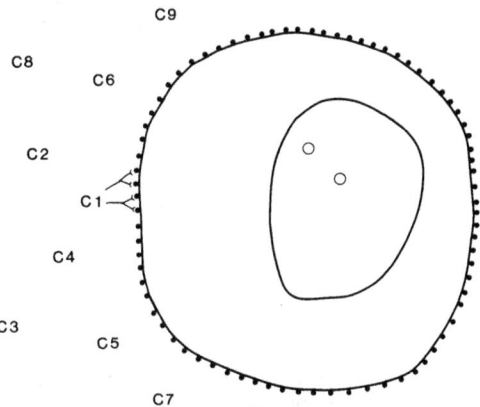

*Figure 3.* In antibody-dependent complement-mediated cytotoxicity either two IgG molecules or a single IgM molecule trigger activation and/or binding of each of the nine complement components found in normal serum. Insertion of C7-C9 in the tumor cell membrane increases permeability and induces osmotic lysis.

osmotic lysis of the tumor targets. B lymphocytes probably do not participate directly in tumor killing. The specific immunoglobulins which they produce, however, can bind to tumor cells and permit antibody-dependent complement-mediated and antibody-dependent cell-mediated cytotoxicity (ADCC). Binding of specific IgM or IgG immunoglobulin to antigens at the tumor cell surface can activate the complement components available in serum and ultimately produce membrane damage and tumor cell death (Figure 3). Alternatively, IgG immunoglobulins mediate ADCC. In this

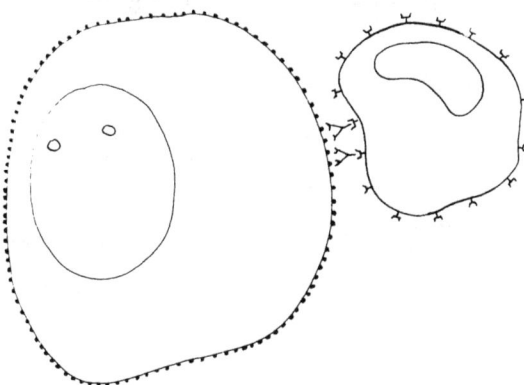

*Figure 4.* In antibody-dependent cell-mediated cytotoxicity (ADCC), specific IgG antibodies bind to antigens on the tumor cell surface. Effector cells which bear receptors for the Fc portion of IgG can then bind to tumor target. Several cell types can act as effectors including null lymphocytes, monocytes, macrophages, activated T cells and polymorphonuclear leukocytes.

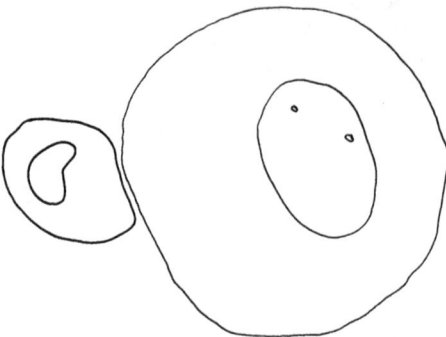

*Figure 5.* Macrophage-mediated cytotoxicity for tumor cells is observed after monocytes and macrophages have been activated with lymphokines, endotoxin or interferon. Activated macrophages bind selectively to tumor cells, but do not utilize conventional antibodies or antigen receptors to facilitate adherence.

reaction, antibody acts as a bridge between tumor cell surface antigens and effector cells which bear receptors for the Fc portion of the IgG molecule (Figure 4). A number of different effector cell types can mediate ADCC. These include activated macrophages, polymorphonuclear granulocytes and 'K' lymphocytes which are found among the null cell population. Macrophages which have been activated by treatment with lymphokines, endotoxin or interferon can also destroy tumor in the absence of antibody, although the reaction proceeds more slowly than it does in the presence of specific antiserum [8]. Discrimination of tumor cells from benign tissue is achieved by recognition of an alteration in cell membrane structure that is shared by a wide variety of tumor cells, rather than by recognition of distinctive antigens that are unique to particular neoplasms (Figure 5). Finally, certain null

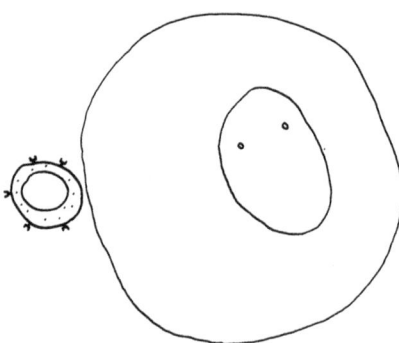

*Figure 6.* Natural killer (NK) cells bind to tumor cells and produce membrane damage. Many NK cells are large granular lymphocytes that bear receptors for the Fc-portion of the IgG molecule, but that do not require antibody to mediate tumor cell killing.

cells can mediate 'natural killing' and 'NK' cells are found in normal donors who have not been intentionally exposed to tumor products [9]. Morphologically the NK cells are large lymphocytes with cytoplasmic granules (Figure 6). Receptors for the Fc protion of the IgG molecule can be found on the cell surface, but antibody is not required for 'natural killing' or 'spontaneous cytotoxicity'. Different tumors vary in their susceptibility to NK cells and to mechanisms by which these lymphocytes recognize neoplastic cells is not known.

Most immunological mechanisms of tumor cell killing have been studied in cell culture and their relative importance in determining host resistance to cancer *in vivo* is still not well defined. From work in animal systems it is apparent that these mechanisms in aggregate can only control growth of a relatively small number of tumor cells [10]. Modest resistance to tumor growth is not simply a function of poor immunocompetence, but also reflects a careful balance of immunoregulatory (helper and suppressor) mechanisms [11]. Interaction of T cells with tumor-specific antigen may suppress as well as stimulate the human immune response. The release of soluble tumor antigen in ever increasing amounts may induce T suppressor cells in animal systems [12] and a similar phenomenon may be observed in man [11]. In addition, the peripheral blood monocytes of cancer patients can suppress the proliferation and differentiation of both T and B lymphocytes nonspecifically [11]. Acute phase reactants and immunoregulatory peptides have also been detected in serum or ascites fluid. These factors may limit the ability of the host to recognize and eliminate tumor cells by T or B cell mechanisms [13].

In addition to the effect exerted by the underlying neoplasm, a number of other factors can suppress the host's response including malnutrition, surgical procedures, radiotherapy and chemotherapy [13]. Consequently, immunotherapy utilizing immunostimulants, interferon, lymphocytes or antibodies must often be administered to immunocompromized patients. Given an immunodepressed host and the complexity of immunoregulatory mechanisms, it is not surprising that many well-intentioned attempts to provide immunotherapy have been unsuccessful.

*1.2. Distinctive properties of epithelial ovarian carcinoma*

Analysis of the immune response to ovarian carcinoma must consider a distinctive pattern of tumor growth, metastasis and recurrence, as well as the impact of currently available treatment. Epithelial ovarian carcinomas are thought to arise from modified peritoneal mesothelial cells which cover the surface of the ovary and which line cysts that are found immediately beneath the ovarian surface. Malignant ovarian tumor cells can invade the cyst wall to grow within the ovarian stroma or can form excresences on the ovarian surface. In theory, tumor antigens that are shed from the surface of the ovary into the peritoneal cavity should be cleared rapidly by subdiaphragmatic lymphatics, enter retrosternal lymph channels and appear promptly in the venous circulation [14]. Antigens that remain within cyst fluid can establish a concentration gradient favoring diffusion of small antigenic molecules into surrounding tissue. Levels of some antigens within ovarian cyst fluid exceed those in serum by 10–1000-fold [15]. With local invasion of the cyst wall, antigens of higher molecular weight could escape into the abundant lymphatics and microvasculature of the ovary. Clearance of antigen from ovarian carcinomas might differ from that of tumors that arise at some other sites. Antigen shed from malignancies of the colon or lung should follow a somewhat different pattern of clearance. A majority of these tumors arise from the mucosal epithelium that lines the luminal surface of tubular structures. For antigen to gain access to the vascular compartment, tumor must actually erode the basement membrane and invade the submucosa. Antigen shed from the bulk of the tumor should pass into the lumen of the bowel or bronchus to be expelled with sputum or feces. Free egress of antigen would preclude development of a concentration gradient across the basement membrane. From this analysis, one would predict that tumor-associated antigens of high molecular weight should appear in the venous circulation only with relatively advanced lesions of the colon or lung, whereas antigens associated with ovarian carcinomas could appear in peripheral blood when tumor was still localized to the ovary and amenable to cure by surgery.

Ovarian carcinoma can metastasize by several routes. Tumor generally spreads along the peritoneal surface and occasionally through retroperitoneal lymphatics. Hematogenous metastases are uncommon. As intraperitoneal tumor growth progresses, blockade of diaphragmatic lymphatics decreases the outflow of interstitial fluid that exudes from tumor tissue. Ascites then accumulates within the peritoneal cavity [16]. Ovarian tumor cells can grow either within the ascites or within implants on the peritoneal surface. Single cells or small clumps of tumor within ascites can interact directly with inflammatory cells which are often present in large numbers. Nutrients required for tumor growth must traverse the ascites. Metabolic waste products and the remnants of degenerating cells accumulate within the proteinaceous fluid. The microenvironment within ascites might well affect tumor cell kinetics and the expression of tumor-associated antigen. Nutrients may be supplied more directly and catabolites removed more readily from vascularized tumor growing within small nodules. Access of immunoglobulins and viable leukocytes, however, could be impeded as large areas of tumor become necrotic or small nests of tumor are encased by dense fibrous tissue following chemotherapy or radiotherapy. The frequent association of ascites with ovarian carcinoma has permitted studies of host–tumor interaction in ascitic fluid that could not be performed as readily with other tumor types. Analysis of the immune response to ovarian carcinoma and development of strategies for effective immunotherapy must, however, consider growth of vascularized tumor as well as tumor in ascitic form.

Regional spread of tumor within the peritoneal cavity is particularly important in the management of patients with ovarian carcinoma. Following successful surgical cytoreduction, chemotherapy can produce complete tumor regression in a majority of patients with Stage III disease [17]. The disease-free interval can often exceed two years [18], suggesting that a very small tumor burden remains following treatment. Even with the most effective regimens tumor generally recurs within five years and recurrence is usually observed within the peritoneal cavity. Death is frequently related to small bowel dysfunction and malnutrition leading to infection rather than to destructive visceral metastases. Recognition of this fact has prompted the intraperitoneal administration of chemotherapy or radioactive colloids to provide high local concentrations of drug in the vicinity of residual tumor. Direct contact between tumor cells and immunostimulants can produce regression of cutaneous nodules of metastatic melanoma and other neoplasms [19, 20]. Intraperitoneal administration of immunotherapeutic agents can provide direct contact between immunological reagents and tumor cells that float free in ascites or are immediately adjacent to the serosa. Access to the peritoneal cavity can also permit the lavage of tumor-associated antigen and immunosuppressive factors from the compartment in which tumor is growing.

## 2. ANTIGENS

### 2.1. Ovarian tumor-associated antigens

A variety of antigens can be associated with tumors including histocompatibility antigens, differentiation antigens and oncofetal antigens. Histocompatibility antigens and tissue differentiation antigens are shared with normal adult tissues. Oncofetal antigens are expressed during embryonic development, repressed in normal adult tissue and reexpressed in neoplasms. Histocompatibility antigens are found on most normal tissues regardless of histologic type. These cell surface antigens permit recognition and destruction of transplanted tissues from genetically disparate donors. In an outbred population such as our own, the large number of alleles for genes that encode histocompatibility antigens minimizes the chance that allografts will be accepted between unrelated individuals. Tissue differentiation antigens are generally associated with cells of a single histological type but can be found in similar tissues from unrelated individuals. Differentiation antigens appear during fetal development or during renewal of certain tissues in the adult. One family of antigens appears in thymus dependent or 'T' lymphocytes during maturation in the thymus. Morphologically, cells at each stage of development can be identified with antisera against a panel of lymphocyte-associated differentiation antigens. Monoclonal expansion of cells bearing distinctive combinations of thymic differentiation antigens have been documented in the T cell leukemias and lymphomas. Normal tissue differentiation antigens are likely to be associated with solid tumors as well.

Using animal systems it has been possible to demonstrate specific antigens that mediate resistance to tumor transplants in genetically identical 'syngeneic' recipients [10]. Tumor-specific transplantation resistance antigens are thought not to be histocompatibility, differentiation or oncofetal antigens in that they cannot be detected in subpopulations of adult or embryonic tissue. Rather, they are distinctive antigens induced during transformation of cells by chemicals, viruses or irradiation. Each chemically induced tumor exhibits unique antigens, whereas virus-induced tumors bear common antigens encoded by the oncogenic virus. Consequently, a common or shared antigen is detected in tumors induced by an oncogenic virus, whereas immunization with tumors induced by the same chemical will generally not confer resistance to transplantation, even if the tumors appear similar morphologically. Given the obvious ethical constraints against tumor transplantation in man, as well as the fact that tumors bear histocompatibility antigens which would inhibit tumor growth in allogeneic recipients, it has been very difficult to document the existence of tumor-specific transplantation resistance toward human cancer. Some apparently specific determinants have been identified serologically on tumors from patients with malignant melanoma [21]. Actually proving that these antigens are not histocompatibility, differentiation or oncofetal antigens is a difficult process of exclusion. Shared virus-induced antigens have been detected in Burkitt's lymphoma and nasopharyngeal carcinoma but it is not clear whether these antigens elicit host response or mediate resistance to tumor growth. Consequently, the existence of tumor-specific antigens in man remains unresolved. Whether or not there are truly specific antigens, those differentiation antigens or oncofetal antigens, which are associated with human cancer might still prove useful for diagnosis or therapy.

*2.2. Oncofetal antigens*

Among the oncofetal antigens, CEA, has been the best studied (see Chapter 2, Section 2). Antigen activity can be detected in the serum of patients with a variety of tumors including carcinomas of the colon, rectum, stomach, pancreas, lung, breast, prostate, bladder, cervix, endometrium and ovary [22]. Approximately 50% of patients with ovarian carcinoma will have abnormal serum levels in excess of 2.5 ng/ml at some time during the course of their disease [23]. In ovarian carcinoma, CEA activity has been associated with a glycoprotein of 375,000 daltons [24], whereas the CEA isolated from colorectal carcinomas exhibits a molecular weight of approximately 200,000 daltons [22]. Consequently, CEA may not be a single molecule, but rather a family of closely related glycoproteins that share similar determinants.

As in the case of colorectal carcinoma, CEA levels are not useful in screening populations for occult ovarian carcinoma. Elevations of CEA are generally modest and occur in advanced stages of ovarian cancer. Modest elevations of CEA are also observed in individuals without apparent malignancy, including heavy smokers and patients with hepatic or inflammatory bowel disease.

Some investigators have found CEA useful for monitoring disease recurrence. Elevated CEA levels generally fall within 8 weeks following complete surgical resection of ovarian tumor [24]. CEA levels can remain elevated for up to 4 months following radiotherapy reflecting a more gradual elimination of tumor. Persistent elevations of CEA following surgical treatment or radiotherapy have been associated with persistent disease [25]. Gradually rising levels of CEA can precede clinical recurrence by as much as 8 months. Rapidly rising levels of CEA are often associated with disease recurrence, although CEA-negative clones can progress in the absence of elevated serum levels of the antigen. Critical studies, in which CEA has been used to prompt 'second look' operations have not been performed and the utility of the marker for determining the response to chemotherapy remains to be established.

CEA is most often produced by tumors of mucinous histology [23, 24, 26], but investigators disagree with regard to the proportion of serous tumors that are associated with elevated serum levels of the antigen [23, 24, 27, 28]. In contrast to colorectal carcinoma where CEA is most frequently associated with moderately well-differentiated tumors, poorly differentiated epithelial ovarian carcinomas are more frequently associated with the marker than are well-differentiated neoplasms [23, 28].

Germ cell tumors can also produce modest elevations of serum CEA, but AFP and HCG have proven to be more useful markers (see Chapter 2, Sections 3 and 4 & Chapter 4, Section 4). Alpha fetoprotein is a glycoprotein of 69,000 daltons that is expressed during fetal development and appears in the maternal circulation during the third trimester of normal pregnancy, it appears as well as in the serum of patients with hepatocellular disease and in the rare immunodeficiency state, ataxia telangiectasia [29]. The marker has proven most useful in following patients with hepatoma and germ cell tumors of the testis. AFP is associated with virtually all endodermal sinus tumors studied and with a majority of embryonal carcinomas [30]. AFP is not associated with ovarian choriocarcinomas. In contrast hCG is produced by choriocarcinomas and embryonal carcinomas, but not by endodermal sinus tumors [30]. In these rare neoplasms oncofetal antigen expression parallels histological differentiation and may aid in diagnosis as well as in monitoring response to therapy. Following excision of tumors, positive values persist for 5–7 weeks, consistent with a half life for AFP of 6 days. In patients with the more common epithelial ovarian carcinomas, modest elevations of AFP and hCG may occur [24], but these antigens have not proven to be useful as single markers.

Different investigators have utilized combinations of markers to monitor disease recurrence. Elevated CEA and placental alkaline phosphatase proved complimentary in detecting disease and in following its course [31]. Using CEA, AFP and hCG in combination more than 85% of ovarian or cervical carcinoma patients had at least one marker elevated [24]. Levels were greater with invasive cancer than with noninvasive cancer and were substantially greater than in controls. Levels of the antigens returned to normal within eight weeks after surgery and within 12 weeks after radiation therapy. However, other investigators [32] have not found any consistent correlation between ovarian tumor burden and placental lactogen, CEA, hCG or AFP when used alone or in combination.

## 2.3. Differentiation antigens and 'tumor-specific' antigens

More precise correlations might be achieved by measuring levels of antigens that can be found only in ovarian tissue. Over the last decade there have been many attempts to develop antibodies against antigens that would be found only in ovarian epithelial carcinomas [33–57]. Heteroantisera have usually been raised by injecting animals with human ovarian tumor tissue obtained at laparotomy or with ovarian carcinoma cell lines established in tissue culture. For must studies tumor tissue or cell lines have been homogenized, sonicated and centrifuged at high speed to remove organelles and cell membrane fragments. In some cases, tissue homogenates have been extracted with perchloracetic acid to obtain glycoproteins that are particularly high in carbohydrate. The clarified supernatant or extract has generally been injected into rabbits, often with an adjuvant to boost antibody titer. Antisera have been absorbed exhaustively with normal tissues or with tissue extracts. Following absorption, antibodies and putative antigens have been studied by immunodiffusion in gel. Specificity has been established by the presence or absence of precipitin lines which form between wells that contain antiserum and wells that contain extracts of tumors or normal tissues.

Only a few reports have utilized the more sensitive techniques of indirect immunofluorescence. Most investigators have attempted to show that absorbed heteroantiserum fails to react with extracts of normal ovary, but only a few reports have considered the fact that ovarian carcinomas are thought to arise from the surface epithelium of the ovary which represents but a small fraction of the cells included in tissue homogenates used for precipitation or absorption. Few heteroantisera have been tested against tumors that arise from nonovarian tissues. Possibly the most useful information has concerned cross reactions between ovarian tumors from different individuals. One antigen has been limited to the tumor from a single individual [39], some have been found in 10% of patients [40] whereas others are more widely distributed. Antisera raised against serous cystadenocarcinomas have often reacted with tumors of both serous and mucinous histology. Some antisera prepared against mucinous tumors have produced antisera which will react only with mucinous tumors.

Antigens associated with epithelial cells at other sites in the body have been detected in ovarian carcinoma. Secretory component of IgA has been detected in cyst fluid [41] and a thermostable antigen of 365,000 daltons has been found in endocervical glands, bronchial serous glands and bile duct canniliculi as well as in columnar epithelium of ovarian neoplasms [42]. Mucinous cysts contain antigens that cross-react with normal gastric mucosa [43]. In several cases, antisera have been produced which recognize moieties that resemble carcinoembryonic antigen (CEA) or normal colonic antigen (NCA) [44]. Not surprisingly, even the antigens that are relatively specific for ovarian carcinoma are found within the cytoplasm, rather than at the cell surface. Cell surface antigens may prove particularly important for immunorecognition or immunotherapy *in situ*. Immunodiagnostic tests might, however, be based upon detection of antigens that are either shed from the cell surface, secreted from cisternae of endoplasmic reticulum or released following breakdown of degenerating tumor cells. As Cantarow and associates have pointed out, early detection requires markers that are (1) present in serum, (2) detectable in patients with localized disease and (3) specific for ovarian cancer. Monitoring requires markers that (1) are present in serum and (2) reflect accurately the amount of tumor present [45].

At present heteroantisera have been utilized to isolate several antigens but radioimmunoassays exist for only two ovarian tumor associated antigens: OCAA [46, 47] and OCA [48–51]. Neither is sufficiently specific to meet Cantarow's requirements for early detection, but both may prove useful for monitoring advanced disease. OCAA is found in the cytoplasm of serous and mucinous cystadenocarcinomas, but has not been associated with benign cystadenomas or the surface epithelium of normal ovary [46, 47]. OCAA is a high molecular weight glycoprotein that is soluble in perchloracetic acid and exhibits beta electrophoretic mobility. The antigen is unrelated to AFP or ferritin but shows partial cross-reactivity with CEA [47]. About 70% of the ovarian carcinoma patients with advanced disease have OCAA levels greater than 10 ng per ml of serum. Approximately 30%–33% of advanced colon, breast and cervical carcinoma patients have similar levels of OCAA by radioimmunoassay [47]. Although not specific for ovarian carcinoma, the OCAA assay may hold promise for monitoring the progression or regression of disease under treatment. Among 15 patients followed serially for one to 26 months by Bhattacharya and Barlow, OCAA levels correlated with clinical disease in approximately 60%. In two patients rising OCAA levels preceeded clinical recurrence by 3.5 to 4 months [47].

OCA is another high molecular weight glycoprotein which is associated with serous, mucinous and 'epidermoid' carcinomas of the ovary. OCA was originally purified by Knauf and Urbach from a perchloroacetic acid extract of a saline homogenate of ovarian tumor tissue utilizing its affinity for the lectin concanavalin-A and its lack of affinity for antibodies directed against normal ovary or against normal female serum [48]. Antibodies raised in rabbits against partially purified OCA were then used to extract OCA from the serum of patients with ovarian cancer. OCA shares determinants with CEA, although the two molecules differ in mobility on electrophoresis in polyacrylamide gel or agar [49]. With the development of a radioimmunoassay, no correlation was found between serum levels of OCA and CEA. Among 77 ovarian cancer patients, 28% had elevated CEA levels, whereas 60% had elevated OCA titers. OCA could be detected in serum from 10% of normal individuals and from 10% of patients with benign ovarian disease, but levels were not elevated in pregnancy [50]. If one accepts normal levels below 1.8 nanograms per ml and abnormal levels above 1.9 ng/ml, the antigen is elevated in 78% of Stage I ovarian carcinoma patients and in a similar fraction of patients with more advanced disease [51].

In an attempt to separate OCA from CEA activity definitively, a 70,000 dalton moiety NB/70K was isolated from OCA [52]. NB/70K is stable in $0.6\,M$ perchloracetic acid, binds to concanavalin-A, and migrates on electrophoresis with an alpha mobility. This antigen does not cross-react with normal serum, normal ovary, normal lung or CEA. A radioimmunoassay has been developed for NB/70K and it remains to be seen whether this antigen will provide more precise identification of ovarian cancer patients. Hollinshead had found an ovarian tumor-associated antigen of 78,000 molecular weight which reacted with serous, mucinous and undifferentiated carcinomas, but not with a variety of other neoplastic and normal adult or fetal tissues [53]. The relationship of the two antigens is not certain.

The observation that ascites from patients with ovarian carcinoma contains sizeable amounts of antigen–antibody complexes has permitted a different approach to the isolation of tumor-associated antigen. Dorsett *et al.* detected IgG and C3 on the surface of ovarian tumor cells from ascites, but found little free antibody in ascitic fluid [54]. When immunoglobulins were isolated from antigen–antibody complexes in ascites, specific binding to the cytoplasm and surface membrane of ovarian carcinoma cells could be demonstrated by indirect immunofluorescence. Imunoglobulin did not bind to normal ovaries or nonovarian tissues. Approximately 70% of ovarian effusions contained specific immunoglobulin complexed with antigen(s) [55]. The antibodies did not react with CEA, ferritin or alpha fetoprotein. Using the antigen from antigen–antibody complexes, a 64,000 dalton moiety has been obtained by Stolbach and associates, which is distinct from albumin and which has been designated immunogenic ovarian tumor antigen (IOTA) [56]. Antibodies against IOTA bound to cells from each of 9 ovarian carcinomas, but not to normal ovaries, benign ovarian tumors or eight nonovarian cancers. Injection of antigen into rabbits produced an antibody that could be absorbed with normal ovarian tissue and that would bind to ovarian tumor cells. Using the rabbit antibody, 11 of 19 ovarian carcinoma fluids contained antigen, compared to 2 of 13 fluids from patients with nonovarian malignancy [57].

Application of somatic cell hybridization to the production of monoclonal immunoglobulins has revolutionized the production of heteroantisera against a variety of antigens [58]. Mice can be immunized with human tumor cells. Under ordinary circumstances, spleen cells from these animals which produce antibody would die within a few weeks in tissue culture. Fusion of immune spleen cells with a murine myeloma line has permitted formation of stable somatic cell hybrids. Each hybridoma can grow progressively *in vitro* or *in vivo* to produce essentially unlimited amounts of a single, homogenous antibody that does not require absorption. Hybridomas can be selected and cloned to obtain antibodies of virtually any desired specificity, avidity and subclass found in immune murine serum.

Recently, monoclonal antibodies have been prepared against cell surface determinants of human ovarian carcinoma. A murine IgGl monoclonal antibody (OC125) has been developed which reacts with each of six epithelial ovarian carcinoma cell lines and with cryopreserved tumor tissue from 12 of 20 ovarian cancer patients [59]. By contrast, the antibody does not bind to a variety of nonmalignant tissues, including adult and fetal ovary. OC125 reacts with only one of fourteen cell lines derived from nonovarian neoplasms and has failed to react with sections from 12 nonovarian carcinomas. Preliminary data indicate the OC125 binds to a cell surface antigen of >100,000 daltons [60]. The antigen does not co-precipitate CEA [59]. Additional evidence against CEA-like activity has been obtained by studying the reactivity of OC125 with a larger panel of ovarian tumors [61]. OC125 reacts with a majority of malignant serous cystadenocarcinomas and benign serous cystadenomas as well as a majority of undifferentiated tumors. No reactivity could be obtained with mucinous cystadenocarcinomas and cystadenomas, many of which should synthesize CEA. It is not yet known whether the antigen recognized by OC125 can be detected in peripheral blood of ovarian cancer patients, but the monoclonal technology should prove quite useful for the development of tests to detect and monitor ovarian cancer.

Antigens useful for diagnosis must both be specific and appear in blood at early stages of the disease. At present, radioimmunoassays exist for only two ovarian tumor-associated antigens. One can detect shed tumor products in approximately 60%–70% of patients with Stage I or II disease. In the case of OCA, however, antigen can also be detected in approximately 10% of normal individuals without apparent malignancy. Use of monoclonal antibodies may permit the identification of epitopes or antigenic determinants that would not be found in normal adult serum or plasma. Nevertheless, tests for following known ovarian malignancy might be based upon detecting antigens that are found on normal ovarian tissue, as the first step in therapy of advanced disease generally involves bilateral total salpingo-oophorectomy. For serotherapy, either tumor-specific or organ-specific antibodies could prove useful, provided that they did not bind to antigens found on non-ovarian tissues or in serum or plasma. Antigens that remain fixed to the cell surface may be particularly appropriate targets for serotherapy as well as for the delivery of toxins, drugs or isotopes using specific antibodies. Cell surface antigens are also likely to be appropriate targets for immunolocalization using antibodies that have been labelled with trace amounts of radioisotope.

CEA associated with tumors has been used as a target for radionuclide scanning, using a conventional anti-CEA heteroantiserum labelled with $^{131}$I [62]. Among 13 patients with ovarian carcinoma, each of the 13 primary tumors could be localized. Metastases were identified in 6 of 9 cases, whereas only two of these six cases showed metastases by more conventional techniques, including CT scan and ultrasound. Successful localization of tumor depended upon a tumor size greater than 2 cm and a CEA content greater than 150 nanograms per gram of tissue. Administration of radiolabelled normal goat serum failed to produce an image suggesting that this effect was indeed due to binding of antibody to tissue, rather than to nonspecific trapping of antibody or antigen–antibody complexes within the tumor. Given large quantities of homogeneous monoclonal reagents with high affinity for other antigens associated with ovarian carcinomas, even more precise localization of small tumors may be possible.

## 3. IMMUNOCOMPETENCE

### 3.1. Immunocompetence of ovarian cancer patients

The immuncompetence of ovarian cancer patients is compromised by their underlying malignancy, by malnutrition, and by the treatment that they receive. In many studies, general immunocompetence has been measured rather than specific reactivity with tumor cells or pathogenic microorganisms. Levels of T cells have been measured *in vitro* by 'E' rosette formation. Lymphocyte response to mitogens or to lymphocytes from other donors has been taken as an index of T cell function. The ability to develop contact allergy to dinitrochlorobenzene or dinitrofluorobenzene as well as the ability to recall delayed cutaneous reactivity to protein antigens such as purified protein derivative of old tuberculin (PPD) reflects not only T cell reactivity, but also the ability of monocytes to migrate to the site of antigen deposition. B cells have been enumerated, immunoglobulins measured and the specific humoral response monitored following immunization with novel antigens such as keyhole limpet hemocyanin. In some studies, it has been possible to measure specific reactivity of lymphocytes or antibodies with tumor cells. However, there have been only a few reports where reactivity with autologous tumor has been studied, rather than reactivity with cell lines established from the tumors of other patients.

### 3.2. Nonspecific parameters of immunocompetence

When immunocompetence has been assessed prior to therapy, defects in B cell numbers and function were found in patients with ovarian carcinoma [63]. Peripheral blood lymphocytes which bear surface immunoglobulins were reduced, the proliferative response to pokeweed mitogen was diminished and the formation of antibody was decreased following immunization with keyhole limpet hemocyanin. At this stage of disease, T cell function was relatively intact. Similar B cell defects are observed in chronic lymphocytic leukemia, multiple myeloma and some cases of non-Hodgkin's lymphoma, but B cell function is generally intact in patients with solid tumors prior to treatment [13].

In addition to the immunological defects associated with the underlying malignancy, various therapeutic modalities can further compromise the immunocompetence of the host. Both T and B cell levels were decreased in the peripheral blood of patients undergoing total abdominal or pelvic irradiation [64]. Lymphocytes are among the few cell types which undergo interphase death following exposure to ionizing radiation. Lymphoid tissues including the thymus need not be radiated directly to produce immunosuppression. Lymphocytes may be damaged as they pass beneath the radiation portal. Cell-mediated cytotoxicity (CMC) of peripheral blood mononuclear cells for allogeneic tumor targets has been observed following delivery of approximately 1000 R. Decreased CMC persisted for 4–6 weeks, particularly in patients with Stage I or Stage II ovarian carcinoma. Other immune functions eventually recover following radiotherapy. By three years after pelvic irradiation, DNCB reactivity has returned to normal limits, as have circulating lymphocyte counts and immunoglobulin levels [65].

Chemotherapeutic agents are also immunosuppressive [13]. Intermittent chemotherapy generally compromises immunological function less than continuous treatment. Among the alkylating agents, cyclophosphamide is generally more immunosuppressive than 2-phenylalanine mustard. At very low dosage, cyclophosphamide affects B cells and monocytes to a greater extent than T cells. At higher dosage, both B and T cell levels are reduced. Suppressor T cells may be more susceptible to low doses of cyclophosphamide than are T cells with helper phenotype and function. Doxorubicin (Adriamycin®) has had little effect upon reactivity to contact allergens or upon the ability of peripheral blood lymphocytes to proliferate in response to mitogens or to histoincompatible cells. In murine systems, doxorubicin has decreased T cell-dependent production of antibodies, but has had little impact on other T cell-mediated reactions, or upon the antitumor activity of macrophages. Cis-dichlorodiaminplatinum (II) (CDDP) can suppress human lymphocyte reactivity to mitogens both *in vitro* and *in vivo*. In mice, CDDP inhibits allograft rejection, graft *versus* host disease and the humoral response to sheep erythrocytes. Little is known regarding the immunosuppressive properties of hexamethylmelamine, another agent used against ovarian carcinoma.

Surgical procedures and anesthetic agents suppress the immune response nonspecifically [13]. Both T and B cell levels are reduced transiently. Lymphocyte proliferation in the presence of mitogens or protein antigens is reduced maximally at approximately one week and generally returns to normal within a month. Reactivity to skin test antigens recovers within two to three weeks. The stress of surgery may stimulate release of hormones including glucocorticoids, as well as the synthesis of acute phase reactants. In patients undergoing elective hysterectomy, use of general anesthetics has been associated with lymphopenia, leukocytosis and elevated plasma cortisol, whereas little change in leukocyte counts or cortisol levels has occurred when the same procedures were performed under epidural anesthesia. Levels of acute phase reactants are increased following operative stress. In addition, suppressor macrophages have been detected following surgical trauma.

In patients with advanced ovarian cancer, reactivity to the contact allergen dinitrofluorobenzene as well as recall of delayed cutaneous reactivity to skin test antigens is reduced. Decreased reactivity may reflect defects in monocyte chemotaxis as well as T cell function. Some 60% of patients with Stage III and IV disease were unable to respond to dinitrofluorobenzene and 64% were anergic to a battery of seven protein antigens. Prognosis appeared related to immunocompetence judged by both assays [66]. When *in vitro* assays were evaluated, the percentage of lymphocytes in gradient-derived cell suspensions and the absolute lymphocyte count were more useful in predicting prognosis of gynecologic cancer patients than were mitogen stimulation, mixed lymphocyte reactivity or T and B cell number [67]. Poor prognosis correlated with a low percentage of lymphocytes which remained at the interface of a Ficoll-Hypaque gradient. The decrease in lymphocyte percentage reflected both a decrease in lymhpocyte number and alteration in lymphocyte density [67].

Local factors within ascitic fluid may be particularly important in regulating growth of tumor as single cells or small clumps in suspension. Levels of 'E' rosettes and zymosan (C') rosettes as well as natural killer activity are lower within ascites than in peripheral blood [68]. Adherent and nonadherent suppressor cells have also been isolated from the tumor-associated lymphocytes of patients exhibiting decreased natural killer function [68]. Recent studies suggest that nonadherent nonphagocytic lymphocytes may be important suppressors of NK [69]. Ascites also contains a humoral suppressor of natural killer activity.

When compared to ascitic fluid associated with hepatic cirrhosis, ovarian carcinoma fluid contains higher levels of fibrinogen, total protein, antithrombin III, anti-trypsin activity, fibrin-split products and plasminogen activator [70]. Nonspecific suppressor factors have been detected in the serum [71] or ascites [72-77] which can inhibit the *in vitro* response of normal lymphocytes to phytohemaglutinin. One macromolecular fraction obtained from ascites inhibits the development of murine antibody producing cells *in vitro* [75]. A similar fraction of ascites suppresses natural killer activity, but not antibody-dependent cell-mediated cytotoxicity [76]. A lower molecular weight fraction has also been described which stimulated production of plaque forming cells, but not mixed lymphocyte reactions. Suppression of T cell responses has been observed with ascites from 12 of 26 patients with ovarian carcinoma. Both the response to phytohemaglutinin and to allogeneic lymphocytes has been inhibited by a factor of 40-80,000 daltons and of pK 4.4 to 4.8 [72]. The factor migrates with albumin and alpha-globulin, but is separable from albumin by affinity chromatography. A similar moiety can be purified from nonmalignant effusions, suggesting that the factor is produced by the host in response to malignancy, rather than by the tumor itself. The factor is noncytotoxic and inhibits proliferation of both B and T lymphoblastoid lines, but not cell lines derived from nonlymphocytic tissue [73]. Lymphoblastoid cell lines either absorb or destroy the activity at 37 °C, but not at 4 °C. A low molecular weight moiety, similar to immunoregulatory peptide, could not be isolated from this preparation. Factors isolated from ovarian carcinoma ascites are similar to the glycoprotein of pI 3.0 and molecular weight 50,000 isolated by Tamura et al. from ascites of a patient with gastric carcinoma. By immunodiffusion and immunoelectrophoresis this substance is indistinguishable from human alpha-1 acid glycoprotein and suppresses proliferation of lymphocytes to mitogens and alloantigens in vitro. One or more of these factors may help to account for the decreased proliferation of lymphocytes from the peripheral blood of patients with ovarian carcinoma [78] and particularly for the decrease in reactivity of tumor-associated lymphocytes isolated from ascites.

Monocytes and macrophages within ascites might either inhibit or stimulate tumor growth. Inhibition or stimulation of tumor growth may depend upon the state of macrophage activation, the ratio of macrophages to tumor cells and the accessibility of tumor cells to direct contact with macrophages. Macrophages that have been activated by pretreatment with lymphokines, endotoxins or interferon can kill tumor cells nonspecifically. In addition, activated macrophages can destroy tumor cells that have been coated with specific antibody. Conversely, macrophages can secrete factors which stimulate proliferation of antigen-triggered B lymphocytes and which stimulate proliferation of a variety of tumors [79]. Depletion of macrophages from ovarian tumor ascites has decreased the formation of ovarian tumor colonies in clonogenic assays [80, 81]. Removal of plastic adherent, phagocytic cells reduced clonogenicity in eight of nine specimens. Clonogenicity could be restored by adding macrophages to a feeder layer in the same cultures [82]. The addition of indomethacin to cultures decreased clonogenicity by inhibiting $PGE_2$ and $PGF_2$ production. In this assay, macrophages were separated from tumor cells by agar suggesting that stimulation of tumor growth was mediated by a diffusable substance, possibly a prostaglandin. When excessive numbers of adherent cells were added to cultures, clonogenicity of tumor declined [83].

Mantovani et al. [84] have isolated mononuclear cells from the peripheral blood and ascites of ovarian carcinoma patients and have obtained peripheral blood and peritoneal washings from patients with benign gynecologic disorders. Peripheral blood and tumor-associated macrophages from cancer patients were significantly less cytotoxic than controls against the SV40 transformed TU5 kidney line. Ovarian tumor cells from different patients differed with regard to susceptibility to macrophage cytotoxicity: seven patients were susceptible, four were resistant. In those cases where tumor was resistant, addition of macrophages stimulated tumor growth. Of four autologous combinations, macrophages were inhibitory in two of the four cases, suggesting that the susceptibility of tumor cells may be important as well as the number of macrophages and their functional status [84]. In additional studies [85], macrophages isolated from human ovarian carcinoma ascites either stimulated or inhibited tritiated thymidine incorporation into tumor cells depending upon the cell line used as target, the effector to target ratio, the incubation time, and the presence or absence of exogeneous antibody. No cytostatic activity was observed against the TLX9 lymphoma or the K562 leukemia line in the absence of antibody. However, 8 of 12 ascites preparations exerted ADCC activity against TLX9. Eight out of 12 inhibited line E cells at an effector to target ratio of 35:1. Significant stimulation was observed in 11 of 22 patients at an effector to target ratio of 7:1 [85]. Peripheral blood monocytes from patients with advanced ovarian cancer had decreased ability to kill tumor and an impaired capacity to mature *in vitro* into macrophages. Interferon, lymphokines, and endotoxin enhanced the cytotoxic activity of peritoneal cells from patients with ovarian cancer in a manner comparable to controls. Two of four patients had similar responsiveness in tumor relative to ascites. Interferon augmented the cytolytic activity of ascites and tumor-associated lymphocytes for killing K562. Lysis of autologous as well as allogeneic cells was increased. The ability of tumor-associated macrophages to respond to inductive stimuli provides at least one rationale for the use of bacterial immunostimulants or interferon to treat ovarian carcinoma. As T inducer (helper) cells regulate the activity of macrophages, suboptimal activation of peritoneal cells suggests that T inducer function may either be inadequate or offset by suppressor cells or substances in ascites.

*3.3. Evidence for specific immune response to ovarian cancer*

Several investigators have sought specific interactions of human ovarian carcinoma cells with lymphocytes or antibodies. Extracts of tumor have failed to stimulate lymphocyte proliferation in tissue culture, despite reactivity of lymphocytes with mitogens [86]. Migration of leukocytes from each of eight patients with mucinous or serous cystadenocarcinomas was inhibited by autologous tumor extracts [87]. Leukocyte migration was not inhibited by extracts from squamous cell carcinoma of the cervix, leiomyosarcoma of the uterus or a mixed mesodermal tumor. However, reactivity to both serous and mucinous extracts was observed with leukocytes from five of seven patients with ovarian carcinoma [87] consistent with the presence of the same antigen in both histological types. Potassium chloride extracts were particularly effective in leukocyte migration inhibition (LMI) [88]. Potassium chloride proved superior to saline, perchloroacetic acid or deoxycholate for solubilizing tumor membrane associated antigen. LMI in the presence of ovarian tumor extracts was observed with leukocytes from 11 of

17 patients with ovarian carcinoma compared to 3 of 17 patients with other nonovarian tumors [88]. Reactivity was not related to disease stage. Ovarian patients showed minimal reactivity to extracts of breast, colon or endometrial carcinoma. The antigen appeared to be of high molecular weight on Sephadex® G-200 chromatography. Approximately 20 times more concentrated control extract was required to produce LMI with leukocytes from patients with breast or colon cancer. LMI has also been observed by Melnick and Barber in six of seven patients with serous cystadenocarcinomas. No inhibition was observed with cells from patients with endometrial carcinoma, teratocarcinoma or benign ovarian neoplasms [89]. Leukocyte migration *enhancement* (LME) was found in the presence of autologous plasma in 15 of 18 cancer patients, including five ovarian patients with persistent disease, but in only 4 of 15 controls. Amniotic fluid and pregnancy plasma enhanced autologous leukocyte migration in pregnancy [90, 91]. Cancer plasma, but not amniotic fluid enhanced leukocyte migration in different gynecologic cancers. Only one patient among 18 showed immune complexes in plasma by the Raji cell assay. No apparent correlation of LME with IgG, C3, or protein was found. By adding autologous tumor homogenate to autologous plasma, however, LME was converted into LMI. Anti-IgG antibody also decreased LME, suggesting that an immunoglobulin which could react with tumor-associated antigen was responsible for stimulating migration of leukocytes.

Peripheral blood lymphocytes from patients with ovarian carcinoma and cervical carcinoma can destroy ovarian and cervical carcinoma lines respectively [92, 93, 94]. The cytotoxic effect was expressed within the first 72 hours of culture. Peripheral blood lymphocytes from normal individuals also destroyed tumor cells, but cytotoxicity was expressed only after 96 hours. In all, 47 of 54 patients with ovarian carcinoma in DiSaia's series lysed an allogeneic ovarian tumor cell line in the first 72 hours. Some 37 of 42 patients with cervical carcinoma had peripheral blood lymphocytes that lysed a cervical carcinoma cell line. Cytotoxic lymphocytes also lysed a fetal gut cell line. Interestingly, lymph node lymphocytes from patients with tumor were not effective. Earlier studies by the Hellstroms had documented blocking factors in the serum of patients with progressively growing tumor that inhibited lymphocyte-mediated cytotoxicity *in vitro*. No blocking activity could be detected in DiSaia's studies, but Patillo *et al.* [95, 96] demonstrated blocking factor(s) in the serum of 18 advanced ovarian carcinoma patients. In eight of these patients, blocking factor decreased concomitant with achieving a complete clinical response to chemotherapy. In 10 patients blocking factors persisted and were associated with disease progression.

Antibodies that would lyse a human ovarian carcinoma cell line in the presence of guinea pig complement have been found in serum from five of eight patients with ovarian carcinoma [97]. Ovarian neoplasms also contained IgG, IgA and IgM, whereas only IgG could be detected in sections of normal ovary [98]. Prior to treatment, 68% of sera from 14 ovarian cancer patients were not cytotoxic for ovarian tumor cultures, 26% showed weak clumping and only 6% damaged cells markedly [99].

Despite isolation of IOTA from 'immune complexes' in ascites, conflicting data exist with regard to the prevalence of tumor-specific or nonspecific complexes in peripheral blood. Fulton *et al.* [100] attempted to precipitate all immune complexes with polyethylene glycol and assayed their content of immunoglobulin by radial immunodiffusion. Ovarian carcinoma patients in relapse had higher serum immune complex levels than did patients in remission who, in turn, were comparable to controls. Sequential studies in three patients indicated an increase in immune complexes which antedated clinical evidence of recurrence. By contrast, no complexes were detected when immune complexes were measured by Clq binding, Clq binding inhibition or Raji cell assay [101]. If complexes are present, they are likely to contain antibodies from immunoglobulin classes and subclasses that do not fix complement. The presence of immune complexes has also been confirmed by Clayton *et al.* [102], where higher levels have been found during relapse than in clinical remission. The reappearance of immune complexes antedates the detection of disease by more conventional methods. Whether or not the immune complexes contain tumor-associated antigens remains to be determined. Regardless of their antigen content, immune complexes with IgG can block Fc receptors of K cells and macrophages. Either specific or nonspecific immune complexes might affect the ability of patients to respond to serotherapy if ADCC is an important effector mechanism.

## 4. IMMUNOTHERAPY

### 4.1. Immunotherapy of ovarian carcinoma

Traditionally, immunotherapy has been divided into two categories – active and passive. In active immunotherapy, bacterial immunostimulants and tumor cell vaccines have been given directly to the cancer patient to stimulate endogenous immunity, whereas in passive immunotherapy, antibodies, lymphocytes or extracts of lymphoreticular cells have been transferred from putatively immune donors to the cancer patient to provide exogenous immunity. Both approaches have been tried in ovarian carcinoma. Nevertheless, most experiences, to date, has been with active immunotherapy using nonspecific immunostimulants with or without allogeneic tumor cells as a vaccine. Recently, trials have been initiated with specific heteroantisera. Monoclonal antibodies should soon be available to permit a more thorough evaluation of specific serotherapy. There has been no systematic attempt to use passive transfer of lymphoreticular cells.

## 4.2. Active immunotherapy of human ovarian carcinoma

In the early years of this century, Dr William B. Coley used toxins isolated from *Streptococcus pyogenes* and *Serratia marcescens* to treat a variety of malignant diseases. Mixed toxins were generally administered subcutaneously or intravenously, although in one patient Coley's toxins were administered intraperitoneally. Each of seven patients reviewed by Nauts [103] appeared to benefit from treatment with increased performance status and with either a decrease in ascites or objective regression of a tumor mass. In four of these seven cases, survival exceeded 10 years, despite the documentation of widespread disease prior to immunotherapy [103].

More recent trials have utilized immunostimulants including Freund's adjuvant, Bacillus Calmette-Gerin (BCG) and *Corynebacterium parvum*. Graham and Graham [104, 105] treated a total of 232 patients with gynecologic malignancies, using vaccines containing Freund's complete adjuvant (CFA) which included heat-killed mycobacteria within a water-in-oil emulsion. CFA was mixed either with intact, living tumor cells or with a DNA-protein extract of tumor. Among those who received vaccines were 48 patients with ovarian carcinoma. Vaccination caused persistent ulceration at the site of injection, but few systemic symptoms. Patients who failed to react to the vaccine seemed to have a worse prognosis than those who developed local tissue reactions, but there was no significant effect of vaccination on tumor growth.

BCG, the tuberculosis vaccine, has been administered to ovarian cancer patients by a variety of routes including intradermal [106-108] intralymphatic [109] and intraperitoneal [109, 110] injection. BCG has been given alone or in combination with an allogeneic tumor cell vaccine [107]. In one pilot study [107] ten patients with stage III-IV ovarian carcinoma were treated with alkylating agents and a vaccine consisting of $10^7$ allogeneic irradiated tumor cells and $2 \times 10^6$ Glaxo BCG split between four intradermal sites. Chemotherapy was administered midway between inoculations. Survival of treated patients was compared retrospectively to an historical control group treated with chemotherapy alone. Actuarial survival was significantly prolonged at $p = 0.005$. Median survival was estimated in excess of 24 months, compared with a 24-month survival of approximately 10% of patients. Patients were chosen who exhibited 'static' disease for at least three months. The immunotherapy did not appear to help two patients with progressive disease who were eliminated from pilot data prior to statistical analysis. As Brandes [111] has noted, however, even if one accepts the censored data, both the controls and patients who received immunotherapy were given a variety of different chemotherapeutic agents rather than any standard treatment regimen. Stage and grade of disease may also not be comparable. Without concurrent, randomized controls who received similar therapy, it is not possible to judge the efficacy of treatment.

The Southwest Oncology Group has conducted a concurrently controlled, randomized trial in patients with Stage III and Stage IV ovarian carcinoma comparing chemotherapy with cyclophosphamide and doxorubicin to a combination of similar chemotherapy with BCG administered by scarification [112]. With follow-up available on 121 patients, 18% of those who had received the combination treatment with immunotherapy and chemotherapy had a pathologically proven complete response to treatment, whereas only 3% of the patients receiving chemotherapy alone had experienced a similar response ($p<0.01$). The sum of complete & partial responses for combination therapy (56%) was not significantly different ($p = 0.12$) from the CR + PR rate for chemotherapy alone (43%). The median survival duration of patients receiving the combination (22.3 months) was significantly better ($p<0.03$) than that for patients who received chemotherapy alone (13.7 months).

Phase I studies have documented the side effects associated with *C. parvum* intraperitoneally [113–116], intravenously [117, 118] and subcutaneously [119]. Toxicity was evaluated in 341 courses of intravenous *C. parvum* and included chills, malaise, fever, nausea, vomiting and headache in a majority. Alterations in blood pressure, fever in excess of 38.6 °C, diarrhea and chest pain were found in a minority of patients [120]. Intraperitoneal administration of *C. parvum* has been complicated by chills, fever, mild nausea and abdominal pain. Decreases in blood pressure have been observed in patients who have been treated concomitantly with anti-hypertensive medication [115, 121].

In early studies [119], patients received *C. parvum* subcutaneously in escalating doses over 10–14 days. Cyclic chemotherapy with cyclophosphamide, doxorubicin and 5-fluorouracil (CAF) was then begun and repeated monthly. Maintenance *C. parvum* was given weekly during chemotherapy. Although pretreatment immune function was better in patients who had a good response to *C. parvum* and CAF (10 out of 12 were PPD positive) than in patients who had a poor response to the combination (4 out of 12 were PPD positive), immune function was not significantly improved during therapy. In a subsequent randomized study [122], immunotherapy plus CAF chemotherapy was compared to CAF chemotherapy alone in Stage III and IV ovarian carcinoma patients who had failed to respond to single agent chemotherapy with or without radiotherapy. The addition of intravenous *C. parvum* to CAF did not improve response rate, duration of remission or survival of advanced ovarian carcinoma patients.

More encouraging results have been obtained by Gall et al. [120] who treated 45 patients with Stage III disease following a maximal surgical effort to resect residual tumor. All patients received melphalan with or without *C. parvum* intravenously. Forty-five patients treated with a combination of chemotherapy and immunotherapy were compared to a group of 63 patients at other institutions who received melphalan alone. With a follow-up of 29–48 months, objective response to the combination treatment was 53% compared to 29% of patients receiving 2-PAM alone. The progression-free intervals were 16 and 6 months respectively. These data require confirmation in a concurrently controlled, randomized study. Monitoring of immunological parameters during the trial with melphalan and *C. parvum* indicated that patients whose disease remained stable had better delayed cutaneous reactivity, but that *C. parvum* did not affect primary delayed hypersensitivity to dinitrofluorobenzene, delayed hypersensitivity recall to standard reagents, 'E' rosette levels, C3 rosette levels, mitogen reactivity or total lymphocyte counts.

Direct contact between tumor cells and immunostimulants might achieve more convincing results. Webb et al. [114] administered intracavitary *C. parvum* to five ovarian cancer patients with malignant ascites or pleural effusion. Ascites regressed in each of the patients, but no definite effect was seen against solid tumor masses. In a subsequent study [116] eight patients with ovarian carcinoma with ascites refractory of chemotherapy were treated with 7–14 mg of *C. parvum* intraperitoneally on days 0, 7, 28 and then monthly. Three had no benefit, two experienced partial resolution, and three had complete resolution of ascites for 2, 6, and 13+ months. Again, no effect was seen on solid tumor masses. Monitoring of the ascites indicated that tumor cell numbers decreased by days 7–15. This observation was associated with a marked increase in polymorphonuclear leukocytes and a more modest increase in the number of macrophages. Natural killer cells in peripheral blood were not altered consistently. Pretreatment levels of natural killer activity in the peritoneum were usually low and were not altered by intraperitoneal *C. parvum* administration. In one patient with high levels of tumor-associated natural killers in ascites, *C. parvum* treatment actually decreased anti-tumor activity. The tumoricidal activity of macrophages was not enhanced and at 14–21 days following the first *C. parvum* treatment actually decreased.

By contrast the administration of *C. parvum* intraperitoneally to 12 patients without ascites, but with peritoneal implants of tumor that had resisted chemotherapy, resulted in the complete regression of nodules in 2 and partial regression in 3 [115]. Responses were confirmed by laparotomy or laparoscopy. In 3 of 8 patients natural killer activity was increased and in 6 of 8 antibody-dependent cell-mediated cytotoxicity was augmented. The difference in results between different studies may relate to the presence of inhibitors in ascites or to larger tumor burdens.

Interferons are glycoproteins produced by a variety of cells in response to viral infection or after treatment with certain chemicals [128]. Once formed, interferons can, in turn, inhibit viral replication in other cells and inhibit the proliferation of tumor cells, as well as normal tissues. Immunological resistance to tumor growth can also be affected by interferon which boosts 'natural killing' and macrophage mediated cytotoxicity. Preliminary data of Epstein [124] suggests that interferon derived from human leukocytes might inhibit ovarian tumor growth, particularly when cells are in the ascitic form. In three of four patients, interferon had a greater effect on cells taken directly from ascites than on cells dissociated from solid tumor [125]. One possible explanation for this observation is that interferon acts by reducing the ability of tumor-associated macrophages to stimulate clonogenic tumor growth, rather than by inhibiting proliferation of tumor cells by any direct interaction. There are anecdotal reports that the intravenous injection of interferon inhibits tumor growth in patients with ovarian cancer [126].

*4.3. Passive immunotherapy of human ovarian cancer*

Trials of serotherapy have also been undertaken in patients with ovarian cancer [127]. Antiserum has been prepared in rabbits by the injection of a macromolecular extract of human ovarian carcinomas. Seven patients have been treated with nonabsorbed, sterile, pyrogen-free rabbit heteroantiserum. In four patients reactivity of heteroantiserum with autologous tumor-associated antigens could be demonstrated by electrophoresis and in one the rabbit heteroantiserum bound to tumor cells by indirect immunofluorescence. The patients received from 45 to 200 cc of antiserum. Intravenous injection produced abdominal fullness and nausea when given as a bolus, but side effects were not observed when the heteroantiserum was given as a slow drip. Rabbit IgG persisted in the circulation for greater than 100 hours in five of six patients. Only mild side effects of rash and fever were observed. A trial has been begun [128] where radiotherapy and chemotherapy have been administered with or without serotherapy to Stage III ovarian carcinoma. Patients receive intraperitoneal $^{32}$P delayed split total abdominal irradiation and melphalan with or without the administration of 150–200 ml of ovarian anti-tumor serum. With follow-up of approximately two years, 4 of 6 patients in the combination plus serotherapy are disease-free compared to 6 of 7 patients treated by the radiation–melphalan combination alone. Three patients experienced hives and one had joint pain complicating antibody administration. The specificity of the antiserum has not been well characterized and it is not certain that the antibody reacts with a cell surface antigen. Finally, it is not clear that host-effector mechanisms, either complement, or antibody-dependent cell-mediated cytotoxicity, would be adequate to eliminate tumor cells.

### 4.4. Immunotherapy of murine ovarian carcinoma

Work with a murine ovarian carcinoma model suggests that the outcome of serotherapy might be improved by concomitant treatment with immunostimulants. The murine ovarian tumor (MOT) is a teratocarcinoma which arose spontaneously in a C3HeB/FeJ mouse and has been passed in ascites form [129]. Originally the tumor would not grow in allogeneic mice. With repeated passage, however, the tumor has lost expression of H-2 major histocompatibility antigens [130]. The murine ovarian carcinoma, like human ovarian cancer, grows progressively within the abdominal cavity, studs serosal surfaces, blocks diaphragmatic lymphatics, and produces ascites [131, 132].

A substantial amount of information has been gathered concerning the response of the murine ovarian carcinoma to chemotherapy and radiotherapy. The tumor responds to doxorubicin [133-135] and to methotrexate [135], particularly when the methotrexate is administered at high dosage with calcium leukovorin rescue [135]. Intraperitoneal administration of doxorubicin is more effective than intravenous injection [133, 134]. This observation appears to relate to higher levels of drug within the peritoneal cavity and relatively lower levels systemically. The tumor is marginally responsive to CDDP in some studies [136], but not in others [134, 137].

Total abdominal irradiation with up to 600R failed to alter the mortality which follows the intraperitoneal injection of $10^6$ cells [138]. On the other hand, intraperitoneal injection of $^{125}$IUDR starting 24 hours after the intraperitoneal injection of $10^6$ tumor cells may eliminate up to five logs of ovarian carcinoma [139]. The antitumor activity of the isotope may relate to the intranuclear incorporation of $^{125}$IUDR, with the release of densely ionizing low energy Auger electrons. The radioresponsiveness of the tumor to an agent that is incorporated during DNA synthesis suggests that a very small number of cells must be noncycling, consistent with Ozol's observation that the tumor shows a doubling time of 22 hours with a cell loss of 9% [134]. That $^{131}$IUDR failed to affect tumor growth is consistent with the fact that this isotope decays without the emission of Auger electrons or the development of a charge transfer reaction. Na$^{125}$I or nonradioactive IUDR were not toxic. Recently the intraperitoneal injection of $^{211}$Astatine-tellurium colloid ($^{211}$At) (5-50 millicuries) prolonged survival of mice given $10^6$ murine ovarian tumor cells intraperitoneally [140]. By contrast chromic $^{32}$phosphate failed to affect the growth of tumor. $^{211}$At emits alpha particles which are directly ionizing. The radiobiological effects are largely independent of oxygen and tumor is destroyed within several cell diameters of the emission.

The murine ovarian carcinoma responds to passive as well as active immunotherapy. Studies of serotherapy have been undertaken with heteroantiserum prepared in rabbits. When the murine ovarian carcinoma is grown in ascites form, a small population of host inflammatory cells is found in association with the majority of murine ovarian carcinoma cells. Injection of the mixed population into rabbits results in the appearance of antibodies that will bind to the tumor [141-143] and in some cases to spermatozoa, embryonic germ cells, and cells of preimplantation embryos [144]. Intraperitoneal injection of nonabsorbed antiserum 24 hours after the intraperitoneal injection of $10^4$ tumor cells into syngeneic mice resulted in 30-40% long-term survival, but there were early deaths apparently related to the toxicity of antibodies directed against normal tissue antigens [142]. Multiple doses of nonabsorbed antiserum proved lethal [143]. Absorption of heteroantiserum with spleen removed most antitumor activity. An antiserum (SG200) was subsequently produced by immunizing rabbits with a partially purified freeze-thaw extract of whole ascites tumor cells that had been partially purified by exclusion on a Sephadex G200 column. Three daily doses of SG200 produced 20% survival after the intraperitoneal injection of $10^6$ tumor cells. Against $10^4$ cells, 90% survival was obtained with treatment on days 1, 2, 6 and 7 following transplantation. Once again absorption with spleen cells substantially reduced the ability of SG200 to bind to MOT *in vitro* or to affect tumor growth *in vivo* [146], suggesting that at least some of the antibodies in the heteroantiserum recognized tumor-associated antigens that were also present on normal tissues.

A more specific heteroantiserum has been raised by immunizing rabbits with purified populations of murine ovarian carcinoma cells that had been freed from contaminating host leukocytes and erythrocytes [145]. Heteroantisera from rabbits immunized with the purified tumor cell suspensions consistently retained antitumor activity against the murine ovarian carcinoma *in vivo* and *in vitro*. Appropriately absorbed antisera failed to bind to fetal tissues or to adult spleen, ovary and kidney cells. However, even the more specific heteroantiserum exhibited only modest antitumor activity in mice that had received $10^6$ murine ovarian carcinoma cells intraperitoneally 24 hours prior to the initiation of serotherapy.

The success of serotherapy must depend, at least in part, upon the ability of the antibody to recruit and trigger host effector mechanisms, including complement-dependent cytotoxicity and antibody-dependent cell-mediated cytotoxicity (ADCC). Work with the SG200 heteroantiserum suggested that ADCC might be particularly important in the murine ovarian carcinoma model. Intraperitoneal administration of silica 24 hours following intraperitoneal tumor transplantation abrogated the antitumor activity of SG200 antiserum [143], consistent with the possibility that macrophages that phagocytize silica contributed to the destruction of tumor in the presence of specific heteroantiserum. Antitumor activity was also abrogated by treating twice with 250R total body irradiation, starting 24 hours before treatment with antiserum and just prior to transplantation of the tumor. Abrogation of the therapeutic activity of heteroantiserum depended upon the dose of irradiation: 400R total body irradiation was more effective than 150 or 250R [146]. Total abdominal irradiation (250R twice) had much less effect on the therapeutic activity of serum. Taken together, these studies suggest that phagocytic peritoneal cells with radiosensitive precursors are required to assure optimal antitumor activity of heteroantiserum.

In an attempt to augment serotherapy, administration of heteroantiserum has been combined with the injection of immunostimulants which would attract and activate peritoneal cells. Intraperitoneal administration of *C. parvum* can cure mice that have been given $10^4$ or $10^5$ murine ovarian carcinoma 24 hours earlier [137, 147, 148]. Nevertheless, *C. parvum* is no longer consistently effective following the intraperitoneal injection of $10^6$ tumor cells. Silica blocks the antitumor activity of *C. parvum* suggesting that activated macrophages may be important effectors [137]. Immunotherapy with a combination of *C. parvum* and specific heteroantiserum is significantly more effective than treatment with either single agent in prolonging the survival of mice that have received an intraperitoneal injection of syngeneic murine ovarian carcinoma cells. *In vitro* a combination of *C. parvum* activated peritoneal cells and specific heteroantiserum has proven significantly more effective than either single component in destroying $^{51}$Cr labelled MOT cells in the absence of complement. Activation of peritoneal cells to produce lysis of tumor in the presence of specific antiserum peaked 3–7 days after a single injection of *C. parvum* and declined to baseline over three to four weeks. With repeated intraperitoneal injections of *C. parvum* at appropriate intervals, activation of peritoneal cells could be prolonged and augmented. Among the routes tested, only intraperitoneal administration of *C. parvum* was effective, although activation of peritoneal cells in collaboration with heteroantiserum was observed over a broad range of intraperitoneal dosage. These data suggest that the administration of *C. parvum* by appropriate doses, routes and schedules can attract and activate a population of peritoneal effectors that mediate antibody-dependent cytotoxicity more effectively than resident peritoneal cells [148]. Approximately 90% of the effector activity is associated with adherent peritoneal cells, predominantly macrophages. If however, nonadherent lymphocytes are purified by removal of B cells and T cells, the null cell population is also effective in producing tumor lysis in the presence of specific heteroantiserum. Intact IgG is required; FAB$_2$ fragments fail to mediate tumor lysis. Adherence of antibody-coated tumor to monolayers is blocked by antigen–antibody complexes or aggregated IgG, but not by trypan blue or 2-deoxyglucose. The latter inhibitors can, however, prevent killing of tumor. All of these data are consistent with a model for ADCC in which IgG immunoglobulin acts as a bridge binding antibody-coated tumor to activated macrophages and null lymphocytes ('K' cells) which bear receptors for the Fc portion of IgG. Doses, routes, and schedules of *C. parvum* administration which augment serotherapy *in vivo* appear to stimulate ADCC *in vitro*. The observation that intraperitoneal injection of *C. parvum* in patients with ovarian cancer also stimulates ADCC [115, 121], suggests that it may also be possible to augment serotherapy in human ovarian cancer with immunostimulants. The development of monoclonal reagents with specificity for human ovarian cancer [59] may provide sufficient quantities of high titered specific heteroantiserum to permit such trials.

Alternatively, monoclonal antibodies may be used as a carrier for toxins, drugs or isotopes. Using the relatively crude SG200 antiserum as a carrier, it has been possible to prolong the survival of mice given $10^6$ murine ovarian carcinoma cells intraperitoneally with conjugates in which methotrexate is bound to immunoglobulin using a carbodiamide or mixed anhydride reaction [149]. Development of a monoclonal antibody against the murine ovarian carcinoma may provide a useful model for examining a variety of agents that may prove useful in treating cancer. With the development of monoclonal antibodies against human ovarian carcinoma the most promising conjugates could be evaluated in clinical trials.

## 5. CONCLUSION

From the preceeding discussion it appears that a number of different antigens can be associated with human ovarian carcinomas. Some antigens are shared with normal adult or fetal tissues, whereas others may be restricted to neoplastic ovarian tissues. Oncofetal antigens have not provided reliable markers for screening populations to detect occult ovarian carcinoma, but may prove useful in selected patients for monitoring persistent or recurrent disease. CEA has been elevated most frequently in sera from patients with epithelial ovarian carcinomas, particularly those of mucinous histology. AFP and hCG have proven useful in monitoring certain germ cell tumors. Despite the limitations of oncofetal antigens, the unique biology of ovarian carcinoma may facilitate the appearance of shed tumor products in the peripheral blood, permitting early immunodiagnosis of the malignancy. At least one shed tumor-associated antigen can be detected in the peripheral blood of a majority of patients with surgically resectable Stage I ovarian cancer. More specific markers will, however, be required to provide a useful screening test. Development of monoclonal antibodies against tumor-associated antigens should facilitate the search for more specific markers.

Early in the course of ovarian carcinoma the patient's own ability to make specific antibody is decreased. Immunocompetence is further compromised by surgical treatment, radiotherapy and chemotherapy as well as malnutrition. Peripheral blood lymphocytes from patients with advanced disease are altered in concentration, density and function. Delayed cutaneous reactivity is decreased *in vivo*. Not only T cell function, but also natural killing and macrophage mediated cytotoxicity are reduced. Changes are particularly marked among tumor-associated lymphocytes and macrophages in ascites. Both cellular and humoral suppressors have been found in ascites fluid.

Cell-mediated immunity to ovarian carcinoma cell lines or extracts has been documented *in vitro* using 72-hour microcytotoxicity, LMI and LME. Antibodies have also been detected, either free or in complex with antigen in peripheral blood and ascites of patients with ovarian carcinoma. Additional work will be required to define the specificity of these assays in larger numbers of patients using autologous tumor cells and extracts. Little is known of factors which regulate specific immunity to tumor-associated antigens.

Attempts to administer immunotherapy have met with modest success. Following encouraging early studies with Coley's toxins, other nonspecific immunostimulants have been administered to ovarian cancer patients, often in combination with cytotoxic chemotherapy. Systemic administration of BCG and *C. parvum* have improved response rates and survival in some studies, though not in others. Several investigators have observed antitumor activity when *C. parvum* has been administered intraperitoneally to assure direct contact with residual tumor deposits.

Trials of serotherapy have been initiated. Work with an animal model suggests that the efficacy of serotherapy might be improved by the concomitant administration of immunostimulants and antibody. Future trials will almost certainly utilize monoclonal antibodies which might either be used unaltered or be conjugated with cytotoxic drugs, toxins or isotopes to achieve complete elimination of tumor.

REFERENCES

1. Black PH: Shedding from the cell surface of normal and cancer cells. Adv Cancer Res 32:75–199, 1980.
2. Ohanian SH, Schlager SI: Humoral immune killing of nucleated cells: Mechanisms of complement-mediated attack and target cell defense. CRC Critical Reviews in Immunology 1:165–209, 1981.
3. Ritz J, Pesando JM, Notis-McConarty J, Schlossman SF: Modulation of human acute

lymphoblastic leukemia induced by monoclonal antibody *in vitro*. J Immunol 125:1506, 1980.
4. Stackpole CW, Jacobson JB: Antigenic modulation. Handbook of Cancer Immunology 2:55–159, 1978.
5. Benacerraf B, Unanue FR: Textbook of Immunology. Baltimore: Williams and Wilkens, 1979.
6. Reinherz EL, Schlossman SF: Regulation of the immune response-inducer and suppressor T-lymphocyte subsets in human beings. New England J Med 303:370–373, 1980.
7. Henney CS: Mechanisms of tumor cell destruction. In: Mechanisms of tumor immunity. Green I, Cohen S, McCluskey RT (eds). New York: John Wiley and Sons, 1977, pp 55–86.
8. Nathan CF, Murray HW, Cohn ZA: The macrophage as an effector cell. New Engl J Med 303:622–626, 1980.
9. Herberman RB, Ortaldo JR: Natural killer cells: Their role in defenses against disease. Science 214:24–30, 1981.
10. Bast RC Jr, Rapp HJ: The immunology of animal tumors. In: Immunological Diseases. Samter M (ed). Boston: Little Brown and Company, 1978 (3rd ed), pp 359–388.
11. Broder S, Waldmann TA: The suppressor cell network in cancer. New Engl J Med 299:1281–1284; 1335–1344, 1978.
12. Perry LL, Greene MI: T cell subset interactions in the regulation of syngeneic tumor immunity. Fed Proc 40:39–44, 1981.
13. Bast RC Jr: Effects of cancers and their treatment on host immunity. In: Cancer Medicine. Holland JF, Frei E III (eds). Philadelphia: Lea and Febiger, 1982 (2nd ed), pp1134–1174.
14. Knapp RC, Berkowitz RS, Leavitt T Jr: Natural history and detection of ovarian cancer. In: Gynecologic Oncology. Buchsbaum HJ (ed). Maryland: Harper and Row, 1980, Vol. 4, pp 1–14.
15. Van Nagell JR, Donaldson ES, Gay EC, Sharkey RM, Rayburn P, Goldenberg DM: Carcinoembryonic antigen in ovarian epithelial cystadenocarcinomas. The prognostic value of tumor and serial plasma determinations. Cancer 41:2335–2340, 1978.
16. Feldman GB, Knapp RC, Order SE, Hellman S: The role of lymphatic obstruction in the formation of ascites in a murine ovarian carcinoma. Cancer Res 32:1663–1666, 1972.
17. Parker LM, Griffiths CT, Yankee RA, Canellos GP, Gelman R, Knapp RC, Richman CM, Tobias JS, Weiner RS, Frei E III: Combination chemotherapy with adriamycin-cyclophosphamide for advanced ovarian carcinoma. Cancer 46:669–674, 1980.
18. Longo DL, Young RC: The natural history and treatment of ovarian cancer. Ann Rev Med 32:475–490, 1981.
19. Bast RC Jr, Zbar B, Borsos T, Rapp HJ: BCG and cancer. New Engl J Med 290:1413–1420; 1458–1469, 1974.
20. Bast RC Jr, Bast BS, Rapp HJ: Critical review of previously reported animal studies of tumor immunotherapy with nonspecific immunostimulants. Ann New York Acad Sci 277:60–93, 1976.
21. Oettgen HF, Hellstrom KE: Tumor immunology. In: Cancer Medicine. Holland JF, Frei E III (eds). Boston: Lea and Febiger, 1982 (2nd ed), pp 1029–1067.
22. Zamcheck W, Kupchik HZ: Summary of clinical use and limitations of the carcinoembryonic antigen assay and some methodological considerations. In: Manual of Clinical Immunology. Rose NR, Friedman H (eds). Washington D.C.: American Society for Microbiology, 1980 (2nd ed), pp 919–935.
23. Stall KE, Martin EW: Plasma carcinoembryonic antigen levels in ovarian cancer patients: A chart review and survey of published data. J Reprod Med 26:75–79, 1981.
24. Donaldson ES, Van Nagell JR, Pursell S, Gay EC, Meeker WR, Kashmiri R, Van de

Voorde J: Multiple biochemical markers in patients with gynecologic malignancies. Cancer 45:948-853, 1980.
25. Khoo SK, Whitaker S, Jones I, Mackay E: Predictive value of serial carcinoembryonic antigen levels in long-term follow-up of ovarian cancer. Cancer 43:2471-2478, 1979.
26. Marchand A, Ferroglio CM, Pascal R, Richart RM, Bennett S: Carcinoembryonic antigens in human ovarian neoplasms. Cancer Res 35:3807-3810, 1975.
27. Khoo SK, Whitaker S, Jones ISC, Mackay EV: Carcinoembryonic antigen in patients with residual ovarian cancer. Clinical and pathological correlations. Gynecol Oncol 7:288-295, 1979.
28. Van Nagell JR, Donaldson ES, Gay EC, Sharkey RM, Rayburn P, Goldenberg DM: Carcinoembryonic antigens in ovarian epithelial cystadenocarcinomas. The prognostic value of tumor and serial plasma determinations. Cancer 41:2335-2340, 1978.
29. McIntire KR, Waldmann TA: Measurement of alpha fetoprotein. In: Manual of Clinical Immunology. Rose NR, Friedman H (eds). Washington D.C.: American Society for Microbiology, 1980 (2nd ed), pp 936-943.
30. Van Nagell JR Jr, Donaldson ES, Hanson MB, Gay EC, Pavlik EJ: Biochemical markers in the plasma and tumors of patients with gynecologic malignancies. Cancer 48:495-503, 1981.
31. Malkin A, Kellen JA, Kickrish GM, Bush RS: Carcinoembryonic antigen (CEA) and other tumor markers in ovarian and cervical cancer. Cancer 42:1452-1456, 1978.
32. Stanhope CR, Smith JP, Britton JC, Crosley PK: Serial determination of marker substances in ovarian cancer. Gynecol Onc 8:284-287, 1979.
33. Levi MM, Parshley MS, Mandl I: Antigenicity of papillary serous cystadenocarcinoma tissue culture cells. Am J Obstet Gynecol 102:433-439, 1968.
34. Levi MM: Antigenicity of ovarian and cervical malignancies with a view toward possible immunodiagnosis. Am J Obstet Gynecol 109:689-698, 1971.
35. Gall SA, Walling J, Pearl J: Démonstration of tumor-associated antigens in human gynecologic malignancies. Am J Obstet Gynecol 115:387-393, 1973.
36. Dorsett BH, Ioachim HL: Common antigenic component in ovarian carcinomas: Demonstration by double diffusion and immunofluorescence techniques. Immunol Communic 2:173-184, 1973.
37. Ioachim HL, Dorsett BH, Sabbath M, Andersson BS, Barber HRK: Antigenic and morphologic properties of ovarian carcinoma. Gynecol Onc 1:130-142, 1973.
38. Order SE, Thurston J, Knapp R: Ovarian tumor antigens: A new potential for therapy. Natl Cancer Inst Monogr 42:33-43, 1975.
39. Imamura N, Takahashi T, Lloyd KO, Lewis JL, Old LJ: Analysis of human ovarian tumor antigens using heterologous antisera: detection of new antigenic systems. Int J Cancer 21:570-577, 1978.
40. Lloyd KO: Ovarian cancer antigen OVC-2. In: Compendium of Assay for Immunodiagnosis of Human Cancer. Herberman RB (ed). Amsterdam: Elsevier, North Holland Inc, 1978, p 533.
41. Klein JL, Gall SA, Dawson JR: Quantitation of secretory component levels in cyst fluids, ascitic fluids and sera from ovarian adenocarcinoma patients. J Natl Cancer Inst 61:57-60, 1978.
42. Burton RM, McGrew TL, Barrows GH, Beyerle MP, Fortwengler HP, Day TG, Kuhns JG, Espinosa E: Occurrence of a thermostable antigen of ovarian carcinoma in normal tissues and secretions. Cancer 43:2385-2391, 1979.
43. Bara J, Malarewics A, Loisillier F, Burtin P: Antigens common to human ovarian mucinous cyst fluid and gastric mucosa. Br J Cancer 36:49-56, 1977.
44. Axelsen NH: WHO-Collaborative study on ovarian tumor associated antigens. 1979.

45. Cantarow WD, Stolbach LL, Bhattacharya M, Chatterjee SK, Barlow JJ: The value of tumor markers in cancer of the ovary. Int J Rad Oncol Biol Phys, in press.
46. Bhattacharya M, Barlow JJ: Ovarian tumor antigens. Cancer 42:1616–1620, 1978.
47. Bhattacharya M, Barlow JJ: Ovarian cystadenocarcinoma-associated antigen (OCAA). In: Compendium of Assays for Immunodiagnosis of Human Cancer. Herberman RB (ed). Amsterdam: Elsevier, North Holland Inc, 1979, pp 527–431.
48. Knauf S, Urbach GI: Purification of human ovarian tumor-associated antigen and demonstration of circulating tumor antigen in patients with advanced ovarian malignancy. Am J Obstet Gynecol 127:705–711, 1977.
49. Knauf S, Urbach GI: The development of a durable antibody radioimmunoassay for detecting ovarian tumor-associated antigen fraction OCA in plasma. Am J Obstet Gynecol 131:780–787, 1978.
50. Knauf S, Urbach GI: OCA, ovarian tumor associated antigen. In: Compendium of Assays for Immunodiagnosis of Human Cancer. Herberman RB (ed). Amsterdam: Elsevier, North Holland Inc, 1979, pp 537–539.
51. Knauf S, Urbach GI: A study of ovarian cancer patients using a radioimmunoassay for human ovarian tumor associated antigen OCA. Am J Obstet Gynecol 138:1222–1223, 1980.
52. Knauf S, Urbach GI: Identification, purification and radioimmunoassay of NB/70K, a human ovarian tumor-associated antigen. Cancer Res 41:1351–1357, 1981.
53. Hollinshead A: Skin test to identify TAA and TAA hyperimmune antisera for use in ELISA. In: Compendium of Assays for Immunodiagnosis of Human Cancer. Herberman RB (ed). Amsterdam: Elsevier, North Holland Inc, 1979, pp 543–551.
54. Dorsett BH, Ioachim HL, Stohlbach L, Walker J, Barber HRK: Isolation of tumor-specific antibodies from effusions of ovarian carcinomas. Int J Cancer 16:779–786, 1975.
55. Dorsett BH, Ioachim HL: Ovarian tumor related factors in peritoneal effusions. In: Compendium of Assays for Immunodiagnosis of Human Cancer, Herberman RB (ed). Amsterdam: Elsevier, North Holland Inc, 1979, pp 559–561.
56. Stolbach LL, Cantarow WD, Gronin WJ, Dorsett B, Ghandbir L, Hamm J, Ioachim H, Kelloway K, McLaughlin M, Walker J, Barber HRK: Dissociation and characterization of ovarian cancer antigen (Ag) and antibody (Aby) from immune complexes. Proc Amer Assoc Cancer Res 21:239, 1980.
57. Cantarow WD, Gronin WJ, Dorsett B, Gandbhir L, Hamm J, Ioachim H, Kelloway K, McLaughlin M, Walker J, Stolbach L, Barber HRK: Characterization of ovarian cancer antigen and antibody from immune complexes. Fed Proc 39:474, 1980.
58. Kohler G, Milstein C: Continuous cultures of fused cells secreting antibody of predefined specificity. Nature 256:495–497, 1975.
59. Bast RC Jr, Feeney M, Lazarus H, Nadler LM, Colvin RB, Knapp RC: Reactivity of a monoclonal antibody with human ovarian carcinoma. J Clin Invest 68:1331–1337, 1981.
60. Sang D, Bast RC Jr, Lazarus H, Terhorst C, Knapp RC: Unpublished data.
61. Kabawat S, Bast RC Jr, Colvin RB, Welch W, Knapp RC: Unpublished data.
62. Van Nagell JR Jr, Kim E, Casper S, Primus FS, Bennett S, Deland FH, Goldenberg DM: Radioimmunodetection of primary and metastatic ovarian cancer using radiolabeled antibodies to carcinoembryonic antigen. Cancer Res 40:502–506, 1980.
63. Mandell GL, Fisher RI, Bostick F, Young RC: Ovarian Cancer: A solid tumor with evidence of normal cellular immune function but abnormal B cell function. Am J Med 66:621–624, 1979.
64. Kohorn EI, Mitchell MS, Dwyer JM, Knowlton AH, Klein-Angerer S: Effect of radiation on cell-mediated cytotoxicity and lymphocyte subpopulations in patients with ovarian carcinoma. Cancer 41:1040–1048, 1978.

65. Halili M, Bosworth J, Romney S, Moukhtar M, Ghossein A: The long term effect of radiotherapy on the immune status of patients cured of a gynecologic malignancy. Cancer 37:2875–2878, 1976.
66. Nalick RH, DiSaia PJ, Rea TH, Morrow CP: Immunocompetence and prognosis in patients with gynecologic cancer. Gynecol Oncol 2:81–92, 1974.
67. Check IJ, Hunter RC, Rosenberg KD, Herbst AL: Prediction of survival in gynecological cancer based on immunological tests. Cancer Res 40:4612–4616, 1980.
68. Mantovani A, Allvena P, Sessa C, Bolis G, Mangioni C: Natural killer activity of lymphoid cells isolated from human ascitic ovarian tumors. Int J Cancer 25:573–582, 1980.
69. Allavona P, Introna M, Mangioni C, Mantovani A: Inhibition of natural killer activity by tumor associated lymphoid cells from ascites ovarian carcinomas. J Natl Cancer Institute 67:319–325, 1981.
70. Svanberg L, Astadt B: Coagulative and fibrinolytic properties of ascites fluid associated with ovarian tumors. Cancer 35:1382–1387, 1975.
71. Veda K, Toyokawa M, Nakamori H, Sako H, Umesaki N, Nakade J, Lee T, Sugawa T: The prognostic value of serum immunosuppressive effect in patients with ovarian cancer. Obstet Gynecol 53:480–483, 1979.
72. Hess AD, Gall SA, Dawson JR: Inhibition of *in vitro* lymphocyte function by cyst and ascitic fluids from ovarian cancer patients. Cancer Res 39:2381–2389, 1979.
73. Hess AD, Gall SA, Dawson JR: Partial purification and characterization of lymphocyte-inhibitory factor(s) in ascitic fluid from ovarian cancer patients. Cancer Res 40:1842–1851, 1980.
74. Hess AD, Gall SA, Dawson JR: Inhibition of human lymphoblastoid cell line proliferation by ascites fluid from ovarian cancer patients. Cancer Res 40:4455–4500, 1980.
75. Badger AM, Cooperband SR: An immunostimulatory substance in the ascites fluid of patients with cancer metastatic to the peritoneum. Cell Immunol 45:15–25, 1979.
76. Badger AM, Oh SK, Moulten RF: Differential effects of an immunosuppressive fraction from ascites fluid of patients with ovarian cancer on spontaneous and antibody-dependent cytotoxicity. Cancer Res 41:1133–1139, 1981.
77. Tamura K, Shibate Y, Matsuda Y, Ishida N: Isolation and characterization of an immunosuppressive acidic protein from ascitic fluids of cancer patients. Cancer Res 41:3244–3252, 1981.
78. Robinson E, Sher S, Mekori T: Lymphocyte stimulation by phytohemagglutinin and tumor cells of malignant effusions. Cancer Res 36:1548–1551, 1974.
79. Salmon SE, Hamberger AW: Immunoproliferation and cancer: A common macrophage derived promoter substance. Lancet 1:1289–1290, 1978.
80. Hamberger AW, Salmon SE, Kim MB, Trent JM, Soehnlen BY, Alberts DS, Schmidt HJ: Direct cloning of human ovarian cancer cell in agar. Cancer Res 38:3438–3444, 1978.
81. Hamberger AW, Salmon SE, Alberts DS: Development of a bioassay for ovarian carcinoma colony forming cells. In: Cloning of Human Tumor Stem Cells. Salmon SE (ed). New York: Alan R Liss, 1980, pp 63–73.
82. Buick RN, Fry SE, Samon SE: Effect of host-cell interactions on clonogenic carcinoma cells in human malignant effusions. Br J Cancer 41:695–704, 1980.
83. Buick RN, Salmon SE: Variables in the demonstration of human tumor clonogenicity: Cell interactions and semi-solid support. In: Cloning of Human Tumor Cells. Salmon SE (ed). New York: Alan R Liss, 1980, pp 127–134.
84. Mantovani A, Polentarutti N, Peri G, Shavit ZB, Vecchi A, Bollis G, Mangioni C: Cytotoxicity of tumor cells of peripheral blood monocytes and tumor associated macrophages in patients with ascites ovarian tumors. JNCI 64:1307–1315, 1980.
85. Mantovani A, Peri G, Polentarutti N, Bolis G, Mangioni C, Spreafico F: Effects of *in vitro*

tumor growth of macrophages isolated from human ascitic ovarian tumors. Int J Cancer 23:157-164, 1979.
86. Chatterjee J, Barlow JJ, Allen HJ, Chung WS, Piver S: Lymphocyte response to autologous tumor antigen(s) and phytohemagglutinins in ovarian cancer patients. Cancer 3:956-962, 1975.
87. Chen SY, Koffler D, Cohen CJ: Cell mediated immunity in patients with ovarian carcinoma. Am J Obstet Gynecol 115:467-470, 1973.
88. Feiferman I, Gleicher N, Cohen CJ, Koffler D: Leukocyte migration in ovarian carcinoma: Comparison of inhibitory activity of tumor extracts. JNCI 59:1593-1597, 1977.
89. Melnick H, Barber HRK: Cellular immunologic responsiveness to extracts of ovarian epithelial tumors. Gynecol Onc 3:77-86, 1975.
90. Gleicher N, Beers P, Cohen CJ, Kerengi TD, Gusberg S: Leukocyte migration enhancement as an indicator of immunologic enhancement. Am J Obstet Gynecol 136-124, 1980.
91. Gleicher N, Beers P, Cohen CJ, Kerengi TD, Gusberg SB: Leukocyte migration enhancement as an indicator of immunologic enhancement. III. Common denominators of pregnancy and malignancy. Am J Obstet Gynecol 136:5-10, 1980.
92. DiSaia PJ, Rutledge FN, Smith JP, Sinkovics: Cell mediated immune reaction to two gynecologic malignant tumors. Cancer 28:1129-1137, 1971.
93. DiSaia PJ, Sinkovics JG, Rutledge FN, Smith JP: Cell mediated immunity to human malignant cells. Am J Obstet Gynecol 114:979-989, 1972.
94. DiSaia PJ: Immunological aspects of gynecological malignancies. J Reproductive Med 14:17-20, 1975.
95. Patillo RA, Story MT, Ruckert CF: Expression of cell-mediated immunity and blocking factor using a new line of ovarian cancer cells *in vitro*. Cancer Res 39:1185-1191, 1979.
96. Patillo RA, Ruckert ACF, Story MT, Mattingly RF: Immunodiagnosis in ovarian cancer: Blocking factor activity. Am J Obstet Gynecol 133:791, 1979.
97. DiSaia PJ, Nalick RH, Townsend DE: Antibody cytotoxicity studies in ovarian and cervical malignancies. Ob Gyn 42:644-650, 1973.
98. Garcia JA, Klein JL, Kotteh WH, Dawson JR, Gall SA: Immunologic studies on the cystic effusions of ovarian epithelial neoplasms. Am J Obstet Gynecol 129:281-284, 1977.
99. Halbrecht I, Komlos L: Cytotoxic effects of various sera on primary cultures of placentas and ovarian tumors. Obstet Gynecol 38:594-598, 1971.
100. Poulton TA, Crowther ME, Hay FC, Nineham LJ: Immune complexes in ovarian cancer. Lancet ii:72-73, 1978.
101. McLaughlin PJ, Price MR, Baldwin RW, Vasey D, Symonds EM: Immune complexes in ovarian cancer. Lancet ii:271, 1978.
102. Clayton LA, Gall SA, Dawson JR, Creasman WT: Immune complexes in ovarian cancer. Proc Soc Gyn Oncol 12:21-22, 1981.
103. Nauts HC: Beneficial effects of acute concurrent infection, inflammation, fever on immunotherapy (bacterial toxins) in ovarian and uterine cancer. Cancer Research Institute Monograph 17:1-122, 1977.
104. Graham JB, Graham RM: The effect of vaccine on cancer patients. Surg Gyn Obstet 109:131-138, 1959.
105. Graham JB, Graham RM: Autogenous vaccine in cancer patients. Surg Gyn Obstet 114:1-4, 1962.
106. Sonkin R, Coudagras M, Blondon J: Traitement des cancers génitaux par la polycimoitherapie. Multiple sequential chemotherapy in patients with advanced gynecological cancer. (Fr) J Gyn Obst Biol Repr 1:61-69, 1972.
107. Hudson CN, Levin L, McHardy JE, Poulton TA, Curling OM, Crowther M, English PE,

Leighton M: Active specific immunotherapy for ovarian cancer. Lancet 2:877–879, 1976.
108. Alberts DS: Adjuvant Immunotherapy with BCG of Advanced Ovarian Cancer: A preliminary report. Salmon SE, Jones SE (eds). Amsterdam: Elsevier, North Holland, Biomedical Press, 1977, pp 327–337.
109. Mangan C, Jeqlum KA, Sedlacek TV, Giuntoli RC, Wheeler JE, Rubin E, Mikuta JJ: Intralymphatic BCG in the treatment of gynecologic malignancies: A Phase I Study. Cancer 40:2933–2940, 1977.
110. Papaioannou AW, Polychronis AB, Agoustis AW, Coco HI, Trichopoulas DB: Maximal cytoreduction, chemotherapy and contact nonspecific immunotherapy for Stage III ovarian cancer.
111. Brandes LJ: Immunotherapy for ovarian cancer. Lancet 2:1195, 1976.
112. Alberts DS, Mason NL, O'Toole R, Neff J, Hilgers R, Carlin D, Moon TE: A randomized trial doxorubicin and cyclophosphamide plus BCG versus doxorubicin and cyclophosphamide therapy in advanced ovarian cancer. Immunotherapy of Human Cancer. Terry WD, Rosenberg S (eds). New York: Excerpta Medica, 1982, pp 343–352.
113. Chang VST, Suit HD, Wang CC, Raker J, Weymuller E, Kaitman S: A preliminary study of intralesional, intralymph node, intravenous and intraperitoneal *Corynebacterium parvum* treatments in patients with advanced cancer. Cancer 42:1912–1915, 1978.
114. Webb HE, Oaten SE, Pike CP: Treatment of malignant ascitic and pleural effusions with *Corynebacterium parvum*. Brit Med J 1:338–340, 1978.
115. Bast RC Jr, Berek JS, Obrist R, Griffiths CT, Berkowitz R, Hacker NF, Parker L, Lagasse LD, Knapp RC: Intraperitonal immunotherapy of human ovarian carcinoma with *Corynebacterium parvum*. Proc Amer Soc Clin Oncol 1:38, 1982.
116. Mantovani A, Sessa C. Peri G, Allvena P, Introna M, Polentarutti N, Mangioni C: Intraperitoneal administration of *Corynebacterium parvum* in patients with ascitic ovarian tumors resistant to chemotherapy: Effects on cytotoxicity of tumor associated macrophages and NK cells. Int J Cancer 27:437–446, 1981.
117. DiSaia PJ, Rich WM: Value of immune monitoring in gynecologic cancer patients receiving immunotherapy. Am J Obstet Gynecol 135:907–916, 1979.
118. Gall SA, DiSaia PJ, Schmidt H, Mittelstaed L, Newman P, Creasman W: Toxicity manifestations following intravenous *Corynebacterium parvum* administration to patients with ovarian and cervical carcinoma. Am J Obstet Gynecol 132:555–560, 1978.
119. Rao B, Wanebo HJ, Ochoa M, Lewis JL, Oettgen HF: Intravenous *C. parvum*. An adjuvant to chemotherapy for resistent advanced ovarian cancer. Cancer 39:514–526, 1977.
120. Gall SA, Creasman WT, Blessing JA, Whisnant JK, DiSaia PJ: Chemoimmunotherapy in primary stage III ovarian epithelial cancer. Immunotherapy of Human Cancer. Terry WD, Rosenberg S (eds). New York: Excerpta Medica, 1982, pp 337–342.
121. Bast RC Jr, Berek JS, Obrist R, Griffiths CT, Berkowitz R, Hacker NF, Parker L, Lagasse LD, Knapp RC: Intraperitoneal immunotherapy of human ovarian carcinoma with *Corynebacterium parvum*. Cancer Res, in press.
122. Wanebo HJ, Ochoa M Jr, Gunther U, Ishi T, Lewis JF Jr, Oettgen HF: Randomized chemoimmunotherapy trial of CAF and intravenous *C. parvum* for resistant ovarian carcinoma. Preliminary results. Proc Amer Assoc Cancer Res 18:225, 1977.
123. Stewart WE, II (ed): Interferons and their Actions. Cleveland, Ohio: CRC Press, 1977.
124. Epstein LB, Shen J-T, Abele JS, Reese CC: Sensitivity of human ovarian carcinoma cells to interferon and other antitumor agents as assessed by an *in vitro* semi-solid agar technique. Ann NY Acad Sci 350:228–244, 1980.
125. Epstein LB, Shen J-T, Abele JS, Reese CC: Further experience in testing the sensitivity of human ovarian carcinoma cells to interferon in an *in vitro* semi-solid agar culture system:

Comparison of solid and ascitic forms of tumor. In: Cloning of Human Tumor Stem Cell. Salmon SE (ed). New York: Alan R Liss, Inc, 1980, pp 277–290.
126. The Biology of the Interferon System. Amsterdam: Elsevier, Biomedical, Press 1981.
127. Order S, Rosenshein NB, Klein JL, Lichter AS, Ettinger DS, Dillon MB, Leibel SA: New methods applied to the analysis and treatment of ovarian cancer. Int J Rad Oncol Biol Phys 5:861–873, 1979.
128. Order SE, Rosenshein N, Klein JL, Leibel S, Torres JPY, Ettinger D: The integration of new therapies and radiation in management of ovarian cancer. Cancer 48:590–596, 1981.
129. Fekete E, Ferrigno MA: Studies on a transplantable teratoma of the mouse. Cancer Res 12:438–440, 1952.
130. Verhaelen CPJ, Fisher RI, Apella E, Ramanathan L: Lack of histocompatibility antigens on a murine ovarian teratocarcinoma. Cancer Res 41:3186–3191, 1981.
131. Feldman GB, Knapp RC, Order SE, Hellman S: The role of lymphatic obstruction in the formation of ascites in a murine ovarian carcinoma. Cancer Res 32:1663–1666, 1972.
132. Feldman GB: Lymphatic obstruction in carcinomatous ascites. Cancer Res 35:325–332, 1975.
133. Ozols RF, Locker GY, Doroshow JH, Grotzinger KR, Myers CE, Young RC: Pharmacokinetics of adriamycin and tissue penetration in murine ovarian cancer. Cancer Res 39:3209–3214, 1979.
134. Ozols RF, Grotzinger KR, Fisher RI, Myers CE, Young RC: Kinetic characterization and response to chemotherapy in a transplantable murine ovarian cancer. Cancer Res 39:3202–3208, 1979.
135. Ozols RF, Locker GY, Doroshow JH, Grotzinger KR, Myers CE, Fisher RI, Young RC: Chemotherapy for murine ovarian cancer: A rational for IP therapy with adriamycin. Cancer Treat Rep 63:269–273, 1979.
136. Finkler N, Cohen CJ: A study of distribution patterns and improved therapeutic techniques in the treatment of ovarian neoplasms with cis-diamminedichloroplatinum. Proc Soc Gyn Onc 12:30–35, 1981.
137. Verhaelen CPJ, Fisher RI: Requirements for successful immunotherapy and chemoimmunotherapy of a murine model of ovarian cancer. Cancer Res 41:980–983, 1981.
138. Order SE, Donahue V, Knapp R: Serologic immunotherapy and interaction with radiation. In: Interaction of Radiation and Host Immune Defense Mechanisms, in Malignancy. Bond VP (ed). Brookhaven National Laboratory (Publ 50418), 1974, pp 363–372.
139. Bloomer WD, Adelstein SJ: 5-$^{125}$I-iododeoxyuridine as prototype for radionuclide therapy with Arger emittors. Nature 265:620–621, 1977.
140. Bloomer WD, McLaughlin WH, Neirinckx RD, Adelstein SJ, Gordon PR, Ruth TJ, Wolf AP: Astatine-211-tellurium radiocolloid cures experimental malignant ascites. Science 212:340–341, 1981.
141. Reif AE: An experimental test of two general relationships to describe the absorption of antibodies by cells and tissues. Immunochem 3:267–278, 1966.
142. Order SE, Donahue V, Knapp R: Immunotherapy of ovarian carcinoma: An experimental model. Cancer 32:573–579, 1973.
143. Michaelson J, Artzt K, Bennett D, Caldwell J, Heath JK: A cell surface antigen, TER, expressed by embryos and germ cells. J Immunol 123:2436–2438, 1979.
144. Order SE, Kirkman R, Knapp R: Serologic immunotherapy: Results and probable mechanism of action. Cancer 34:175–183, 1974.
145. Bast RC Jr, Knapp RC, Donahue VC, Thurston JG, Mitchell AR, Feeney M, Schlossman SF: Specificity of heteroantisera developed against purified populations of intact murine ovarian carcinoma cells. J Natl Cancer Inst 64:365–372, 1980.

146. Order SE, Donahue V, Knapp R: Serologic immunotherapy and interaction with radiation. In: Interaction of Radiation and Host Immune Defense Mechanisms in Malignancy. Bond VP (ed). Brookhaven National Laboratory (Publ 50418), 1974, pp 363–372.
147. Knapp RC, Berkowitz RS: *Corynebacterium parvum* as an immunotherapeutic agent in an ovarian cancer model. Am J Obstet Gynecol 128:782–786, 1977.
148. Bast RC Jr, Knapp RC, Mitchell AK, Thurston JG, Tucker REV, Schlossman SF: Immunotherapy of a murine ovarian carcinoma with *Corynebacterium parvum* and specific heteroantiserum. 1. Activation of peritoneal cells to mediate antibody dependent cytotoxicity. J Immunol 123:1945–1951, 1979.
149. Burstein S, Knapp RC: Chemotherapy of murine ovarian carcinoma by methotrexate-antibody conjugates. J Med Chem 20:950–952, 1977.

# 7. Lymph Node Metastases from Gynecologic Cancer – Biological Concepts and Therapeutic Implications

ARLAN F. FULLER, Jr.

## 1. INTRODUCTION

The prognostic and therapeutic importance of lymph node metastases in gynecologic oncology is founded upon biological principles that are only now in evolution. Developments in immunology, tissue transplantation, and tumor biology, among many fields, have led to reappraisal of long-held tenets in clinical oncology and alternative approaches to the therapy of patients with regional metastases. Although the ominous prognostic significance of nodal metastases has long been recorded, only within the past decade have they been regarded as more than the result of passive trapping or 'filtering' of tumor cells by lymph nodes.

The establishment of a metastasis, regardless of site, is the product of a multifactorial process involving multiple events, each necessary, but none independently sufficient for distant tumor spread. The tumor cells must effectively penetrate an adjacent vessel, embolize to a distant site and then implant and acquire an independent blood supply, all the while maintaining viability in the presence of host defenses, whether in lymphatic or hematogenous channels. Although the establishment of lymphatic metastasis may be anatomically and immunologically distinct from that of a hematogenous metastasis, review of features common to both may provide information about tumor metastases in general and their interrelationships in specific.

The available experimental data provides, at best, an imperfect understanding of the pathophysiologic processes involved in the establishment of regional lymph node metastases. Viewed within the context of data derived from the diagnosis and treatment of gynecologic malignancy, this evidence now permits re-evaluation of a strict anatomic approach to the problem of nodal metastases in gynecologic oncology.

*Griffiths, C. T. and Fuller, A. F. (eds.), Gynecologic Oncology.*
© *1983, Martinus Nijhoff Publishers, Boston. ISBN 0-89838-555-5.*
*Printed in The Netherlands.*

## 2. HISTORICAL CONSIDERATIONS OF THE ANATOMIC HYPOTHESIS

More than a century ago, Virchow recognized the anatomic relationship between a primary tumor and its regional draining nodes and postulated that the lymph nodes represented efficient filters which cleared the afferent lymph of particulate material, including tumor cells [1]. The constant relationship between the lymphatic drainage from the primary site and the pattern of metastases among these nodes supported this anatomic concept of tumor spread and provided the basis for Halsted's approach to the surgical management of carcinoma; en bloc resection of the primary tumor and its regional nodes along with intervening lymphatic channels, potentially permeated with tumor cells [2, 3]. Subsequent controversy over lymphatic permeation *versus* embolization carried on until pathologic studies demonstrated the absence of tumor cells in intervening lymphatic channels and confirmed the concept of discontinuous, embolic spread of tumor cells to the regional nodes [4, 5, 6].

The emphasis upon elucidation of anatomic pathways of lymphatic spread from primary carcinomas, coupled with the improved results of en bloc resection of carcinomas at the turn of the century, led quite naturally to an anatomic concept of lymphatic metastases. This concept was further supported by Virchow's view of the regional node as a passive filter and by continued improvement in survival as lymph node dissections became more extensive.

These same observations influenced the early surgical treatment of carcinoma of the cervix by Wertheim in 1889 and later, carcinoma of the vulva by Bassett in 1912. Wertheim's lymphadenectomy was a selective procedure, with excision of grossly enlarged nodes only; his skepticism of the need to remove intervening lymphatics indicated his belief in tumor embolization at a time when the theory of permeation was widely accepted. Sixty-two of his first 250 cases (25%) had enlarged, histologically positive nodes. Forty-one of the 62 patients survived the operation; all but 5 (12%) developed recurrent carcinoma while 71% of the negative node patients remained disease-free. In this series of patients Wertheim demonstrated the prevalence of pelvic nodal metastases associated with resectable cervical carcinoma and indicated the overwhelmingly adverse effect of such extensive nodal disease on prognosis. Although he did not attribute the advantage of the abdominal approach to resection of enlarged pelvic nodes, he did prove that some patients so treated could be cured and that nodal extension of disease beyond the cervix had to be considered by those advocates of a vaginal approach [7].

In his text published in 1934, Meigs (Figure 1) reviewed the experience with invasive carcinoma of the cervix treated by his predecessors at the

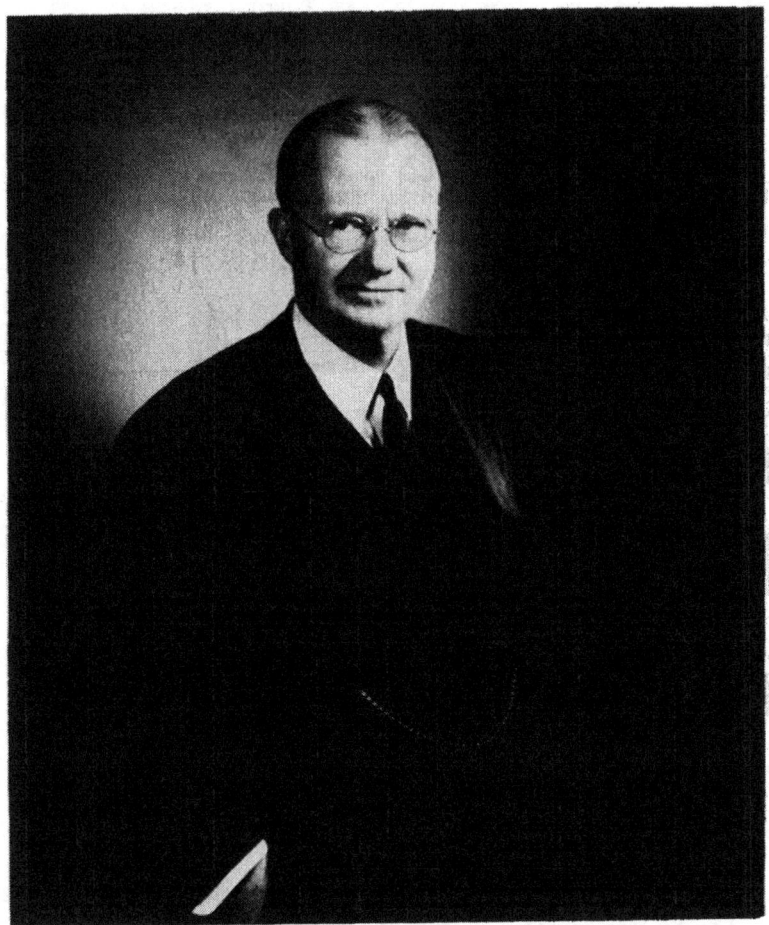

*Figure 1.* Joe Vincent Meigs, M.D., first professor of gynecology at the Massachusetts General Hospital. Dr Meigs was responsible for association of the Massachusetts General Hospital and the Vincent Memorial Hospital which continues to this day as the gynecologic service of the Massachusetts General Hospital.

Massachusetts General Hospital and described a progression of nodal involvement from pericervical (parametrial) to hypogastric, obturator, sacral, iliac, and inguinal sites. He emphasized the need for removal of all the pelvic nodes, and the failure of radium therapy to treat nodes beyond those most proximal to the cervix [8]. Meigs cited Shields Warren's correlation of histologic grade of cervical carcinoma with pelvic nodal metastases at autopsy and concluded that these metastases were the source of failure after radium treatment of poorly differentiated tumors [9].

Meigs' interest in lymph node metastases led to a general study of 707 patients with various gynecologic neoplasms (Figure 2) and later an inten-

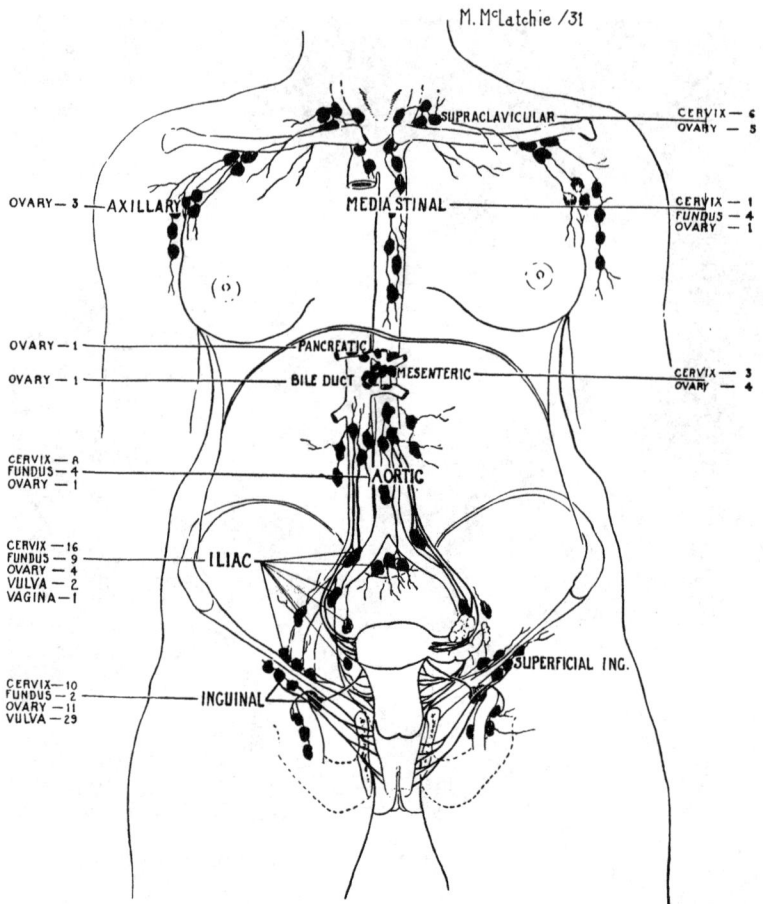

*Figure 2.* Distribution of metastases to lymph nodes as reported by Meigs [8]. These 150 nodal metastases were identified in 707 patients with gynecologic cancers (396 cervical, 122 endometrial, 131 ovarian, 37 vulvar, 20 vaginal and 1 tubal). Reprinted from Meigs [8], with permission.

sive study of 102 additional cases of cervical carcinoma. In the former study he reported on patients at all stages of disease, although clinical information was incomplete. Nevertheless, Meigs was able to identify 150 instances of nodal metastases (Table 1). Pelvic (iliac or regional) nodal metastases were detected, largely by clinical exam, in 8% of patients with cervical carcinoma and para-aortic (aortic, mesenteric, bile duct, and pancreatic) metastases in 3%. The presence of pelvic and para-aortic nodal metastases were also recognized in endometrial carcinoma (8% and 3%), in ovarian carcinoma (3% and 5%, with an additional 4% 'regional'), and in vulvar carcinoma (5% and 0%; 80% inguinal). Based upon this study, Meigs developed a

Table 1. Lymph node metastases identified by Meiqs in 707 patients.

| Metastases to | Lymph nodes | | | | | |
|---|---|---|---|---|---|---|
| | Cervix | Body of uterus | Ovary | Vulva | Vagina | Total |
| Supraclavicular | 6 | 0 | 5 | 0 | 0 | 11 |
| Axillary | 0 | 0 | 3 | 0 | 0 | 3 |
| Inguinal | 10 | 2 | 11 | 29 | 0 | 52 |
| Pancreatic | 0 | 0 | 1 | 0 | 0 | 1 |
| Common bile duct | 0 | 0 | 1 | 0 | 0 | 1 |
| Aortic | 8 | 4 | 1 | 0 | 0 | 13 |
| Iliac | 16 | 9 | 4 | 2 | 1 | 32 |
| Mesenteric | 3 | 0 | 4 | 0 | 0 | 7 |
| Mediastinal | 1 | 4 | 1 | 0 | 0 | 6 |
| Regional | 16 | 1 | 5 | 1 | 1 | 24 |
| | 60 | 20 | 36 | 32 | 2 | 150 |

0 = no metastases.
Reprinted from Meigs [8] with permission.

schematic distribution of regional metastases from the genital viscera (Figure 3); generally, this remains valid today.

In his detailed study of 102 patients previously treated with a 'modified Wertheim' hysterectomy or radiation therapy, there were 240 sites of metastatic disease subsequently identified of which 41 (17%) represented nodal disease. Half of these metastases were pelvic recurrences in iliac nodes, one-quarter were para-aortic nodal recurrences, and the remainder were in the inguinal (7), supraclavicular (3) or mediastinal nodes (1). Central recurrences were more prevalent with low grade tumors and distant nodal metastases as well as intra-thoracic metastases were associated with high grade tumors. Proper denominators indicating number of patients at risk were not available, however, for statistical comparison. In this survey of the 'state of the art' in the early 1930s, Meigs made a substantial contribution to knowledge of the pattern of spread of gynecologic cancer, much of which has recently been rediscovered, and prepared the foundations for his future clinical work in the surgical therapy of carcinoma of the cervix and endometrium [10, 11].

## 3. THE ANATOMIC HYPOTHESIS

As a consequence of the anatomic theory of passive filtration of tumor emboli, it was presumed that the appearance of more distant metastases was

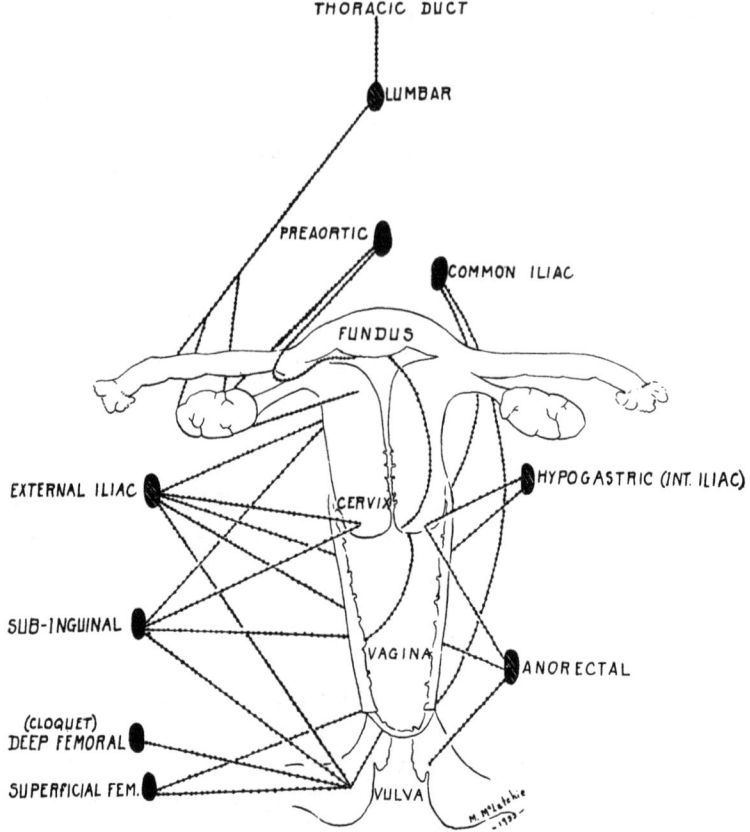

*Figure 3.* Schematic diagram indicating the regional nodes of gynecologic cancers by site. The dotted lines extend from the primary tumors along lymphatic channels to the region involved. (From Meigs [8].)

the result of either bypass of regional nodes clogged with metastatic cells from the primary site or embolization of malignant cells from the metastasis itself through its efferent vessels. This explanation of distant metastases is still presented in textbooks today [12]. Failure of operative treatment in patients with nodal metastases presumably resulted from the surgeon's inability to remove every nodal metastasis. Failure of radiation therapy for nodal metastases was a consequence of disease too bulky to be effectively sterilized with tolerable doses of radiation. There evolved two new guidelines in the therapy of nodal disease in gynecologic malignancy, particularly cervical carcinoma; first, radiation therapy might be preferable to surgical treatment, since it would not 'miss' occult nodal metastases hidden in the pelvis [13] and, second, the combination of lymphadenectomy and pelvic radiation therapy in either sequence might improve survival in patients with nodal metastases [14]. What was discovered in prospective studies, however, was that surgical and radiotherapeutic treatment provided equivalent survivals in Stage I cervical carcinoma [15, 16, 17]. Studies of combined therapy achieved no greater success at the additional cost of severe morbidity among survivors [18, 19]. In fact, the survival of patients with nodal metastases at post-radiation lymphadenectomy was near zero [20, 21].

*3.1. Hypothesis for the immunologic role of the regional lymph node*

The concept of separation of the lymphatic from the vascular system by at least one echelon of intervening lymph nodes was effectively challenged in the late 1960s by Fisher and associates [22]. They demonstrated in a series of experimental studies that tumor cells injected through lymphatic channels *in vivo* rapidly appeared in the systemic circulation. Fisher proposed an alternative hypothesis for the presence of nodal metastases. He stated that although the regional lymph node might be responsible in part for the initiation of an immune response, constant exposure to cells or surface antigens shed from the progressively enlarging tumor mass could provoke local anergy or immunosuppression. Progressive nodal tumor growth would then mirror systemic immunosuppression in the host and indicate the presence of occult systemic metastases which might appear only after effective local and regional tumor control. The occurrence of long-term survivors after excision or irradiation of nodal metastases would indicate that some tumors metastasize to regional nodes but do not have the cellular capacity requisite for systemic metastases (Section 4). Alternatively, removal of gross nodal disease in these patients might swing the tumor–host immunological balance in favor of the host.

This alternative hypothesis does provide an explanation for the clinical events, outlined above, indicating that nodal metastases signify systemic extension of disease. The hypothesis is predicated upon the immunogenicity of spontaneous human tumors, the pivotal role of the regional node in the immune response to carcinoma, and the concept of tumor dormancy, that occult systemic metastases can be held in check for long periods of time by host defenses before clinical metastases appear.

*3.2. The common pathway hypothesis for metastasis*

A second, less complex alternative, moreover, might be considered in the process of metastasis itself (Figure 4), that the processes of tissue invasion, vessel invasion, cell detachment and intravessel survival, are common to both routes of spread. Lymphatic metastases, therefore, would be predictive

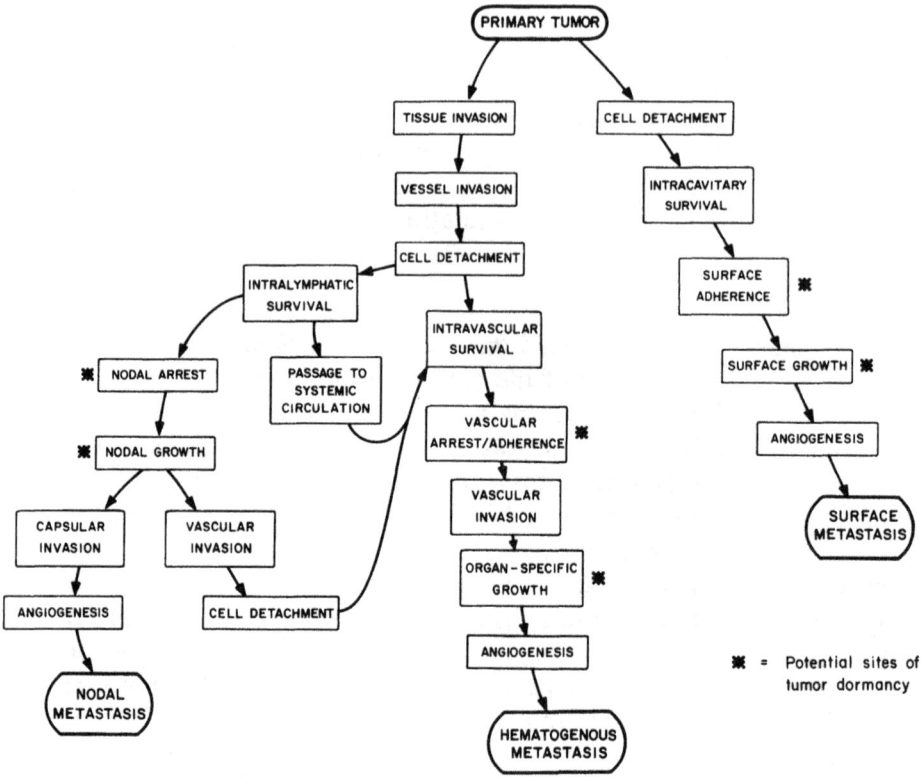

*Figure 4.* Steps in dissemination of tumor cells from the primary site through the three major pathways of lymphatic, hematogenous and surface metastasis. Note that lymphatic to vascular passage of tumor cells may occur either early, with immediate passage to the systemic circulation from lymphatic channels or late, as a result of vascular invasion from nodal tumor growth. Tissue invasion is not a prerequisite of surface metastasis and this may explain the lack of visceral or surface invasion by many well-differentiated ovarian carcinomas. This also supports the observation of visceral invasion by those poorly differentiated ovarian cancers which spread to lymph nodes. Tumor dormancy may be the result of the tumor cells' inability to grow at that site or the effect of host factors on proliferation [43].

of hematogeneous metastases in the sense that they indicate a high likelihood that the remaining functions needed for hematogenous metastasis had been acquired by the tumor capable of metastasizing to the regional node. This alternative skirts the issue of tumor immunology and is based on the concepts of tumor heterogeneity which have been promulgated through the experimental studies of Fidler and associates [23]. These workers have shown that a primary tumor, though it may be monoclonal, consists of subclones of cells, presumably generated by epigenetic mechanisms, which are heterogenous in their potential for metastases. Pressures from the host environment or those generated by various therapeutic modalities may preferentially select tumor cells with different metastatic potentials. In this case the presence of lymph node metastases may only indicate that the first few steps in the acquisition of the capacity for hematogenous dissemination have been completed.

The 'immunologic' and 'common pathway' alternatives are not, of course, mutually exclusive; the former may be operative in the case of more immunogenic tumors such as those associated with oncogenic viruses (refer to Dr. Aurelian's chapter), the latter may explain dissemination of less immunogenic, spontaneously occurring tumors, perhaps endometrial carcinoma.

4. MECHANISMS OF TUMOR METASTASIS

The appearance of a metastatic focus distant from the primary site of tumor necessitates that a subset of cells within the population of the primary parent tumor has acquired *all* of those functions of the appropriate pathway outlined in Figure 4. Each step in this pathway represents the acquisition of a distinct function necessary, but not in itself sufficient to produce tumor dissemination. Relative proportions of cells with these metastatic capabilities may be influenced by pressures from the host environment as well as by therapeutic intervention; much of the pioneering work in this field has been carried out by Fidler and his associates at the Frederick Cancer Research Center and has recently been reviewed in detail [24, 25].

*4.1. Local invasion*

The association of lack of tumor differentiation and tissue as well as vessel (lymphatic and vascular) invasion has been well documented since the work of Warren [8] in multiple studies involving cervical [26, 27, 28], endometrial [29–31], vulvar [32, 33] and tubal carcinomas [34]. Local tumor invasion may be aided by mechanical pressure from the expanding tumor, release of lytic enzymes and reduced intercellular adhesiveness [24]. Distinct subclones may exist, moreover, with high and low metastatic potential; the former subclone demonstrates enhanced ability to invade blood vessel walls *in vitro* and produce large numbers of pulmonary metastases *in vivo* [23]. Although local tissue factors may influence the extent and direction of tissue invasion, for example, the lateral rather than anteroposterior extent of tumor in cervical carcinoma and the absence of direct arterial invasion, there is little evidence to support the concept that the tumor directly invades lymphatic but not small venules in its path of invasion. Norris, in a meticulous study of cervical carcinoma, reaffirmed the difficult

## 4.2. Intravascular and transcoelomic survival

In spite of its adverse prognosis, not *all* patients with documented lymphatic or vascular invasion ultimately develop distant metastases, nor do ovarian cancers with surface extension of tumor invariably recur with peritoneal or omental metastases. Fidler has reported that as few as 0.1% of tumor cells entering the systemic circulation may implant and ultimately give rise to distant tumors [24]. Once the tumor has acquired the capacity for vessel (or surface) invasion and detachment, survival may be determined by immune or nonimmune factors (refer to Dr. Bast's chapter). The cellular or tumor immune mechanisms that may be responsible, however, are uncertain. The capacity for 'immune surveillance' as initially postulated by Burnet may have some role in the recognition and control of nascent tumors and their metastases [36], but this concept is being increasingly disputed; appropriate effector cells are lacking, as is evidence for the immunogenicity of spontaneously appearing tumors [37]. For example, athymic nude mice, without demonstrable T cell function, have a low incidence of spontaneous tumors. Other, nonspecific mechanisms of 'surveillance' may

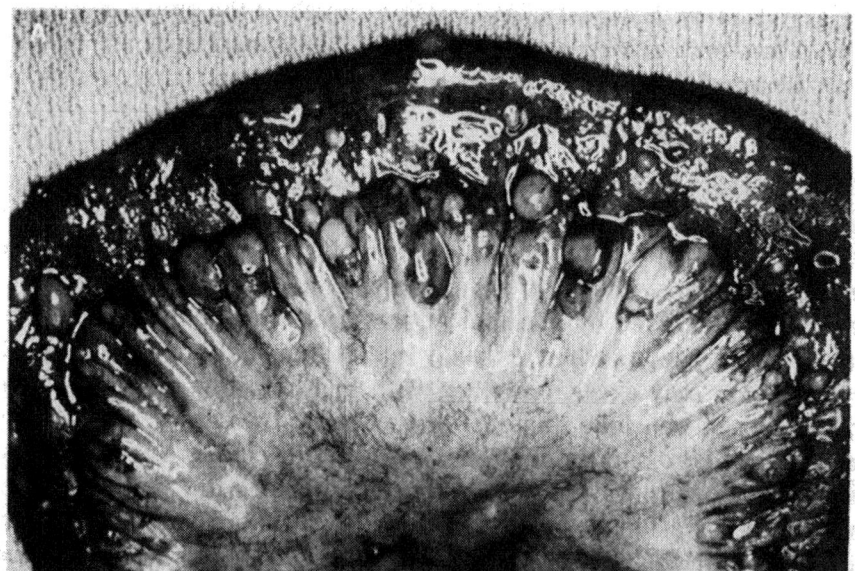

*Figure 5a.* The tumor cells from this primary ovarian cancer have proliferated at the junction of the mesentery and small bowel. This may be the result of exposure of mesentery blood vessels to angiogenesis factor at this point as they enter the serosa of the small intestine.

exist; tumor heterografts are more readily accomplished in immature nude mice who have not yet developed their full complement of natural killer (NK) cells, a subset of small lymphocytes capable of nonspecific cell killing [38, 39]. Further work by Hanna and Fidler have recently demonstrated that these NK cells are responsible for inhibition of hematogenous metastases in various experimental models [40, 41].

With respect to survival of ovarian carcinoma in the peritoneal cavity, Bast and Knapp have identified cell killing by the peritoneal macrophage and its activation by *C. parvum* which may have an important role in the therapy spread of early ovarian carcinoma as well as the therapy of minimal residual intraperitoneal disease (refer to Dr. Bast's chapter).

*4.3. Arrest, invasion and angiogenesis*

Sites of tumor arrest and subsequent growth for ovarian carcinoma are not random and preferential early growth on diaphragmatic surfaces and in omentum have been widely recognized. More advanced disease, as it initially spreads to small bowel, also appears to preferentially invade the junction of small bowel and its mesentery, perhaps because small branching nutrient vessels at this site are more exposed and readily susceptible to tumor angiogenesis (Figures 5a and 5b). It should be noted, moreover, that although surface metastasis is a frequent occurrence with ovarian carcinoma, tissue invasion is not a prerequisite as it is for other modes of spread. Many ovarian tumors have the capacity for tissue arrest, angiogenesis and surface growth, but may still be incapable of parenchymal invasion. It is not sur-

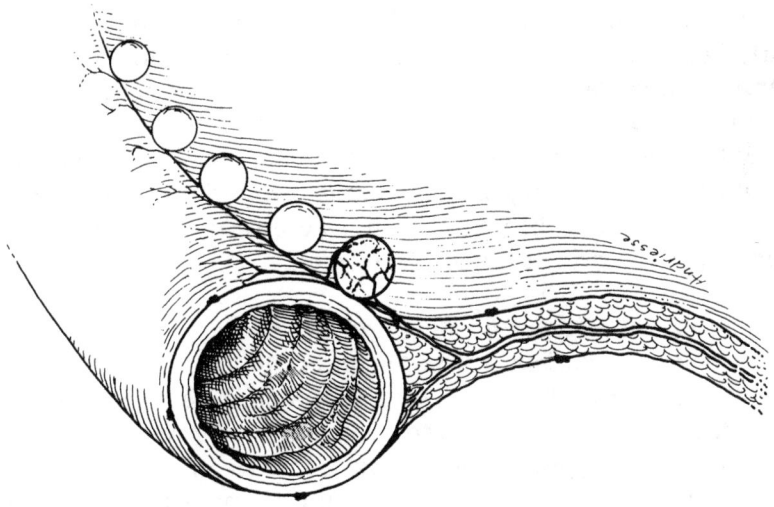

*Figure 5b.* Differential growth of tumor implants may occur because of the availability of nutrient vessels.

prising, therefore, that poorly differentiated tumors may be associated with both parenchymal invasion and nodal metastases.

Hematogenous metastasis, in general, results from endothelial arrest of the tumor cell, adhesion to the vessel wall (possibly aided by local thrombus formation) and then growth of the clump of adherent tumor cells through the vessel wall. Fibrin may either have a role in tumor arrest or in protection of the growing tumor clump from host destruction; there is considerable experimental data and some prospective clinical data indicating that anticoagulation may decrease metastasis formation by one of these means [42]. Localized trauma may also predispose to metastases, either by endothelial damage or by thrombosis and cell arrest and may also be a factor responsible for release from tumor dormancy. Neoplastic dormancy may be characterized by tumor cells either quiescent in resting (Go) state or proliferating in a steady state where the rate of cell renewal equals the rate of cell loss [43].

## 5. PARTICIPATION OF THE REGIONAL LYMPH NODE IN THE HOST RESPONSE TO CANCER

A satisfactory explanation for the appearance of an antigenic tumor progressively growing in the immunocompetent host remains an elusive goal as far as most human tumors are concerned. At varous times investigators have questioned both the antigenicity of spontaneous human tumors and the integrity of the multiple components that constitute the host immune response. Although the regional node has been proposed as a mediator of the early host response to growing tumors, its relation to the host capacity for immune surveillance remains unclear. All of the criticisms of the validity of immune surveillance apply equally well to the role of regional nodes [37]. Moreover, experimental studies supporting these functions have been carried out with antigenic, chemically-induced or virally-induced cancers in animals, whose behavior do not necessarily correspond to that of spontaneously appearing carcinomas in man.

### 5.1. *Experimental evidence for the participation of the regional lymph node in the immune response to cancer*

Resection of a transplantable tumor of syngeneic mice along with its regional draining nodes suppressed in the animal's response to a second tumor transplant, suggesting, according to Fisher and associates, that the nodes were involved with mediation of the primary immune response to this spontaneous cancer [44]. This process appeared to be present only in response to weakly antigenic tumors and appeared to be a transient phenomenon such that in a subsequent study with a chemically induced, strongly antigeneic tumor, antitumor immunity was affected only when the lymphadenectomy was carried out before day seven post transplant [45]. Whether this effect corresponds to the human situation, however, remains uncertain (see Section 5.3).

*5.2. Response of regional lymph nodes to cancer*

If the regional lymph nodes do participate in the host immune response to cancer, it might be expected that they would be exposed to greatest numbers of shed tumor cells or antigens and would exhibit some morphologic or functional changes that would predict the overall host response to that tumor. There is considerable evidence in the growth of the primary cervical carcinoma that a marked lymphocytic response accompanies the earliest recognizable invasion (the 'microinvasive' carcinoma). This reaction is generally not identified in association with overt invasive carcinoma, although a few patients with marked lymphocytic infiltration have been reported. These patients with invasive carcinoma have had few nodal metastases and a correspondingly good prognosis. Hasumi and co-workers carried out a study of 39 patients with circumscribed invasive carcinoma and described a 5% incidence of nodal metastases and 100% survival in patients with extensive lymphocytic infiltration, compared with an 18% incidence of nodal metastases and an 80% survival in a group of 117 controls with similar depths of invasion [46].

Examination of regional lymph node morphology from patients with cervical carcinoma has provided some additional prognostic information. Tsakraklides and associates separated patients into 4 groups based upon the appearance of their regional node. 'Lymphocyte predominance' indicated moderate nodal enlargement with an increased number of small lymphocytes in the cortex, paracortical area, and medullary regions. 'Germinal center predominance' identified nodes that were distinctly enlarged with germinal centers containing large lymphoid cells and mitoses. 'Unstimulated' nodes had small, hypocellular paracortical areas and cortical lymphoid follicles without germinal centers, whereas 'lymphocyte depleted' nodes were hypocellular and fibrotic, often with extensive hyaline deposits and relatively increased numbers of plasmacytes. Only one of 24 patients with the lymphocyte predominant pattern was found to have nodal metastases with an 87% overall 5-year survival. For patients with germinal center predominance, 5 of 20 patients had nodal metastases and 69% survived 5 years. The corresponding values for the 'depleted' nodes were a 33% incidence of nodal metastases and a 5-year survival of 25%. There were not sufficient patients in the 'unstimulated' group to warrant statistical evaluation [47]. A subsequent study by Van Nagell and associates confirmed the association of the lymphocyte predominance pattern with a decrease in nodal metastasis ($p<0.001$) and an increased survival rate ($p<0.0001$) and also noted an association of tumor size with lymph node morphology [48]. Sixty-five percent of patients with lymphocytic predominance had tumors less than 2 cm in size while 86% of patients with germinal center predominance and 100% of patients with lymphocyte depletion had tumors 2 cm size or greater, suggesting that progressive tumor growth is associated with a progressive change in the constituents of the regional node.

Analysis of the lymphocyte subsets present in the regional nodes of patients with gynecologic cancer using monoclonal antibodies has not yet been carried out. Studies performed to date on normal lymph nodes, however, indicate that T and B cells are located within separate compartments in lymph nodes, with restriction of T cells generally to paracortical areas. B cells are present in primary lymphoid follicles while the few T cells identified at this site have been characterized as T4 positive helper/inducer cells. The germinal centers of secondary follicles, moreover, stain positively with T10 antibody, indicating the presence of plasma cells, the terminally differentiated B cell [49, 50]. The morphologic changes seen with the progressive cancer may represent, therefore, a change in the constituents of the regional node from T cell to B cell (plasma cell) predominance. This shift in cellular constituents has been observed in the regional nodes from patients with head and neck cancers [51].

Herr, in a study of patients with bladder cancer, has examined the functional characteristics of regional lymph node cells and documented the presence of cells that suppress the mixed lymphocyte response of normal peripheral blood lymphocytes. Suppression, however, was not present in early invasive cancer and appeared to correlate with progressive, deeply invasive carcinoma [52].

*5.3. Clinical studies of regional nodes in nongynecologic cancer*

A major problem in assessment of the clinical benefit of lymph node dissection in patients with cancer has been the indivisibility of the diagnostic and therapeutic procedures, i.e., distinguishing between negative and positive node patients necessitates lymphadenectomy. As a result, clinical data have been attained by inference; with lymphadenectomy, patients with positive nodes develop regional recurrence and patients with negative nodes generally do not. Similarly inferential conclusions can also be reached following radiotherapy of regional nodes.

In malignant melanoma the efficacy of immediate regional lymphadenectomy in Stage I tumors has been a subject of considerable controversy. Although resection of micrometastatic disease in nodes will prevent regional recurrence, evidence that lymphadenectomy will prevent systemic spread has been absent. Moreover, in addition to lymphadenectomy being an unnecessary procedure, the removal of negative nodes *could* have a negative effect on the immunologic tumor–host relationship. Two prospective randomized studies of Stage I malignant melanoma of the limbs have been carried out with similar results when immediate regional lymphadenectomy was compared with lymphadenectomy performed after the appearance of regional metastases. In both studies the survival of patients with nodal metastases was the same, regardless of timing of the procedure [53, 54].

In breast carcinoma, Fisher has reported the results of 1665 woman with medial-central breast tumors treated in the National Surgical Adjuvant Breast and Bowel Project. These patients have been stratified on the basis of clinical examination of axillary nodes and then randomized to radical mastectomy *vs* total mastectomy with radiation therapy for patients with clinically positive nodes and radical mastectomy *vs* total mastectomy with radiation therapy *vs* total mastectomy alone for patients with clinically negative nodes. Although radiation therapy was given to the ipsilateral chest wall as well as the axillary, supraclavicular and internal mammary nodes, it did not alter the incidence of distant recurrence or death when compared to the outcome of nonirradiated patients, including the total mastectomy patients in whom both the axillary and internal mammary nodes were left intact [55]. In the case of patients with axillary node metastases, at least 40% would be expected to have carcinoma in the untreated internal mammary nodes. Data from this large series of patients does appear to indicate that excision of nodal metastases in breast cancer provides only prognostic and not therapeutic benefit beyond control of regional disease. Extrapolation of this data to treatment of pelvic nodal disease must be approached with caution, however, because of the far greater difficulty in achieving regional disease control in the pelvis than in the axilla, regardless of nodal status.

In addition to the lack of therapeutic benefit from nodal irradiation in patients with medial-central lesions who have a high risk of internal mammary node metastasis, when radical mastectomy patients were compared to those having total mastectomy plus radiation therapy, patients with clinically positive axillary nodes treated with combined therapy had an 18% greater incidence of recurrence and 15% greater mortality at 5 years. This difference was observed *despite* lack of any therapy directed at the internal mammary nodes in the radical mastectomy patients and therefore indicated a potentially deleterious effect of postoperative radiation therapy [56]. This adverse effect of radiation therapy has also been identified in patients with negative axillary nodes in two retrospective studies.

The most recent study demonstrated a decrease in 5-year survival from 94% to 75% in Stage II and III breast cancer patients when postoperative adjuvant radiation therapy was added to radical mastectomy [57]. The relationship between postoperative radiotherapy and adjuvant chemotherapy has also been addressed by Holland and co-workers who demonstrated that the addition of postoperative radiation therapy drastically reduced survival in patients with four or more positive nodes despite the use of adjuvant chemotherapy of equivalent duration. At eight years follow-up, 14 of 27 patients with postoperative radiation therapy and adjuvant chemotherapy had recurred in contrast to nine of 73 patients receiving chemotherapy alone [58].

## 6. NODAL METASTASIS FROM GYNECOLOGIC SITES

### 6.1. Carcinoma of the vulva

Radical vulvectomy and en bloc resection of the inguino-femoral regional nodes which drain that area has been the paradigm for the classical 'Halstedian' approach to cancer extirpation. Basset's advocacy in 1912 of complete resection of the vulva, in light of its complex lymphatic anastomoses, represented a significant advance over previous methods of limited local resection, as substantiated by an improved survival [59], culminating in Taussig's report in 1936 of an 81% 5-year survival with the 'Basset operation' in a selected group of 76 patients [60]. Early concerns with the treatment of vulvar carcinoma were the technical management of locally advanced malignancy and the adequacy of regional lymph node dissection, especially whether or not to subject the patient to the additional morbidity of pelvic node dissection [61]. With a trend toward earlier diagnosis of these cutaneous lesions over the past 50 years, both the size at diagnosis and the prevalence of groin node metastases have progressively decreased at the Massachusetts General Hospital (Table 2). As a result of this trend toward earlier diagnosis, emphasis has shifted to attempts to define the least extensive lesion at risk for nodal metastases in hopes of sparing some individuals the morbidity of regional node dissection.

*Table 2.* Incidence of node metastases by interval of study (MGH-Pondville series).

| Interval | Patients with groin metastases | (%) | Patients with pelvic metastasis | (%) |
| --- | --- | --- | --- | --- |
| 1927–1950 | 38/69 | (55) | 16/69 | (23) |
| 1951–1959 | 25/47 | (53) | | |
| 1960–1972 | 21/60 | (35) | 2/142 | (1.4) |
| 1973–1976 | 8/35 | (23) | | |

From Fuller [61], reprinted with permission.

Any compromise in the application of an otherwise curative surgical procedure in hopes of reducing surgical morbidity must be judiciously founded in knowledge of the anatomy of the region and pathophysiology of early invasive vulvar neoplasia. The crucial questions relevant to the surgical treatment of vulvar cancer once again pertain to the presence of lymph node metastases:
1. What is the maximal *size* of vulvar carcinoma that bears *no* risk of inguino-femoral metastases?
2. What is the maximal depth of *invasion* completely free of risk of nodal metastases?
3. What combination of size, position and depth of invasion permits ipsilateral dissection only?

Review of clinical evidence indicates, first of all, that direct metastases to the pelvic nodes essentially do not occur in the absence of inguino-femoral nodal disease, unless there is tumor extension into the vagina [61]. Primary clitoral tumors specifically do not appear to metastasize directly to pelvic nodes despite the description by Reiffenstuhl of supra- and retropubic lymphatic channels [62]. This discrepancy is probably the result of Reiffenstuhl's choice of stillborns for lymphatic injection as adults show no evidence of this route of dissemination by clinical studies involving lymphography or node dissection [61].

Collective data recently summarized in two articles by Tamimi and DiSaia indicate that even the Stage I tumor ($\leqslant 2$ cm) with $\leqslant 5$ mm invasion still presents substantial risk of groin node metastases [63, 64]. Exclusion of confluent tumors (extent of invasion $>1$ mm), anaplastic tumors, and tumors with lymphatic or vascular invasion greatly reduces this risk, but simultaneously excludes the vast majority of young women with Stage I disease. Tamimi has noted that these patients with early stromal invasion have tongue-like projections with enlargement of cell size and eosinophilic cytoplasm in these projections. He has suggested that patients fulfilling these criteria could safely be treated with superficial ('skinning') vulvectomy and split thickness skin grafting while treatment of more extensive lesions ('microcarcinomas') require standard therapy until further data become available [63]. DiSaia, alternatively, has recommended wide local excision of tumors whose size is $\leqslant 1$ cm with a depth of invasion of 5 mm or less. Based on the knowledge that 3% of 68 patients with invasion of 1–3 mm had nodal metastases in a study from the Mayo Clinic [65], DiSaia has recommended preliminary bilateral dissection of inguino-femoral nodes superficial to the cribriform fascia; if these are positive on frozen section examination then complete radical vulvectomy and bilateral deep groin dissections are carried out, with a pelvic node dissection on the involved side. If the preliminary dissections are negative for tumor, however, the vulvar lesion is widely excised with a 3 cm perimeter of normal tissue along with adequate subcutaneous tissue beneath the lesion. In the first series of 20 patients, 18 had negative nodes, wide local excision, and no evidence of recurrence at a mean follow-up of 39 months (range 14-81). Two patients had ipsilateral nodal metastases only and were treated with the complete radical procedure. Retrospective evaluation revealed that one of these patients had stromal invasion to the 6-7 mm level and both had 1 mm areas of confluent invasion; one of the two was also an anaplastic lesion. All patients undergoing wide local excision maintained their normal sexual response in contrast to the two patients with radical vulvectomy, in whom it was lost [64].

These two approaches actually appear complementary, rather than mutually exclusive; early stromal invasion could be adequately treated with superficial excision and grafting when necessary, while more advanced lesions excluded by Tamimi's criteria could be treated with the local excisional biopsy and superficial groin node dissection to include the sentinel nodes.

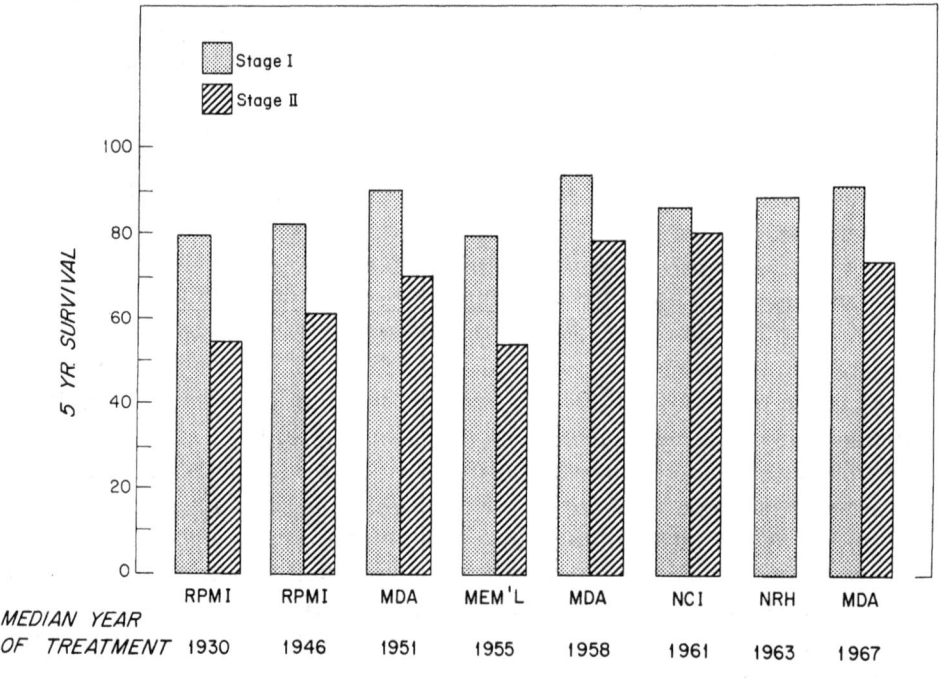

*Figure 6.* Five-year survival, cervical carcinoma Stages I and II. There is no significant improvement in end results of patients treated at the institutions reporting recurrence data: MDA, M.D. Anderson Hospital [68, 69, 70], MEM'L, Memorial Hospital, New York [71, 75], NCI, National Cancer Institute [72], NRH, Norwegian Radium Hospital [73], RPMI, Roswell Park Memorial Institute [74].

As we gain more prognostic information about the tumor–host relationships in this disease, particularly with respect to the recent dramatic decrease in age at onset, and its relationship to herpes simplex and human papilloma viruses, we should be able to more clearly select *only* the patients at risk of nodal metastases for truly radical surgery. At present time this synthesis seems to be a reasonable approach for further scrunity.

*6.2. Carcinoma of the cervix*

'The management of cancer of the cervix uteri requires an understanding of its rate of growth, direction of spread, route and sites of metastases and the effect of surgery or radiation on these events' [66]. Thus Henriksen began the introduction to his discussion of the pelvic lymph nodes in Meigs' *Surgical Treatment of Cancer of the Cervix,* published in 1954. This observation has never been more appropriate than today, as we recognize little improvement in survival within each stage of invasive cervical carcinoma despite refinements in surgical and radiotherapeutic techniques [67]. It will become clear that despite our improved understanding of the anatomic extent of disease and our increasing ability to achieve local control of the primary tumor, that treatment failure as a result of occult metastases will continue to be an increasing problem (Figures 6 and 7) [60–75]. As patients

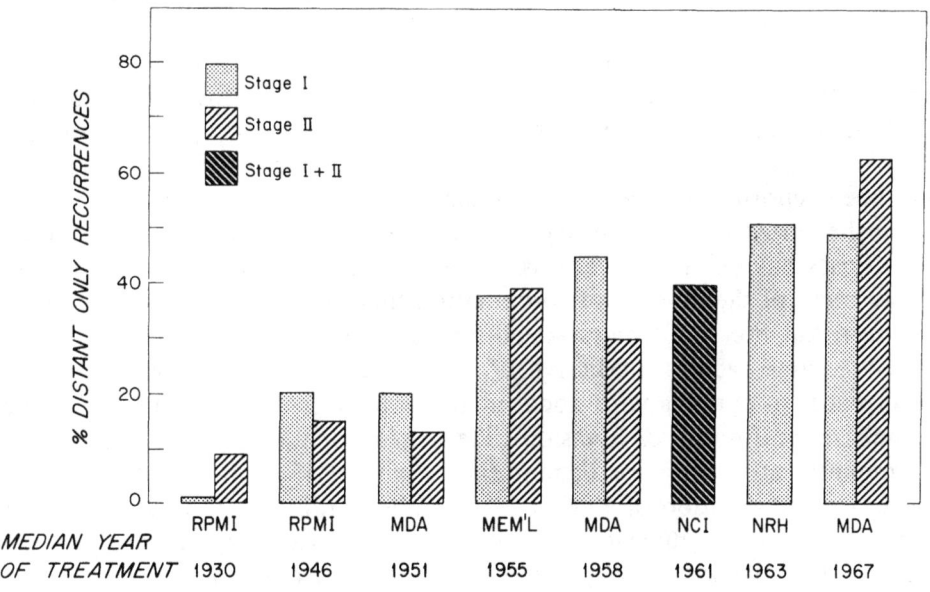

*Figure 7.* Trend in site of recurrence. There is a progressive shift in the percent of recurrences attributed to distant disease alone. MDA, M.D. Anderson Hospital [68, 69, 70], MEM'L, Memorial Hospital, New York [71, 75], NCI, National Cancer Institute [72], NRH, Norwegian Radium Hospital [73], RPMI, Roswell Park Memorial Institute [74].

with lymph node metastases constitue an increasing proportion of patients with recurrent carcinoma, perhaps more attention to Henriksen's admonition can reveal some of the reasons for failure. We have already reviewed some of the basic biology of metastasis and we will review the *direction* and *sites* of nodal metastases as well as the *effect* of our therapeutic modalities on these events, particularly as they relate to the host.

Because patients with less extensive nodal disease have better survival rates than those patients with more extensive metastases, resection of larger numbers of nodes increases the chance of finding microscopic metastases and enlarges the population of positive node patients with individuals with better prognosis because of more limited nodal disease. This shift of 'lower risk' patients with micrometastases into the positive node group improves the survival for the group as a whole and concomitantly removes the same 'higher risk' patients from the negative node group and improves their survival. In fact, more careful sectioning of each node removed in the lymphadenectomy specimen results in the same artefactual shift toward a greater proportion of patients with positive pelvic nodes. Survival by nodal status improves in both groups. One must therefore compare the entire group, regardless of nodal status in a prospective study in order to assess the effect of more extensive lymphadenectomy. This effect is illustrated by Kolbenstvedt's series from the Norwegian Radium Hospital in which nodal dissection under lymphographic control increased the incidence of nodal metastases from 15.1% to 21.1% [76, 77]. It must be assumed, of course, for the purpose of valid comparison, that those factors which are predictive of nodal metastasis, such as primary tumor size, histologic grade and depth of invasion [78] were similar in both groups. At present, survival data have not been reported for these two groups.

Further attempts to improve survival in high risk patients with nodal metastases have included various combinations of radiation and operation. Assessment of the efficacy of combination therapy has been complicated by the fact that the risk factors stated above predicting nodal metastases are also the same factors predictive of local recurrence. When one examines recurrences in patients with nodal metastases compared with tumors of the same size (and depth of invasion), the increased risk of failure occurs predominantly at regional or distant sites (Table 3) [78]. It is not surprising then, that the addition of 4000 R pelvic radiotherapy to the treatment of 32 patients with nodal metastases resulted in a survival curve (Figure 8) identical to that of another 39 patients with similar extent of local and nodal disease [79]: These data confirm observations of Morrow (reporting for the Society of Gynecologic Oncologists) and Zander who have demonstrated a similar lack of effectiveness of postoperative radiation therapy for nodal metastases [80, 81]. Moreover, in the Memorial Sloan-Kettering study there

Table 3. Percent of patients recurring at regional or distant sites by primary tumor size and nodal status. Note that the site of recurrence refers to the most proximal site of recurrence identified.

| Tumor size (cm) | Regional nodes | Number of patients | Local | Regional | Distant |
|---|---|---|---|---|---|
| <2 cm | negative | 137 | 4% | 3% | 0% |
| | positive | 10 | 0% | 30% | 0% |
| 2.0–3.9 cm | negative | 147 | 11% | 4% | 2% |
| | positive | 33 | 18% | 6% | 12% |
| ≥4.0 cm | negative | 64 | 25% | 3% | 3% |
| | positive | 27 | 33% | 19% | 0% |

was no decrease in the frequency of pelvic recurrences in the irradiated group, an effect also reported by Onsrud and associates after postoperative radiation therapy for endometrial carcinoma involving the cervix [82].

Further evidence for the presence of occult systemic metastases and for the effectiveness of this dose of radiation therapy is provided by the results

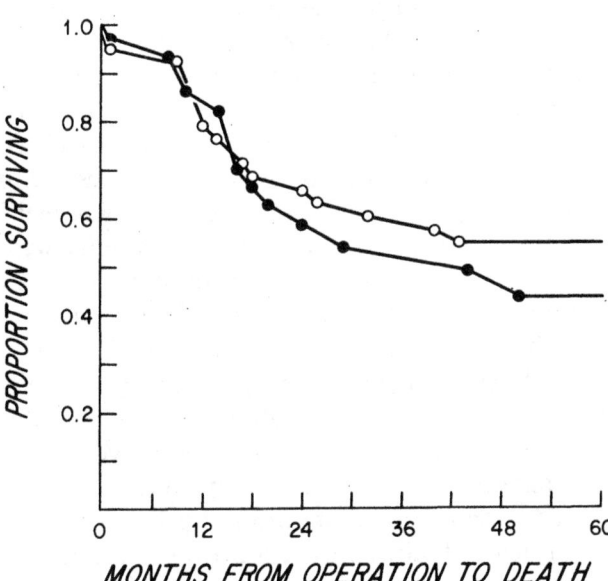

Figure 8. Life table survival curves for patients with lymph node metastases treated with and without postoperative radiation therapy demonstrate no significant difference in survival. Reprinted from [9], with permission.

of postoperative therapy for microscopic parametrial involvement after radical hysterectomy for carcinoma clinically confined to the cervix and upper vagina. Survival did significantly improve with six of seven irradiated patients free of recurrence at six years, in contrast to only nine of 13 unirradiated control patients. Time to recurrence was also prolonged in the one patient who was irradiated and recurred at 65 months in contrast to the four recurrences in controls at 12, 16, 21 and 30 months. The treatment of recurrent carcinoma in this study also indicates the systemic nature of recurrence after diagnosis of nodal metastases at the time of primary surgical treatment. Of 347 patients with negative nodes, 56 patients recurred, and secondary therapy of recurrence including such procedures as pulmonary resection, cured 10 of them, yielding an 18% 5-year salvage after recurrence. In comparison, of 71 patients with positive nodes, 29 patients subsequently recurred and *no* patient was salvaged after recurrence, regardless of site. At present, as far as pelvic lymph node metastases are concerned in invasive carcinoma confined to the cervix and upper vagina, it can be concluded that lymphadenectomy identifies individuals at high risk for regional and distant recurrence and that postoperative radiation therapy directed toward possible microscopic residual disease in these nodal areas has no benefit.

The presence of para-aortic nodal metastases with disease clinically limited to the pelvis was identified more than 50 years ago [8]. Despite early recognition of this extension of disease confirmed by studies, this route of spread had little relevance to clinical practice until Nelson and associates reported their preliminary experience with 13 Stage IIB and III patients, 7 of whom has para-aortic metastases when laparotomy was carried out prior to definitive radiation therapy [83]. Multiple investigators have since confirmed this observation as well as its ominous prognostic significance. In a study of patients with Stage IB-IV disease explored at Roswell Park Memorial Institute, Piver and associates identified 31 patients with para-aortic metastases. All 31 of these patients had been followed 5 years or more and only 3 (9.6%) remained alive at that time. Two of the surviving patients had microscopically positive, clinically negative para-aortic nodal disease and the other patient with Stage IB disease had a solitary 3 × 3 cm node completely resected; each survivor also sustained serious complications from abdominal radiotherapy requiring intestinal surgery. Moreover, because of the association of para-aortic metastases with large, poorly differentiated and locally advanced carcinoma, failure of local primary tumor control was the leading cause of death, followed by death from radiation complications in second place [84]. In locally advanced cervical cancers, although para-aortic nodal metastases may be associated with occult systemic metastases, including positive scalene nodes in half of the patients [85, 86], modification in therapy directed toward this problem must await improvements in our ability to control the primary tumor.

## 6.3. Endometrial carcinoma

The lymphatics of the uterine fundus extend through the mesosalpinx and along the upper edge of the broad ligament anastomosing with afferents from the tube and ovary to terminate in primary nodes in the para-aortic area at the level of the renal vessels. Afferents from the central portion of the corpus, however, transverse the parametrium and drain into iliac nodes, most frequently at the bifurcation of the common iliac vessels. A third channel, inconstant and less readily identified, passes along the round ligament and terminates in ipsilateral nodes in the inguinal canal (Figure 2) [8]. Meigs noted that though the inguinal route of spread was infrequent, the lymph nodes in the pelvis were 'probably involved in more instances than is generally believed' citing the experience of Weibel with a 16% incidence of pelvic node metastases in carcinoma confined to the corpus. His own review (Table 1) confirmed that both routes to pelvic and para-aortic nodes were clinically significant, even when the tumor was confined to the corpus.

Henriksen's detailed autopsy study [87] in 1949 of 64 patients with endometrial carcinoma confirmed these three routes of spread and indicated the presence of nodal metastases in one of eight cases without myometrial invasion, in 8/18 cases with myometrial invasion and a grossly enlarged uterus (= 10 weeks gestational size) and in 28/38 cases with more extensive uterine tumor. Ingersoll and Meigs subsequently presented their autopsy data along with a prospective clinical trial of radical hysterectomy plus pelvic lymphadenectomy for cancer apparently localized to the uterus [11]. In their autopsy series of 46 patients (Table 4), Ingersoll and Meigs identified two of 11 patients (18%) with disease confined to the uterus and nodal metastases (one pelvic, one para-aortic) whereas 25 of 35 patients (71%) with extra-uterine spread were also found to have pelvic nodal metastases, para-aortic metastases, or both. In the prospective group of patients treated with radical hysterectomy and bilateral pelvic lymphadenectomy, two of 21 patients with disease confined to the corpus were found to have pelvic node

*Table 4.* Nodal involvement in carcinoma of the corpus (46 autopsy cases).

|  | Cofined to uterus | Extra-uterine spread |
|---|---|---|
| Number of cases | 11 | 35 |
| Cases with nodal metastases | 2 | 25 |
| Pelvic only | 1 | 1 |
| Para-aortic only | 1 | 11 |
| Pelvic and para-aortic | 0 | 13 |

Adapted from Ingersoll and Meigs [11].

metastases as well as one of four patients with disease extending to the cervix. They concluded, as a result of these investigations, that lymph node metastasis was a definitive possibility in Stage I carcinoma and that, despite the unproven value of lymph node dissections, further surgical exploration should be carried out in good risk patients.

Subsequently, a large number of studies have confirmed both the prevalence of widespread nodal metastases in autopsy series of patients with advanced disease and up to a 28% incidence of pelvic nodal metastases in patients with carcinoma confined to the uterus. These have been collected and reviewed by Plentl and Friedman [88] who have noted that more than one-half of their collected series (predominantly from autopsy) of 142 patients with 258 positive nodes had para-aortic nodal metastases. They also confirmed the tendency for nodal metastases from endometrial carcinoma to occur more frequently in the cephalic pelvic nodes (hypogastric > common iliac > external iliac > obturator), whereas cervical carcinoma was associated with metastases to more caudal nodes (external iliac > obturator > hypogastric > common iliac). The correlation of pelvic nodal metastases with depth of myometrial invasion was evident in a collected series of 600 patients whose lymphadenectomies were done in the course of primary treatment of the neoplasm. Although the overall incidence of nodal metastases was 20.3%, only 0.6% of patients without myometrial invasion and 6.3% of patients with superficial invasion had nodal metastases. In contrast 55% of patients with deep myometrial invasion had nodal involvement.

A strong case has also been made for the presence of concurrent hematogenous metastases in patients with nodal metastases, in light of the prevalence of suburethral vaginal recurrences in these patients who also tend to have poorly differentiated tumors and deep myometrial invasion [89, 90]. The presence of metastases at this site from other tumors which predominantly spread along hematogenous routes (choriocarcinoma and hypernephroma) provided circumstantial evidence for this assumption which is strengthened by evidence that suburethral metastases occur predominantly from the *left* kidney where direct venous, but not lymphatic anastomoses exist [91].

In this last decade, multiple investigators have reaffirmed the association of increasing histologic grade with depth of tumor invasion and increasing depth of invasion with risk of pelvic and para-aortic nodal metastases as well as risk of recurrence in retrospective and prospective studies [92–99]. Increasing awareness that as many as one-half of patients with clinical Stage I disease and deep myometrical invasion may have nodal metastases both at pelvic and para-aortic sites has led to renewal of attempts at anatomic staging and treatment protocols based on surgical rather than clinical staging procedures.

*Table 5.* The effect of postoperative external radiation therapy upon distant metastases and death in low and moderate risk patients with Stage I endometrial carcinoma.

| Histology | Group A (controls) | | | Group B (external RT) | | |
|---|---|---|---|---|---|---|
| | No. of patients | Cancer deaths | Distant metastases | No. of patients | Cancer deaths | Distant metastases |
| G1 and G2 myometrial invasion ≤1/2 | 126 | 2.3% | 1.6% | 131 | 6.9% | 6.9% |
| G1 and G2 myometrial invasion >1/2 | 51 | 7.5% | 3.9% | 32 | 9.5% | 9.4% |
| G3 myometrial invasion ≤1/2 | 36 | 8.3% | 5.6% | 47 | 17.0% | 17.0% |

(Adapted from the data of Aalders, *et al.* [101]).

The most dramatic evidence of the inadequacy of previously accepted treatment of endometrial carcinoma has been provided by the large prospective clinical trial begun in 1968 at the Norwegian Radium Hospital by Kolstad and associates [100, 101]. In this controlled study, which has already accrued 540 patients over 6 years (all available for 5-year follow-up), patients with clinical Stage I endometrial carcinoma who did not have proven metastases at the time of total abdominal hysterectomy and bilateral salpingo-oophorectomy were all treated with postoperative intravaginal radiation therapy (Table 5). Total dose delivered was 6000 R measured at the vaginal surface. Patients were randomly allocated to two groups: 'group A' were controls and received no further treatment; 'group B' received 4000 R via high voltage external radiation therapy with central shielding after 2000 R. Actuarial survival rates in the two groups were virtually superimposable with a slight but insignificantly better survival in those control patients not receiving additional external radiation therapy [101]. Five-year survival in the controls (group A) was 91% and in the patients with additional therapy (group B) the corresponding figure was 89%. Prognostic factors influencing outcome were evenly distributed in both groups and, considered individually, did not influence survival in these two groups. There was, however, a decreased incidence of vaginal or local pelvic recurrence in those patients treated with whole pelvis radiotherapy and a corresponding increase in distant metastases for the same group. Only when the subset of Grade 3 patients were subdivided by depth of myometrial invasion did there appear any significant improvement in survival rate after external radiation therapy. Patients with Grade 3 tumors and myometrial invasion of half or less of the uterine wall who received external radiotherapy recurred almost twice as often as those who were not treated. This difference was accounted for by a greater than three-fold increase in the number of patients with distant metastases (group A, 5.6%, group B, 17.0%). In contrast, among 95 patients with Grade 3 tumors and myometrial invasion involving greater than half of the uterine wall, the incidence of distant metastasis was similar but the rate of vaginal and pelvic recurrence in the control group was more than three times higher (19.6% vs 4.5% in the treated group) and a significantly larger number of controls died from recurrent disease (27.5% vs 18.2%). It was also noted that the mean time to recurrence for the entire treated group B was *shorter* than the corresponding time for untreated controls (22 vs 18 months).

Given the association of deep myometrial invasion with pelvic nodal metastases *and* para-aortic metastases [93, 95, 97, 99] it is not surprising that patients at risk for metastases at both sites have no decrease in incidence of distant metastases after additional regional treatment directed toward pelvic nodes only. This result becomes even more self-evident on review of Creasman's data from peritoneal cytology which indicated that 65% of patients with pelvic nodal metastases also had cytologically positive peritoneal washings [102]. Because of the risks of distant lymphatic metastases (from which Piver has recently reported a series of *no* survivors after para-aortic irradiation [103], hematogenous metastases, and metastases through the peritoneal cavity associated with pelvic nodal metastases, this truly must be considered a systemic disease either on the basis of nodal immunosuppression or because of the *association* of tumor invasion and metastases to nodes with hematogenous and surface metastases. Although a reduced frequency of local recurrence if confirmed may result from external therapy in a small subset of patients, presumably effective systemic therapy, if available, would also improve local control. An important finding as well is the increased incidence of distant metastases after external radiation therapy for Stage I disease in all three other groups with low to moderate risk of nodal metastases (Table 5). Here the potential negative effect of postoperative radiation therapy of patients with limited risk nodal metastases appears evident and indicates the possibility of a deleterious effect upon host immune defenses, an effect previously described by Johnstone after postoperative nodal radiation in the therapy of breast carcinoma with negative nodes [56].

## 6.4. Adenocarcinoma of the Fallopian tube

Tubal carcinoma is a rare lesion first described by Orthmann in 1886 [104]. Undoubtedly precipitated by early invasion into the rich lymphatic investment of the tubal mucosa and the predominance of poorly differentiated tumors, lymphatic metastasis may occur early in the progression of this disease. Meigs noted that metastases in the proximal iliac nodes were commonly the results of extension to the broad ligament and that the predominant lymphatic path of dissemination led to the para-aortic nodes (Figures 2 and 3) [8]. Surface extension of disease through the peritoneal cavity was also a prominent feature of the poorly differentiated, deeply invasion primary. Prevalence of the site of origin of this tumor in distal portions of the tube may well be related to the increased surface area of the mucosa at risk at the ampullary end. The relative rarity of tumors occurring at the cornual end of the tube may also explain the infrequent appearance of inguinal metastasis, apparently the result of lymphatic anastomoses between that portion of the tube and the round ligament. Although, in many cases, anatomic extension to the adjacent ovary can be identified, certainly the distinction between the two primary sites should be made with great care, as it is often a decision based solely upon gross pathologic assessment of extent of disease.

Relying upon the similarity between the tube and the intestine as a hollow, muscular viscus, Schiller and Silverberg have proposed a staging system (Table 6) in which their 76 collectively reviewed cases are stratified well by prognosis for 5-year survival and reasonably well distributed by stage [105]. It is of note that not all patients with Stage 0, (*in situ*) carcinoma have an assured survival, probably because of invasion of lymphatic vessels within the mucosa. Tamimi and Figge have reviewed 15 cases treated at

*Table 6.* Pathologic staging of primary Fallopian tube carcinoma.

| Stage | Extent of disease | Number of cases | 5-year disease-free survival |
|---|---|---|---|
| 0 | Carcinoma *in situ* (limited to the tubal mucosa) | 11 | 82% |
| I | Tumor extending into the submucosa and/or muscularis but not penetrating to the serosal surface of the Fallopian tube | 13 | 53% |
| II | Tumor extending to the serosa of the Fallopian tube | 6 | 16% |
| III | Direct extension of the tumor to the ovary and/or endometrium | 12 | 8% |
| IV | Extension of the tumor beyond the reproductive organs (e.g. other pelvic organs, pelvic soft tissues, peritoneal implants, abdominal viscera) | 34 | 9% |

From Schiller and Silverberg [105].

their institution over an 11-year period [34]. Para-aortic nodal metastases were identified in 5 patients (33%) even though node-bearing areas were not explored in all patients and no patient underwent pelvic node dissection. Two of eight patients with disease apparently confined to the Fallopian tube were found to have para-aortic metastases; one patient with pelvic disease that had been completely resected recurred in para-aortic nodes only. Three additional patients with more advanced disease had distant nodal metastases including two with groin metastases, one of whom also had a positive supraclavicular node. In all, 53% of patients with Fallopian tube carcinoma were found to have nodal metastases at the time of treatment of the primary disease or its recurrence and 73% had high grade tumors. All but one of the patients dead of disease had Grade 3 tumors; the exception was a patient with a Grade 1 tumor who recurred in the para-aortic nodes at 72 months. This report appears to confirm the applicability of Schiller and Silverberg's staging system. Survival by stage indicated a relatively even distribution of patients, with a survival in Stage I of 67% (2 of 3), in Stage II of 33% (1 of 3) and in Stages III and IV of 0% and 50% respectively. The improved survival in Stage IV compared with Stage III is the result of adjuvant chemotherapy in patients with extrapelvic nodal metastases that had been completely resected, while Stage III patients often had residual pelvic disease. Three recurrences in six Stage I and II patients with disease apparently confined to the tube indicate that further extent of disease evaluation needs to be systematically carried out at the time of primary laparotomy; this should specifically include pelvic washings and pelvic node sampling or dissection, as suggested by Tamimi and Figge [34]. In fact, the one patient with tumor confined to the tubal muscularis was the one patient who recurred in para-aortic nodes only despite Grade I histology. In light of their apparent success with adjuvant chemotherapy for Stage IV patients with para-aortic metastasis, the staging system may have to be further revised to accurately reflect the less favorable prognosis of gross residual disease when compared with completely resected extra-pelvic nodal metastases.

*6.5. Ovarian carcinoma*

The significance of nodal metastases in epithelial ovarian carcinoma has long been overshadowed by the presence of massive intra-abdominal tumor unresponsive to therapy. The therapeutic advantage gained by effective cytotoxic chemotherapy has presented both the need to understand the true extent of malignant disease and the wherewithal to control it.

Although the primary route of lymphatic drainage from the ovary to the para-aortic nodes at the renal level and secondary routes to high iliac and inguinal nodes had long been known from autopsy studies of patients with nodal metastases (Figures 1 and 2) [8], Knapp and Friedman in 1974 emphasized the presence of para-aortic nodal metastases in patients with tumors that were poorly differentiated but apparently confined to the ovary [106]. Five of the 26 patients (19%) in their report had histologic evidence of para-aortic nodal metastases. When tumors 8 cm or more in primary size were considered, the incidence was 5/21 (24%); when the primary tumor was undifferentiated the corresponding number was 80%. In fact, para-aortic nodal metastases occurring in the epithelial ovarian tumors were found *only* with those with poorly differentiated histologic pattern. Subsequent reports from multiple investigators [107, 108, 109], have confirmed the presence of para-aortic nodal metastases in patients with disease otherwise confined to the ovary and predominance of nodal metastases with poorly differentiated tumors. One of these reports also identified 3 of 28 (10.6%) patients with pelvic nodal metastases as well [107].

The presence of occult metastases in the majority of patients with ovarian cancer has had little significance in their treatment. For the subset of patients with anaplastic cancers confined to one or both ovaries, however, evaluation of both pelvic and para-aortic sites must be as routine as peritoneal cytology and omental biopsy. The benefits of adjuvant therapy with alkylating agents and the apparently deleterious effects of pelvic radiation therapy in this setting might be explained by this extent of disease [110]. Precise staging and equally precise treatment directed toward the meticulously determined extent of disease will be essential to improved survival. The second major area of impact will be upon those patients having 'second look' procedures, in whom the degree of primary tumor differentiation and prior nodal metastases will determine the need for retroperitoneal exploration.

Until further markers for residual disease can be identified and usefully evaluated, thorough anatomic exploration remains the best means of establishing risk of persistent carcinoma.

## 7. SUMMARY AND CONCLUSIONS

An increasing body of experimental and clinical evidence exists that is inconsistent with the traditional concept that the regional lymph node represents an effective anatomic filter protecting the host from dissemination of primary carcinoma. Review of the multiple steps in the process of lymphatic metastases indicates that many steps are also common to surface and hematogenous metastases also; the appearance of nodal disease may merely indicate the tumor's capacity to spread by these other routes as well. The clinical behavior of endometrial cancer seems to closely follow this course.

The presence of an immunologic response to cancer, mediated by early sensitization of the regional draining node and overcome by the continued progressive growth of the tumor ultimately may result in localized or systemic immunosuppression. The growth of metastatic cancer in the lymph node, therefore, may reflect this tumor-host relationship rather than any anatomically limited spread of malignancy. The immune response to cancer, however, remains largely uncertain as does the existence of *unique* tumor antigens that might be characteristic of a histologic class of tumors. Virally induced or associated tumors which can be more immunogenic, however, may be more likely to elicit this host response and our presently available data for cervical carcinoma confirms this.

Whatever the etiology of the regional node metastasis might be, its prognostic importance is becoming increasingly clear. The functionally intact node does seem to exhibit some protection in that adjuvant radiation therapy may have a deleterious effect upon survival. The positive node, on the contrary, appears to signal the presence of systemic, though often occult, even dormant, disease that necessitates the development of more effective programs of adjuvant therapy.

## REFERENCES

1. Virchow R: Cellular Pathology. London: JA Churchill Ltd, 1863.
2. Paget J: The distribution of secondary growth in cancer of the breast. Lancet 1:571-573, 1889.
3. Halsted WS: The treatment of wounds with special reference to the value of the blood clot in the management of dead spaces. Johns Hopkins Med J 2:255-314, 1890.
4. Heidenhain L: Über die Ursachen der lokalen Krebsrezidive nach Amputation Mammae. Arch Klin Chir 39:97-104, 1889.
5. Stiles HJ: On the dissemination of cancer of the breast. Br Med J 1:1452, 1899.
6. Gray JH: The relation of lymphatic vessels to the spread of cancer. Brit J Surg 26:462-495, 1968.
7. Ballon SC: The Wertheim hysterectomy. Surg Gynecol Obstet 142:920-924, 1976.
8. Meigs JV: Tumors of the Female Pelvic Organs. New York: Macmillan Co, 1934.
9. Warren S: Grading of carcinoma of cervix uteri as checked at autopsy. Arch Path 12:783-786, 1931.
10. Meigs JV: Radical hysterectomy with bilateral lymph node dissection. Am J Obstet Gynecol 62:854-861, 1951.
11. Ingersoll FM, Meigs JV: Lymph node dissection for carcinoma of the endometrium. In: Proceedings of the Second National Cancer Conference. New York: Am Cancer Soc, 1954.
12. Parsons L, Somers SC: Gynecology, 2nd ed. Philadelphia: Saunders, 1978.
13. Selim MA, Kurohara SS, Webster JH: Surgical or radiation therapy for cancer of the cervix Stage I. Obstet Gynecol 38:251-255, 1971.
14. Decker DG, Aaro LA, Hunt AB, Johnson CE, Smith RA: Sequential radiation and operation in carcinoma of the uterine cervix. Am J Obstet Gynecol 92:35-43, 1965.

15. Newton M: Radical hysterectomy or radiation therapy for Stage I cervical cancer; A prospective comparison with five and ten year follow-up. Am J Obstet Gynecol 123: 535-543, 1975.
16. Roddick JR Jr, Greenlaw RH: Treatment of cervical cancer: A randomized study of operation and radiation. Am J Obstet Gynecol 109: 754-764, 1971.
17. Morley GW, Seski JC: Radical pelvic surgery vs radiation therapy for Stage I carcinoma of the cervix (exclusive of microinvasion). Am J Obstet Gynecol 126: 785-798, 1976.
18. Gray MJ, Frick HC: Pelvic lymph node dissection following radiotherapy for cancer of the cervix. Am J Obstet Gynecol 93: 110-114, 1965.
19. Stage AH, Crawford EJ, Robinson LS, Brooks GG: Combined radiologic/operative therapy in the treatment of cervical malignancy. Am J Obstet Gynecol 120: 960-968, 1974.
20. Rutledge FN, Fletcher GH: Transperitoneal pelvic lymphadenectomy following supervoltage irradiation for squamous cell carcinoma of the cervix. Am J Obstet Gynecol 76: 321-334, 1958.
21. Lagasse LD, Smith ML, Moore JG, Morton DG, Jacobs M, Johnson GH: The effect of radiation therapy on pelvic lymph node involvement in Stage I carcinoma of the cervix. Am J Obstet Gynecol 119: 328-334, 1974.
22. Fisher B: The surgical dilemma in the primary therapy of invasive breast cancer: a critical appraisal. Current Problems in Surgery, pp 1-50, 1970.
23. Fidler IJ, Kripke ML: Metastasis results from preexisting variant cells within a malignant tumor. Science 197: 893-895, 1977.
24. Fidler IJ, Gersten DM, Hart IR: Cancer invasion and metastasis. Adv Cancer Res 28: 149-250, 1978.
25. Post G, Fidler IJ: The pathogenesis of cancer metastasis. Nature 283: 139-146, 1980.
26. Piver MS, Chung WS: Prognostic significance of cervical carcinoma. Obstet Gynecol 46: 507-510, 1975.
27. Burghardt E, Pickel H: Local spread and lymph node involvement in cervical carcinoma. Obstet Gynecol 52: 138-145, 1978.
28. Gusberg SB, Yannopoulos K, Cohen CJ: Virulence indices and lymph nodes in cancer of the cervix. Amer J Roentgenol Ther Nucl Med 3: 273-277, 1971.
29. Liu W, Meigs JV: Radical hysterectomy and pelvic lymphadenectomy. Am J Obstet Gynecol 69: 1-32, 1955.
30. Lewis BV, Stallworthy JA, Cowdell R: Adenocarcinoma of the body of the uterus. J Obstet Gynaecol Brit Comm 77: 343-348, 1970.
31. Parsons L, Cesare F: Wertheim hysterectomy in the treatment of endometrial carcinoma. Surg Gynecol Obstet 108: 582-590, 1959.
32. Green TH: Carcinoma of the vulva, a reassessment. Obstet Gynecol 52: 462-469, 1978.
33. Krupp PJ, Lee FY, Batson HWK, Allen P McD, Collins JH: Carcinoma of the vulva. Gynecol Oncol 1: 345-362, 1973.
34. Tamini HK, Figge DC: Adenocarcinoma of the uterine tube: potential for lymph node metastases. Am J Obstet Gynecol 141: 132-137, 1981.
35. Roche WD, Norris HJ: Microinvasive carcinoma of the cervix. Cancer 36: 180-186, 1975.
36. Burnet MF: Immunologic Surveillance. Oxford: Pergamon Press, 1970.
37. Prehn RT: Immunostimulation of the lymphodependent phase of neoplastic growth. J Natl Cancer Inst 59: 1043-1049, 1977.
38. Hanna N: Expression of metastatic potential of tumor cells in young nude mice is correlated with low levels of natural killer cell-mediated cytotoxicity. Int J Cancer 26: 675-680, 1980.
39. Herberman RB, Djeu JY, Kay HD, Ortaldo JR, Riccardo C, Bonnard GD, Holden HT,

Sagnani R, Santoni A, Puccetti P: Natural killer cells: characteristics and regulation of activity. Immunol Rev 11:43-70, 1979.
40. Hanna N, Fidler IJ: Role of natural killer cells in the destruction of circulating tumor emboli. J Natl Cancer Inst 65:801-809, 1980.
41. Hanna N: Inhibition of experimental tumor metastasis by selective activation of natural killer cells. Cancer Res 42:1337-1342, 1982.
42. Zacharski LR, Henderson WG, Rickles FR, et al.: Rationale and experimental design for the VA cooperative study of anticoagulation (warfarin) in the treatment of cancer. Cancer 44:732-741, 1979.
43. Wheelock EF, Weinhold KJ, Levich J: The tumor dormant state. Adv Cancer Res 34:107-140, 1981.
44. Fisher B, Fisher ER: Studies concerning the regional lymph node in cancer – I. Initiation of immunity. Cancer 27:1001-1004, 1971.
45. Pendergrast WJ Jr, Soloway MS, Myers GH, Futrell JW: Regional lymphadenectomy and tumor immunity. Surg Gynecol Obstet 142:385-390, 1976.
46. Hasumi K, Sugano H, Sakamoto G, Masubuchi K, Kubo H: Circumscribed carcinoma of the uterine cervix, with marked lymphocyte infiltration. Cancer 39:2503-2507, 1977.
47. Tsakraklides V, Anastassiades OT, Kersey JH: Prognostic significance of regional node histology in uterine cervical cancer. Cancer 31:860-868, 1973.
48. Van Nagell JR Jr, Donaldson ES, Parker JC, Van Dyke AH, Wood EG: The prognostic significance of pelvic node morphology in carcinoma of the uterine cervix. Cancer 39:2624-2632, 1977.
49. Bhan AK, Nadler LM, Stashenko P, McCluskey RT, Schlossman SF: Stages of B cell differentiation in human lymphoid tissue. J Exp Med 154:737-749, 1981.
50. Poppema S, Bhan AK, Reinherz EL, McCluskey RF, Schlossman SF: Distribution of T cell subsets in human lymph nodes. J Exp Med 153:30-41, 1981.
51. Saxon A, Portis J: Lymphoid subpopulation changes in regional lymph nodes in squamous head and neck cancer. Cancer Res 37:1154-1159, 1977.
52. Herr HW: Suppressor cells in the pelvic lymph nodes regional to bladder cancer. J Surg Oncol 11:289-293, 1979.
53. Sim FH, Taylor WF, Ivins JC, Pritchard DJ, Soule EH: A prospective randomized study of the efficacy of routine elective lymphadenectomy in management of malignant melanoma. Cancer 41:946-948, 1978.
54. Veronesi U, Adamas J, Bandiera DC et al.: Delayed regional lymph node dissection in Stage I melanoma of the skin of the lower extremities. Cancer 49:2420-2430, 1982.
55. Fisher B, Wolmark N, Redmond C, Deutsch M, Fisher ER, and participating NSABP investigators: Findings from NSABP protocol No. B-04: Comparison of radical mastectomy with alternative treatments. II. The clinical and biological significance of medial-central breast cancers. Cancer 48:1863-1872, 1981.
56. Johnstone FRC: Postoperative radiation in the treatment of carcinoma of the breast. Am J Surg 128:276-281, 1974.
57. Nevin JE, Baggerly JT, Laird TK: Radiotherapy as an adjuvant in the treatment of carcinoma of the breast. Cancer 49:1194-1200, 1982.
58. Holland JF, Glidewell O, Cooper RC: Adverse effect of radiotherapy on adjuvant chemotherapy for carcinoma of the breast. Surg Gynecol Obstet 150:811-821, 1980.
59. Basset A: Traitement chirurgical opératoire de l'épitheliome primitif du clitoris. Rev Chir (Paris) 46:546-552, 1912.
60. Taussig FJ: Late results in the treatment of leukoplakic vulvitis and cancer of the vulva. Am J Obstet Gynecol 31:746-754, 1936.
61. Fuller AF: The role of pelvic lymphadenectomy in the treatment of invasive carcinoma of

the vulva. In: Gynecologic Oncology; Controversies in Cancer Treatment. Ballon S (ed). Boston: GK Hall, 1981.
62. Reiffenstuhl G: Lymphatics of the Femal Genital Organs. New York: Lippincott, 1964. Translation of Das Lymphsystem des weiblichen Genitalien.
63. Tamini HK: The treatment of early invasive carcinoma of the vulva. In: Gynecologic Oncology; Controversies in Cancer Treatment. Ballon S (ed). Boston: GK Hall, 1981.
64. DiSaia PV, Rich WM: The treatment of early invasive carcinoma of the vulva. In: Gynecologic Oncology; Controversies in Cancer Treatment. Ballon S (ed). Boston: GK Hall, 1981.
65. Magrina JF, et al.: Microinvasive squamous cell cancer of the vulva. AJOG 134:453–459, 1979.
66. Henriksen E: The lymph nodes and lymph channels of the pelvis. In: Surgical Treatment of Cancer of the Cervix. Meigs JV (ed). London: Grune and Stratton, 1954.
67. Cutler SJ, Myers MH, Green SB: Trends in survival rates of patients with cancer. N Engl J Med 293:122–124, 1975.
68. Jampolis S, Andras EJ, Fletcher GH: Analysis of sites and causes of failures of irradiation in invasive squamous cell carcinoma of the intact uterine cervix. Radiology 115:681–685, 1975.
69. Paunier JP, Delclos L, Fletcher GH: Causes, time of death, and sites of failure in squamous cell carcinoma of the uterine cervix on intact uterus. Radiology 88:555–562, 1967.
70. Nelson AJ, Fletcher GH, Wharton JT: Indications for adjunctive conservative extrafascial hysterectomy in selected cases of carcinoma of the cervix. Am J Roentgenol 123:91–99, 1975.
71. Barker HRK, O'Neil WH: Recurrent cervical carcinoma after treatment by a primary surgical program. Obstet Gynecol 37:165–172, 1971.
72. Ketcham AS, Hoye RC, Taylor PT, Deckers PJ, Thomas LB, Chretien PB: Radical hysterectomy and pelvic lymphadenectomy for carcinoma of the uterine cervix. Cancer 28:1272–1277, 1971.
73. Rampone JF, Klein V, Kolstad P: Combined treatment of Stage IB carcinoma of the cervix. Obstet Gynecol 41:163–167, 1973.
74. Kurohara SS, Vongtama VY, Webster JH, George FW: Post irradiational recurrent epidermoid carcinoma of the uterine cervix. Radiology 111:249–259, 1971.
75. Brunschwig A, Barker HRK: Surgical treatment of carcinoma of the cervix. Obstet Gynecol 27:21–29, 1966.
76. Kolbenstvedt A, Kolstad P: Pelvic lymph node dissection under perioperative lymphographic control. Gynecol Oncol 2:39–59, 1974.
77. Kolbenstvedt A, Kolstad P: The difficulties of complete lymph node dissection in radical hysterectomy for carcinoma of the cervix. Gynecol Oncol 4:244–254, 1976.
78. Fuller AF Jr, Elliott N, Kosloff C, Lewis JL Jr: Radical hysterectomy for Stage IB and IIA carcinoma of the cervix at the Memorial-James Ewing Hospitals, 1959–1977. Obstet Gynecol, in press.
79. Fuller AF Jr, Elliott N, Kosloff MS, Lewis LJ Jr: Lymph node metastases from carcinoma of the cervix, Stages IB and IIA: Implications for prognosis and treatment. Gynecol Oncol 13:165–174, 1982.
80. Morrow CP, et al.: Panel Report: Is pelvic radiation beneficial in postoperative management of Stage IB squamous cell carcinoma of the cervix with pelvic node metastasis treated by radical hysterectomy and pelvic lymphadenectomy. Gynecol Oncol 10:105–110, 1980.
81. Zander J, Baltzer J, Lohek J, Ober KG, Kaufmann C: Carcinoma of the cervix: An attempt to individualize treatment. Am J Obstet Gynecol 139:752–759, 1981.

82. Onsrud M, Aalders J, Abeler V, Taylor P: Endometrial carcinoma with cervical involvement (Stage II): Prognostic factors and value of combined radiological-surgical treatment. Gynecol Oncol 13:76–86, 1982.
83. Nelson JH Jr, Boyce J, Macasget M, Lu T, Bohorquez JF, Micastri AD, Fruchter R: Incidence, significance, and follow-up of para-aortic lymph node metastases in late invasive carcinoma of the cervix. Am J Obstet Gynecol 128:336–340, 1977.
84. Piver MS: The value of pretherapy para-aortic lymphadenectomy for carcinoma of the cervix uteri. Surg Gynecol Obstet 145:17–18, 1977.
85. Ketchan AS, Chretien PB, Hoye RC, Harrah JD, Deckers PJ, Sugarbaker EV, Taylor PT, Rabson AS: Occult metastases to the scalene lymph nodes with clinically operable carcinoma of the cervix. Cancer 31:180–183, 1973.
86. Buchsbaum HJ, Lifshitz S: The role of scalene node biopsy in advanced carcinoma of the cervix uteri. Surg Gynecol Obstet 143:246–248, 1976.
87. Henriksen E: The lyphatic spread of carcinoma of the cervix and body of the uterus. Am J Obstet Gynecol 58:924–939, 1949.
88. Plentl AA, Friedman EA: Lymphatic system of the female genitalia. Philadelphia: WB Saunders, 1971.
89. Way S: Vaginal metastases from carcinoma of the body of the uterus. J Obstet Gynecol Brit Comm 58:558–572, 1951.
90. deMuelenaere GFGO: Vaginal metastases in endometrial carcinoma. Am J Obstet Gynecol 118:168–172, 1974.
91. Whitmore WF Jr, Sogani PC: Solitary vaginal metastases from unsuspected renal carcinoma. J Urol 121:95–97, 1979.
92. Homesley HD, Boronow RC, Lewis JL Jr: Treatment of adenocarcinoma of the endometrium at Memorial-James Ewing Hospitals, 1949–1965. Obstet Gynecol 47:100–105, 1976.
93. Creasman WT, Boronow RC, Morrow CP, DiSaia PJ, Blessing J: Adenocarcinoma of the endometrium: Its metastatic lymph node potential. Gynecol Oncol 4:239–243, 1976.
94. Malkasian GD Jr: Carcinoma of the endometrium: Effect of stage and grade on survival. Cancer 41:996–1001, 1978.
95. Masubuchi S, Fujimoto I, Musubuchi K: Lymph node metastases and prognosis of endometrial carcinoma. Gynecol Oncol 7:36–46, 1979.
96. Yoonessi M, Anderson DG, Morley GW: Endometrial carcinoma: Causes of death and sites of treatment failure. Cancer 43:1944–1950, 1979.
97. Musumeci R, DePalo G, Conti U, Kenda R, Mangioni C, Belloni C, Marzi M, Bandieramonte G: Are retroperitoneal lymph node metastases a major problem in endometrial carcinoma? Cancer 46:1887–1982, 1980.
98. Berman ML, Ballon SC, Lagasse LD, Watring WG: Prognosis and treatment of endometrial cancer. Am J Obstet Gynecol 136:679–688, 1980.
99. Piver MS, Lele SB, Barlow JJ, Blumenson L: Para-aortic lymph node evaluation in Stage I endometrial carcinoma. Obstet Gynecol 59:97–100, 1982.
100. Onsrud M, Kolstad P, Normann T: Postoperative external pelvic irradiation in carcinoma of the corpus Stage I: A controlled clinical trial. Gynecol Oncol 4:222–231, 1976.
101. Aalders J, Abeler V, Kolstad P, Onsrud M: Postoperative external irradiation and prognostic parameters in Stage I endometrial carcinoma. Obstet Gynecol 56:419–426, 1980.
102. Creasman WT, DiSaia PJ, Blessing J, Wilkinson RH Jr, Johnston W, Weed JC Jr: Prognostic significance of peritoneal cytology in patients with endometrial cancer and preliminary data concerning therapy with intraperitoneal radiopharmaceuticals. Am J Obstet Gynecol 141:921–929, 1981.
103. Piver MS, Lele SB, Barlow JJ, Blumenson L: 'Criteria for para-aortic lymph node biopsy

in Stage I endometrial carcinoma' presented at Society of Gynecologic Oncologists Annual Meeting, 1/20/80, Marco Island, Florida.
104. Orthmann EG: A primary papillary carcinoma of the right tube with an ovarian abscess. Z Gynaekol 10:816, 1886, quoted in Kinzel: Am J Obstet Gynecol 125:816–820, 1976.
105. Schiller HM, Silverberg SG: Staging and prognosis in primary carcinoma of the Fallopian tube. Cancer 28:389–395, 1971.
106. Knapp RC, Friedman EA: Aortic node metastases in early ovarian cancer. Am J Obstet Gynecol 119:1013–1017, 1974.
107. Musumeci R, Barfi A, Bolis G, *et al.*: Lymphography in patients with ovarian epithelial cancer: An evaluation of 289 consecutive patients. Cancer 40:1444–1449, 1977.
108. Harbert JC, Rocha L, Smith FP, Delgado G: Efficacy of radionuclide liver and bone scans in the evaluation of gynecologic cancers. Cancer 49:1040–1042, 1982.
109. Piver MS, Barlow JJ, Lele SB: Incidence of subclinical metastasis in Stage I and II ovarian carcinoma. Obstet Gynecol 52:100–104, 1978.
110. Hreshchyshyn MM, Park RC, Blessing JA, *et al.*: Role of adjunctive therapy in Stage I ovarian cancer. Am J Obstet Gynecol 138:139–145, 1980.

# 8. Radiation Therapy of Ovarian Carcinoma

ALON J. DEMBO and RAYMOND S. BUSH

There has been considerable energy devoted to the study of epithelial cancer of the ovary during the last decade. Although the impact of this effort on the overall mortality from the disease has been depressingly small, advances have been made. The principles of surgical, radiotherapeutic and chemotherapeutic management are better understood, even if there is uncertainty about the precise place of each in the overall therapeutic armamentarium. There is also improved understanding of the patterns of spread of the disease and of the prognostic importance of several tumor-related variables. Recognizing the significance of these factors has brought out the complexity of evaluating the results of treatment. This is because results are often reported in a univariate mode, e.g., by stage, or residium, or grade, but not by considering several variables at once in a multivariate manner. A pioneering example of multifactorial analysis in ovarian cancer was presented by Griffiths, but for the most part the multifactorial presentation of treatment outcome has been avoided [1a]. In many ways, however, those techniques of analysis which allow us to take account of several prognostic factors at once provide the clearest understanding of this disease. A valuable perspective on the place of radiotherapy in ovarian cancer can be gained by considering it in the light of these issues. Accordingly this essay will be in three sections, dealing with problems in interpreting results of treatment, the use of prognostic factors in classifying patients for prediction of treatment outcome and choice of therapy, and finally a critical review of a few selected trials of external beam radiation therapy.

1. INTERPRETING TREATMENT RESULTS

*1.1. Objectives of treatment and study end-points*
The treatment of patients with cancer has two principal objectives: to

reduce the threat to life posed by the disease, and to increase the patient's level of ease and comfort. When the threat to life can be removed completely, then we consider the patient cured. Unfortunately there is no method of directly measuring whether an individual patient has been cured, nor the exact proportion of a study population which has been cured. An estimate of the probability of cure can be obtained by determining the proportion of a study population which has the same expectation of survival as that of a matched population of normals [1, 2]. To achieve this, patients in a study population need to have been followed after treatment for many years, and the assessment is made by examining the 'tail' of the survival curve (Figure 1a) [1].

The benefit of noncurative therapy has two components: prolongation of survival, and improved quality of survival. Only the former can be quantitated, for example by estimating the median survival time or by comparing the slopes of the population survival curves (Figure 1b). A dilemma results from evaluating only the survival prolongation component of noncurative therapy. This occurs when a treatment that prolongs survival for some months is far more toxic than the less effective therapy with which it is being compared. At what point do the patient and physician decide that the gains in duration of survival are offset by the reduced quality of that survival resulting from treatment toxicity? There is thus a need to develop scales which measure quality-adjusted survival. An example of this dilemma is found in some ovarian cancer patients presenting with large residuum Stages III and IV, when the relative merits of single agent *vs* combination chemotherapy are weighed.

The end-points we choose to assess cancer therapy are often chosen for their expediency rather than because they measure the two fundamental states of greatest interest to us, namely, cure and palliation [1]. The information yielded by the end-points most commonly used in ovarian cancer trials, is best understood in the context of the phases of clinical investigation of a new anticancer agent or treatment method. The objective of Phase I studies is to establish a safe, tolerable dosage schedule. The frequency and severity of various treatment toxicities constitute the appropriate study endpoints. Once these are known the activity of the agent or method is assessed in Phase II studies for a variety of human tumors. Measurable regression of tumor masses, i.e., tumor response, provides a rapid simple answer to whether the treatment shows activity, and sometimes the frequency with which it does so. Response rates have their greatest utility as end-points in the context of Phase II studies.

The intent of Phase III studies is to compare the efficacy of the new therapy with that of existing treatment methods ('standard therapy'). Greater precision is required to assess treatment activity than in Phase II studies.

The stakes are higher because the 'best arm' of a Phase III study often becomes the new standard therapy. The context of the study should be carefully defined (cure or non-cure) and appropriate end-points selected. The end-point least subject to interpretive bias is the survival time, i.e., the time from diagnosis to death, or to last follow-up. The relapse-free survival (or progression-free survival time), which measures the time to disease relapse (or progression) or death, is more subject to variability and even bias in the detection of recurrence, but it provides an index of outcome earlier than does the survival time. It is a useful end-point for interim reporting because almost all patients who develop recurrent ovarian cancer die of this disease, and the majority of relapses occur within 5 years of initial treatment.

We have proposed previously that the comparison of survival curves is the preferred method of evaluating treatment efficacy in any Phase III study, particularly ovarian cancer [1]. The shape of the curve also gives more information than a survival rate at a given time (e.g., 2, 5, or 10 years); or than a time at which a given proportion of patients are alive (e.g., median or seventy-fifth percentile survival times). Survival curves may be significantly different from each other according to two main patterns as shown in Figure 1. When the difference is in the terminal portions ('tails') of the curves, Figure 1a, it is because there is a difference in the proportion of long-term survivors. Provided that the patients have been observed for an adequate period of time, this type of difference usually indicates different *cure* rates in the two populations. When the tails are at the same level, but the difference is in the initial slope, sometimes seen as a 'shoulder', Figure 1b, then the duration of survival is different even though the proportion of long-term survivors is similar. The therapy which produced a longer duration of sur-

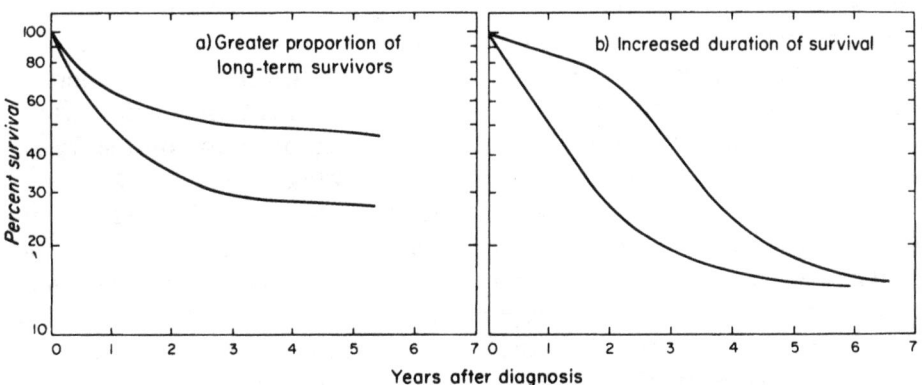

*Figure 1.* Patterns of survival in cancer therapy. (a) Greater proportion of long-term survivors; (b) Increased duration of survival.

vival but did not result in a greater number of cures may be regarded as the superior therapy in a palliative context, provided that the toxicity of the therapy did not abrogate the benefit of prolonged survival. Significantly improved response rates do not necessarily assure the investigator of improved survival curves (as in either Figure 1a or 1b) in the studied patients, particularly if the response times are short or if the proportion of responders is small or if the life expectancy of nonresponders is shortened. Conversely, prolongation of survival can occur even when the effect of the therapy is less than the 50% regression required for a partial response. For example, although responses to second line therapy of ovarian cancer are rarely seen after failures with alkylating agents, we have observed that second-line cisplatin combination chemotherapy prolongs the survival of patients with tumors that have progressed on melphalan therapy [11].

The use of response rates in Phase III studies is inappropriate and misleading, because of their vulnerability to bias, and because they fail to predict for either of the survival patterns in Figure 1. A response rate of 50% does not tell us with any confidence whether any patients have been cured, or whether and for how long the duration of survival of the treated population has been prolonged. In this setting, the fallacy and danger of concluding that a treatment method is superior because of a difference in response rates become obvious. A treatment whose response rate is 70% does not necessarily cure more patients nor keep them alive longer, than a treatment producing a 40% response rate.

For those cancers where cure by chemotherapy does not occur, a case can be made for the value of response rates as Phase III study end-points. That is, regression of tumor can be an index of palliation, provided that the palliative benefit is not outweighed by toxicity. Nevertheless, ovarian cancer is a disease which may be cured by chemotherapy. There is, therefore, no justification for further confusing the complex issue of evaluating treatment efficacy by using inadequate end-points such as response rates to report results. A major reason for the difficulty in deciding whether radiotherapy or chemotherapy constitutes the appropriate treatment choice in certain subsets of patients is that much of the published information on the use of chemotherapy is reported in terms of response rates.

There is one circumstance in which tumor response may be useful as an interim (but *not* definitive) predictor of cure in ovarian cancer. This is the complete response as defined by means of a meticulously performed second-look laparotomy in which there is no gross or microscopic evidence of residual cancer in patients who have had approximately one year of chemotherapy [3]. A large number of these cases may be cured, although the exact proportion in any series must be established by the survival data. Conversely if treatment has not resulted in a complete response, the prospects of cure by subsequent therapy are remote indeed.

It is important to bear in mind that a proportion of patients who had no macroscopic disease after their initial surgical procedure may have been cured by that procedure. The term response should only be applied to situations where the effect of chemotherapy on macroscopic disease is being evaluated.

*1.2. Limitations of staging classifications*

Another obstacle impeding the interpretation of treatment results, stems from the limitations inherent in any classification of patients based solely or principally upon the anatomical extent of their tumor. An objective of staging classifications in cancer is to provide a standard for comparison of subpopulations of patients between different centers. This objective is not realized in ovarian cancer for two reasons. First, there are variations in the technical thoroughness of the staging procedure and in staging conventions. Second, there are other powerful prognostic variables independent of stage whose co-existence diminishes the predictive value of the variable, stage, particularly if there is an imbalance of such factors by stage between centers.

Studies utilizing meticulous exploration of the abdomen have shown that tumor spread into the upper abdomen can be found frequently if care is taken during the examination [19, 20, 21]. The effect of this upper abdominal scrutiny is to classify as Stage III a considerable proportion of patients that would be considered to be Stage I or II at pelvic operation. The consequences are shown in Figure 2, where a diagram to represent these changes in a theoretical population is shown. Two stages only are shown: Stage A, confined to pelvis, and Stage B spread to abdomen. Using 'older' staging techniques half of the patients belong in Stage A (75% cured) and half in Stage B (15% cured). Overall, 45% of patients are cured. With newer staging techniques that explore the upper abdomen, it is discovered that there are in fact 2 equal-size subpopulations of Stage A: a group with a cure rate of 90% in whom there is no detectable evidence of upper abdominal spread, and another group with a cure rate of 60% in whom minimal evidence of gross abdominal spread can be found. When this latter group is classified in Stage B, the cure rate for Stage A becomes 90% and of Stage B

Theoretical Disease

| | Stage A = Pelvis | | Stage B = Abdomen | |
|---|---|---|---|---|
| Old staging: | A=75 | | B=15 | A+B = 45 |
| (% cures) | 90 | 60 | 15 | mean = 45 |
| New staging: | A=90 | | B=30 | A+B = 45 |

*Figure 2.* The effect of reclassifying patients on outcome by stage. Old staging: equal patient numbers in Stages A and B. New staging: one quarter in Stage A, three quarters in Stage B.

30%. The cure rate for Stage A and B combined is still only 45%. This 'improvement' in the cure rate in each stage has resulted from the reclassification of patients and not from the treatment given. The relevance of this example in ovarian cancer is two-fold. Treatment results in a given stage using the newer techniques of classification are sometimes incorrectly compared with those obtained using the older staging technique, resulting in an inflated estimate of the therapeutic benefit of the more recently tested therapy. Second, studies which are confined to one or two stages rather than all stages fail to address the question of whether the observed improvement in treatment has a meaningful impact on the overall outcome of ovarian cancer. The ideal is to study all stages and to report the result obtained for all stages combined.

Certain conventions in staging are also difficult to standardize between centers. Three examples are given. First, when the surgeon detected as the only evidence of disease beyond the pelvis nodules on the liver surface which appeared suspicious but which he did not biopsy, should this patient be classed as Stage III? Should the size (1 mm?, 1 cm?) and number (1?, 5?) of such lesions influence the classification? Another example is the distinction between gross or clinical findings, and microscopic, or pathological findings. This distinction is recognized by the UICC (International Union Against Cancer) with the T, N, M *vs* pT, pN, pM, designations. When the abdominal contents are normal to inspection but biopsy of the omentum or peritoneum shows microscopic spread, is this Stage III? If we accept biopsy evidence for purposes of advancing the stage classification, is cytologic evidence also acceptable? Third, the significance of tumor adherence is well recognized as worsening the prognosis, presumably because it indicates tumor invasion of adjacent structures [6]. The Ovarian Cancer Study Group (National Cancer Institute, M.D. Anderson Hospital, Roswell Park Memorial Institute and the Mayo Clinic) has adopted the convention of advancing the stage if sharp dissection is required to mobilize the lesion [7]. Applying the criterion of the need for sharp rather than blunt dissection to remove the tumor, relies on the technique of the surgeon rather than a definite knowledge of the extent of the tumor to define the stage. What if the surgeon has not specified the technique of dissection he used? Should dense tumor adherence influence the stage differently if there is evidence of prior pelvic inflammatory disease or endometriosis?

The effects of variations in staging conventions applied by investigators to the above situations are almost never addressed, and yet they are not inconsequential. The comments made above with reference to staging technique (Figure 2) apply equally to staging conventions. It may never be possible to standardize both staging technique and conventions between institutions or individuals. The confounding effect of the variations which exist for staging could be minimized if information from the other prognostic variables were used, to reduce the dependence on only one attribute of the disease. This is the subject of the following section.

## 2. THE INTERDEPENDENCE OF THE PROGNOSTIC VARIABLES IN OVARIAN CANCER

Several patient-tumor characteristics are known to predict outcome in patients with epithelial carcinoma of the ovary. The extent to which each influences prognosis and their relative interdependence are issues which require further study. The key to optimizing treatment selection probably lies in the unravelling of this complex problem. To illustrate these points, clinical material will be presented for each of the more important prognostic factors singly, i.e., a univariate representation, and then in various combinations, using different techniques of multivariate representation. The framework for this analysis consists of cure *versus* non-cure situations, and the characterization of patients for optimizing the choice of postoperative treatment. The material is presented as another step towards a functional multivariate classification of ovarian cancer patients.

The following clinical data is taken from the first 430 postoperative patients with all stages studied on prospective treatment protocols at The Princess Margaret Hospital (PMH). Patients were entered on study between April 1971 and September 1976 [1]. The age range at diagnosis was 21 to 79 years, and the median 54 years. These patients have been at risk for 3.6 to 9 years, median 5.8 years, and all had invasive epithelial carcinoma on review of the pathologic material by Dr T.C. Brown, pathologist-in-chief, PMH [5]. The initial surgery was performed at a variety of hospitals before patients were referred to the PMH for postoperative therapy. Only occasionally was meticulous exploration of the upper abdomen carried out, and documentation of findings and tumor residuum was inconsistent.

The actuarial survival rates of the entire population of 430 patients are shown in Figure 3 (a) to (e) with respect to each of the 5 variables: stage, tumor residuum, grade, patient age, pathologic subtype. Some qualifying remarks are required for the information presented in Figure 3. Patients were staged by us on referral from information provided in the operative reports. Where the information was scanty and conclusive contradictory clinical information was present, the latter was used; however, this circumstance occurred infrequently. The relatively high proportion of patients in the lower stages, particularly Stage II probably reflects the lack of adequate intraoperative staging in these cases. Similar problems apply to the definition of residual disease. The term *gross residuum* is used to refer to macro-

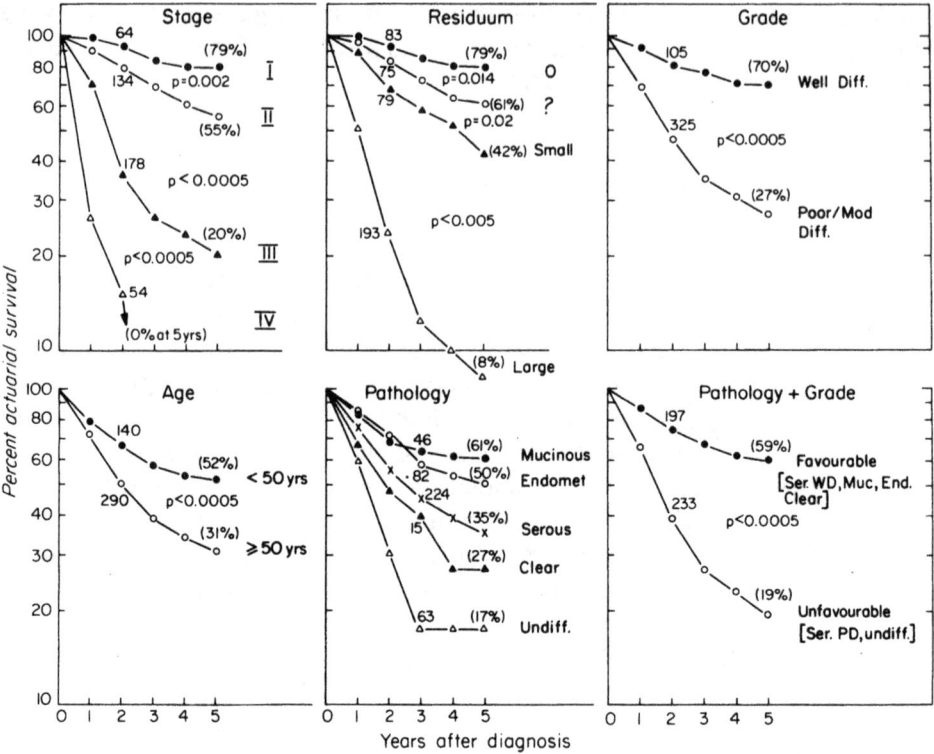

*Figure 3.* Univariate representation of survival in 430 patients by (a) stage; (b) residuum (see text); (c) grade; (d) age; (e) pathology. In (f) pathology and grade have been combined. The non-brackened numbers indicate the numbers of patients in each subset. The bracketed percentages are the respective 5-year survival values. The $p$ values (Gehan-Wilcoxon) refer to a comparison of the survival curves immediately above and below them.

scopic, identified tumor of any size which was not removed. Patients were considered to have no gross residuum if this was clearly implied in the surgical note. In an appreciable number of patients it was uncertain whether all identified disease had been removed. This category is referred to as '?-residuum' or 'uncertain residuum'. Small residuum refers to gross disease not removed but bilateral salpingo-oophorectomy and hysterectomy (BSOH) had been completely performed. Accurate information on the size of residual masses was not available, but in some of the small residuum group as defined herein they exceeded 2 cm in diameter; usually mass size was inferred to be under 2 cm when BSOH was completed. In the large residuum group invariably the residual masses were larger than 2 cm. The group was so defined if residual disease was present when a complete BSOH had not been performed. These definitions for size of residuum will be used throughout this chapter.

Grading and pathologic subtyping were performed by reviewing the material on every case (to be published). *Patients were excluded if stromal invasion was not identified.* Moderately differentiated lesions were grouped with poorly differentiated ones. Unclassified (= undifferentiated) lesions were all too poorly differentiated to permit recognition of the original cellular pattern, but were considered to be epithelial and ovarian in origin.

## 2.1. Univariate representation of outcome

It is evident that classifying patients according to each of the variables in Figures 3a to 3e provides a prediction of outcome. Two questions arise from these data. First, is each of these variables an independent predictor of outcome? For example, it is not apparent whether the worse prognosis of patients over 50 years of age is an intrinsic property of age, or whether it can be explained on the basis of the other variables. Thus the worse prognosis could be because the older patients more often have tumors in the higher stages, with large tumor residua, and less favorable pathology types and grade. This type of question cannot be answered without performing some form of multivariate analysis. The second question is whether one variable is more appropriate than any of the others for purposes of deciding on treatment, and if so, does the information from the other variables contribute materially to the predictive value of that variable. The answer to this question also requires multivariate analysis, but as will be shown, the answer can only be relevant if the context in which the variable is evaluated has been articulated. In other words, unravelling the complex implications of the many prognostic variables of ovarian cancer is the joint responsibility of clinicians and biostatisticians working in consort: neither can do it alone.

## 2.2. Multivariate analysis: the log-rank test

The applicability of the log-rank test has been described in detail by Peto *et al.*, in a paper that is essential reading for clinicians wishing to understand the value of multivariate analysis in clinical trials [8]. The test is based on the proportional hazards model which uses an exponential hazard function rather than the more simplistic linear function used in a multiple linear regression analysis. Log-rank multivariate analysis assesses the prognostic effect of a variable (e.g., treatment) by comparing outcomes of subgroups of that variable (e.g., regimen A *vs* B) while adjusting for the confounding effect of other variables which may be unequally distributed between the groups being compared (e.g., stage, grade, residuum, etc.). The outcome or dependent variable is time-related (e.g., relapse rate). In essence the test performs a retrospective stratification of the patient groups being compared.

In this section we have used the log-rank test to analyze the intrinsic prognostic value of each of the variables shown in Figure 3a to 3e by adjusting each for the confounding effect of the other four, with survival rate as the dependent variable. The adjusted significance levels ($p$ values) obtained were: residual disease $<0.0001$; tumor grade $<0.0001$; stage $= 0.002$; age $= 0.004$; histologic type $= 0.058$. (Since this chapter was written we have had the opportunity to perform this analysis on 808 patients, and to use relapse rate as the dependent variable [35]. The above results were corroborated in the larger sample. However, while adjusted survival rates were significantly different in the two age groups, adjusted relapse rates were not. Thus younger patients were not less likely to experience tumor relapse than older patients, all things being held equal. The shorter survival times in older patients could have been due to intercurrent deaths or less effective treatment of relapse.) In other words, for the example of grade, this analysis has shown that even when we adjust for the higher frequency of early stage, lesser residuum, favorable histology, and younger age presentations that occur in patients with well-differentiated tumors, their survival is still significantly better than that of patients having poorly differentiated tumors.

Nevertheless, a complex relationship exists between histologic subtype and tumor grade. The prognostic significance of grade varies within the different pathology subtypes. (In the analysis of 808 cases undertaken since this chapter was written, the above observations on grade and histologic type were substantiated [35, 36]). In addition, however, we noted that the prognosis of mucinous and endometrioid tumors was intermediate between that of the serous well-differentiated and the serous poorly differentiated and undifferentiated subgroups. The clear-cell subtype accounted for fewer than 5% of our cases, so that it is difficult to be certain as to the best way to group such cases.) In 224 of the 430 patients (52%) the histologic type was serous. For these patients the effect of grade (well vs moderately/poorly differentiated) was highly significant, both in univariate analysis ($\chi^2 = 58.8$ on 1 D.F., $p < 0.0001$) and also when the effect of residuum, stage and age were corrected for by log-rank multivariate analysis ($\chi^2 = 30.8$ on 1 D.F., $p < 0.0001$). In contrast there were 143 patients (33%) with the mucinous, endometrioid and clear-cell pathology subtypes. Within these subtypes, considered either singly or together (as they are here), grade was not of prognostic significance on univariate analysis ($\chi^2 = 1.12$ on 1 D.F., $p = 0.29$) or on multivariate analysis ($\chi^2 = 0.30$ on 1 D.F., $p - 0.59$). This important observation is obscured when the effect of grade is considered for all pathologic types together, since for the two thirds of the patients who have serous and unclassified/undifferentiated tumors, grade is highly significant. Thus, in order to make the most use of histologic information for prognostic purposes cell type and grade have both to be taken into account. The following analysis is oriented in part towards identifying patients with a high likelihood of relapse. For this reason we chose to subdivide the pathology/grade factors with emphasis on the worst subgroups (Figure 3f).

These results apply to the staging practices and pathology criteria used at the PMH. It might differ in other centers. Moreover, the relative importance of each factor may vary for different subgroups of patients from those obtained in the patient population overall. It is critical to appreciate that no statements can be made about the absolute prognostic significance of a variable *in vacuo:* a context must be defined. For instance, concluding that residuum is the most powerful factor may be correct for the population overall but the information is of limited applicability in Stage I, where there is no gross residuum by definition, or in Stage IV, where in our experience no patients were cured regardless of the size of the lesion.

*2.3. The clinical context of multivariate analysis*

Although the value of the information yielded above by multivariate analysis is intuitively appealing, its clinical applicability is not immediately obvious. The log-rank test has identified several independent prognostic factors. The next step is to present the data in a manner which permits us to incorporate this information into the therapeutic decision-making process. Choice of treatment is often based on stage and residuum only. If it were possible to take into account patient age, tumor grade and pathology as well, might this improve the therapeutic outcome?

One way is to examine the relative importance of appropriate variables in a given subgroup of patients for different treatment methods. If for example we consider patients with Stage III minimal residuum presentations we might find that survival is similar whether patients receive either chemotherapy or radiotherapy. It is likely that within the minimal residuum Stage III designation certain factors will be recognized to predict for an increased risk of relapse. If these high risk factors are different for the two treatment modalities it might be possible to improve survival by choosing therapy accordingly. Hypothetically, we might find for chemotherapy that older patients or those with macroscopic residuum larger than 1 cm were rarely cured, but that site of residuum and pathology had little influence on outcome. Conversely we might find that radiotherapy rarely cured patients with visible residual disease in the upper abdomen even if it were smaller than 1 cm or if pathology were unfavorable, but size of pelvic residuum between 1–3 cm and age had only a weakly negative effect on survival. We could then utilize this information by directing patients with upper abdominal disease or unfavorable histology towards chemotherapy, and older patients and those with pelvic residuum to radiotherapy. Multivariate analysis can aid in optimizing treatment selection in this way.

The following analysis is intended to derive for the overall patient population a prognostic classification which uses multiple variables and is presented in the context of choice of postoperative therapy. The subgroups are:
I: Poor prognosis: patients who are rarely cured and should be treated with postoperative chemotherapy.
II: Good prognosis: patients who should be treated with curative intent.
   (a) Low risk – usually cured by operation and require no postoperative treatment.
   (b) Intermediate risk – high cure rates with radiotherapy.
   (c) High risk – only a minority cured by radiotherapy or chemotherapy.

For clinicians, the most important initial decision in choice of therapy is whether the patient has disease that is likely to be cured by postoperative treatment or not. A first approximation at classifying patients in this context is shown in Figure 4, where the 430 cases are divided into two groups based

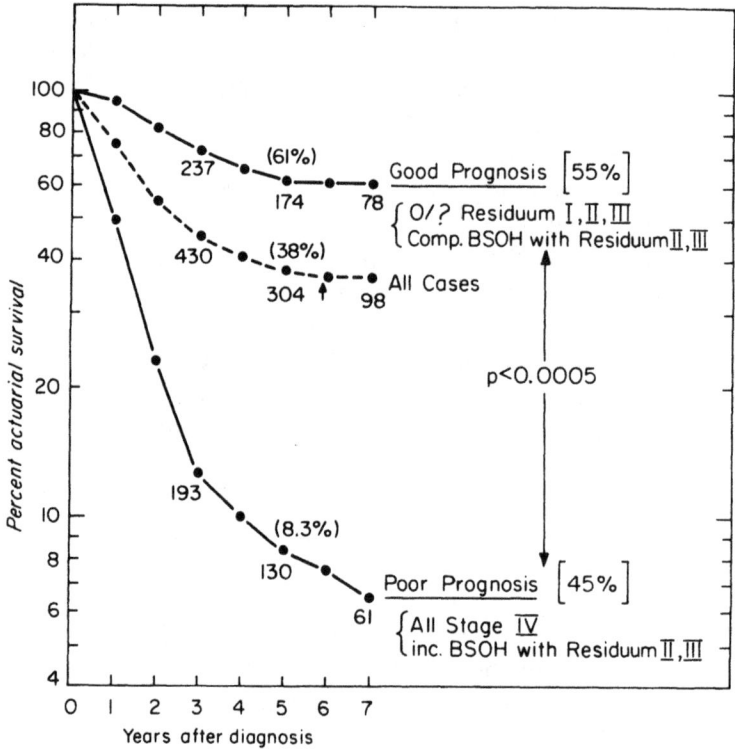

*Figure 4.* PMH Ovarian Cancer Protocols 1971–76, all therapies survival of 430 patients overall and in two prognostic groups. The arrow indicates the median time at risk. See text for explanation.

on the variables stage and residuum [2]. The poor prognosis group (45% of the total) comprises patients who present with FIGO Stage IV and patients with FIGO Stages II and III who have large residual tumor masses. The rationale for this grouping is found in Figures 3a and 3b. There were no long-term survivors in Stage IV (Figure 3a) and very few in the large residuum (BSOH-incomplete) Stage II and III patients (Figure 3b). These factors constitute the definition of the poor prognosis patients shown in Figure 4. The five-year relapse-free survival is under 5% in these patients indicating that a very small fraction only was cured.

The therapy given included radiotherapy for patients with Stage II and some with Stage III disease, and primarily single alkylating agent chemotherapy for the remaining Stage III and IV cases [4]. There are two main avenues of therapeutic endeavor aimed at improving curability of these patients at the present time. The first is cytoreductive surgery, which likely enhances prognosis if the residual lesions are smaller than 1 cm in largest diameter [1a, 1, 9, 10].

It remains to be clarified what proportion of large-bulk Stage III cases is amenable to such surgery, and what impact a policy of aggressive cytoreductive surgery has on overall survival. Combination chemotherapy is the second approach to improve cure rates in the poor prognostic group. Nevertheless, for patients in Stage III and IV with residual tumor masses greater than 1-3 cm, it has *not* been shown that curability is greater with cisplatin and adriamycin containing regimens (or other combinations) than with single agent therapy [1, 11]. For example, Ehrlich has reported a negative second look rate of 13% in such patients treated with cisplatin-adriamycin-cyclophosphamide suggesting an ultimate cure rate of 10% or less [12]. Sturgeon has reported no survival difference between such patients treated in a randomized study from the PMH, comparing single agent and combination chemotherapy [11]. These were also the results in the HexaCAF study reported by Young *et al.* [1, 13]. This poor prognosis group therefore poses the biggest obstacle to improved cure rates in the management of epithelial ovarian cancer. Chemotherapy forms the mainstay of postoperative treatment in these patients. Radiotherapy has at present only a palliative or adjunctive role to play, but this situation may change in the future if successful ways are found of combining irradiation and chemotherapy in an additive or synergistic manner.

Thus, despite the advances in chemotherapy the rationale for categorizing patients as we have done in Figure 4 seems appropriate.

The second, good prognosis group of patients (55% of the total) has in contrast a high likelihood of cure by surgery and/or postoperative therapy. These are patients with Stage I, Stages II and III with no or uncertain gross residual disease, and Stages II and III with small residual masses, i.e., with

*Table 1.* Proposed classification of 430 patients by prognostic category, showing patient distribution and survival.

|   |   | No. | % | % 5-year survival rate |
|---|---|---|---|---|
| A. | Good prognosis | 237 | 55 | 61 |
|    | a. Low risk | 26 | 6 | 96 |
|    | b. Intermediate risk | 159 | 37 | 67 |
|    | c. High risk | 52 | 12 | 25 |
| B. | Poor prognosis | 193 | 45 | 8 |

BSOH completed. Five-year survival is 61% (Figure 4). We have previously presented a subgrouping of patients with good prognosic presentations based on grade, stage and residuum to define a group of patients suitable for the study of methods of adjuvant therapy [5]. The following analysis is oriented towards the selection of postoperative therapy and incorporates the prognostic factors of age and pathology as well. Table 1 shows a summary of the classification developed in this section.

Figure 5 displays a detailed breakdown of treatment outcome, i.e., the proportion of tumor relapses for all treatment methods combined, in each prognostic category for patients with good prognosis Stage II and III presentations. This figure at one time demonstrates the complexity and the value of the multivariate representation of clinical data in tabular form. Our

| FIGO Stage and Residuum | | Serous WD, Muc, End Clear-cell | | | | Serous PD + Unclass. | | | | All Ages and Path. | |
|---|---|---|---|---|---|---|---|---|---|---|---|
| | | <50 yr | | ≥50 yr | | <50 yr | | ≥50 yr | | | |
| II | 0/? Res | 5/20 | (.25) | 11/30 | (.37) | 2/5 | (.40) | 12/23 | (.52) | 30/78 | (.38) |
|    | Small Res (C-BSOH) | 3/10 | (.30) | 7/13 | (.54) | 3/6 | (.50) | 8/9 | (.88) | 21/38 | (.55) |
| III | 0/? Res | 1/4 | (.25) | 1/4 | (.25) | 2/2 | (1.00) | 5/6 | (.83) | 9/16 | (.56) |
|     | Small Res (C-BSOH) | 3/6 | (.50) | 11/15 | (.73) | 4/5 | (.80) | 12/15 | (.80) | 30/41 | (.73) |
| All good prognosis II+III | | 12/40 | (.30) | 30/62 | (.48) | 11/18 | (.61) | 37/53 | (.70) | 90/173 | (.52) |

*Figure 5.* Proportion of relapses in 173 Stage II and III good-prognosis patients by stage, residuum, age, pathology and grade. The high risk subgroups are shaded; the intermediate risk subgroups are unshaded (see text for explanation).

intent in this figure is not to emphasize the minute details of each subset of patients. It is rather to show that by this technique of displaying the data, we can define patient subgroups which use the information that each variable contributes.

The rationale for grouping the patients according to the combined pathology–grade division shown in Figure 5 rather than by grade alone has already been partly alluded to above. First, grade is not of predictive value in our material in the mucinous, endometrioid and clear-cell pathology types. Second, only 25% of all cases are well differentiated. From the univariate representation in Figure 3f, and from a multivariate log-rank analysis, we observed that the prognosis of the unclassified and serous poorly/moderately differentiated pathology categories (unfavorable pathology) is significantly worse than the other pathologic categories combined. (Serous well differentiated, all mucinous, endometrioid and clear-cell types, i.e., favorable pathology.) In fact the survival difference with this grouping is very similar to that found with grade alone (Figures 3f, 3c). However, the proportion of the patients is more evenly distributed using the combined categorization affording it a greater utility, and the prognosis of the unfavorable pathology group (Figure 3f) is slightly worse than for patients with the poorly/moderately differentiated designation (Figure 3c).

Reading from left to right in Figure 5 it can be seen that within each pathologic group, there is a trend for prognosis to worsen with increasing age, and that between pathologic groups there is a striking prognostic gradient. Reading downwards in each column, there is a prognostic gradient by stage and presence of gross residual disease. These trends are most clearly appreciated in the totals columns, i.e., the extreme-right vertical and the bottom horizontal columns. Within the 16 individual subsets, patients appear to fall into two separate groups. The majority of patients (121/173, 69%) belong to subsets in which the proportion of relapses is between 0.25 and 0.54, mean = 0.40. These subsets are not shaded in Figure 5 and constitute an intermediate risk group. The subgroups with the highest proportion of tumor relapse (0.73 to 1.00, mean = 0.81) are enclosed in the shaded area. These comprise approximately 31% of the good prognosis Stages II and III cases, and make up a high risk group. It is apparent from the shaded area in Figure 5 that the prognostic factors stage, residuum, pathology, grade and age have all been taken into account for this definition of a high risk group. Treatment for the patients in Figure 1 consisted of pelvic irradiation alone or followed by chlorambucil, or pelvic plus abdominopelvic irradiation alone or followed by a single alkylating agent (see below [4, 5, 14]).

The high and intermediate risk subgroupings shown in Figure 5 might differ for radiotherapy and chemotherapy, and might be further improved upon by using more precise information on site and size of the macroscopic tumor residuum, and perhaps other factors.

*Table 2.* Proportion of relapses in 237 good-prognosis patients by risk category and FIGO stage.

|  | Low risk | Intermediate risk | High risk | All |
|---|---|---|---|---|
| I W D | 0/26 (0.00) | — | — | 13/64 (0.20)[a] |
| I P D | — | 13/38 (0.34) | — |  |
| II | — | 43/107 (0.40) | 8/9 (0.88) | 51/116 (0.44)[b] |
| III | — | 5/14 (0.36) | 34/43 (0.79) | 39/57 (0.68)[c] |
| All good prognosis | 0/26 (0.00) | 61/159 (0.38) | 42/52 (0.81) | 103/237 (0.43) |

[a] 41% of Stage I low risk.
[b] 8% of Stage II high risk.
[c] 75% of Stage III high risk.

In Stage I the division of patients by grade alone produced a better separation between those patients in whom relapses would or would not occur, than did the composite grade–pathology grouping we used in Stages II and III. Accordingly, we have chosen to continue using grade for purposes of treatment decision making [5]. The situation in Stage I is thus less complex, and tumor grade is the most powerful variable. No relapses have occurred in 26 patients with well-differentiated carcinomas and these constitute the low risk patients in the good prognosis category [5, 15]. In contrast the proportion of relapses in patients with the poorly/moderately differentiated tumors (13/38, 34%) is similar to that found in the intermediate risk group of patients in Stage II and Stage III above. Hence, these patients are all classed together to form the intermediate risk category of the good prognosis patients. The subclassification of the good prognosis patients shown in Figure 4, is summarized in Table 2.

## 2.4. Recommendations for therapy

In Figure 6 the actuarial survival rates are displayed for the three subgroups of good prognosis patients. The low risk group is comprised of Stage I patients with well-differentiated tumors (21/25 Stage IA; 5/26 Stage IB). These make up 11% of the good prognosis patients and 6% of all cases. We currently recommend that no postoperative therapy be given to the Stage IA patients with well-differentiated carcinoma and we are attempting to determine whether any is required for the Stage IB patients with well-differentiated tumors. The single death in this group of patients was due to a late postsurgical complication in a patient who received no postoperative therapy.

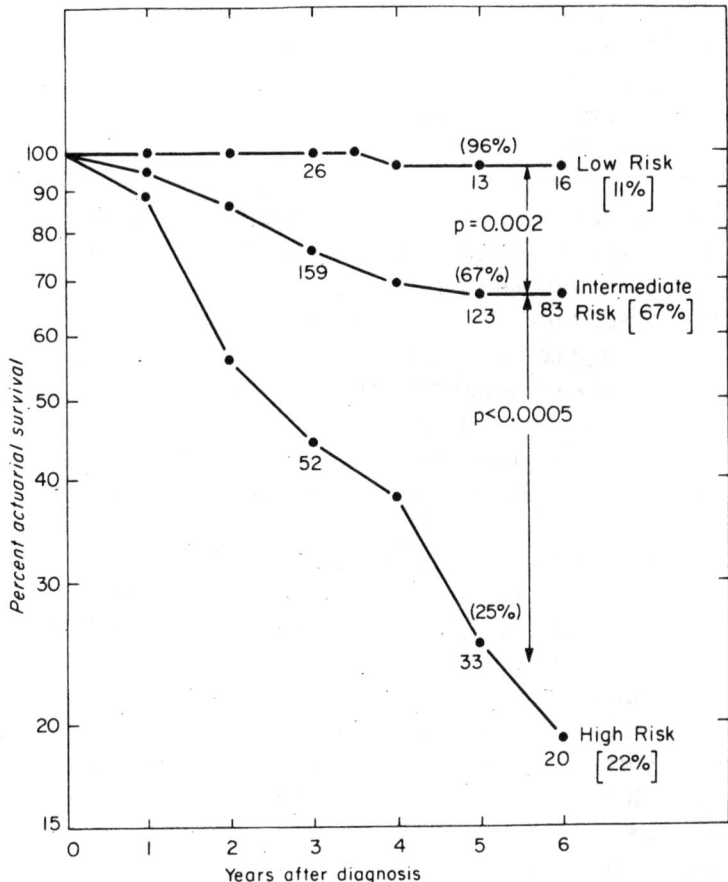

*Figure 6.* Survival by prognostic category in 237 good-prognosis cases referred to in Table 3, for all treatment methods combined.

The intermediate and high risk groups, constituting the remainder of the 237 good prognosis patients, are ones whom we recommend should be treated postoperatively with pelvic plus abdominopelvic irradiation [1, 2, 14-16]. This recommendation is based on the demonstrated superiority of this method over pelvic irradiation alone or with single agent chemotherapy as discussed in Section 3.2.1 below [14]. More recently, reports have appeared suggesting a curative potential of combination chemotherapy (especially cisplatin containing regimens) which is greater than that obtainable with single agent therapy, for 'optimal surgery' patients, namely, those with tumor residua under 2-3 cm in diameter [9, 12, 13, 17, 18]. It is unclear at the present time whether the use of combination chemotherapy in small residuum and no residuum cases will yield similar, inferior or superior results to those obtained with the PMH technique of abdominopelvic irradiation [14, 16]. Direct comparison between the two methods of treatment has not been made in a randomized study and it is almost impossible to know when comparing results between different series whether the patient populations are similar with respect to prognostic variables.

In the PMH series precise information on size of residuum and staging is not available for many patients since meticulous exploration and documentation were usually not performed at the time of the initial laparotomy [14]. From the re-exploration-staging data reported by others, it might be expected that at least a third of the Stage I and II cases would be reclassified as Stage III if careful upper abdominal examination were performed intraoperatively [19, 20]. Moreover, under these circumstances, the category of 'true' Stage II with residual disease is one that appears to be particularly uncommon, because of the frequent presence of extrapelvic metastases [21]. This should be borne in mind in the interpretation of Tables 1 and 2, and Figures 5, 6 and 7, which show results for all treatment methods.

In Figure 7 the survival curves for the good prognosis Stage II and III patients only, separated into the high and intermediate risk groups, are shown for two treatment categories. Those which included abdominopelvic irradiation (AB-PEL) *versus* pelvic irradiation alone or with chlorambucil [4, 5, 14]. Caution should be applied to conclusions drawn from this comparison, as only a portion of the material is randomized. The benefit to abdominopelvic irradiation appears to exist mainly in the intermediate risk group (5-year actuarial survival rate 78%). We therefore have no hesitation in continuing to advocate that pelvic plus abdominopelvic irradiation using the PMH technique should be the treatment of choice for the intermediate risk patients, a group comprising 37% of all patients in this series (Table 3) [16]. (In the expanded series more recently analyzed (see [35]) the 5-year survival of 128 intermediate risk patients treated with abdominopelvic irradiation was 75%, and the intermediate risk group comprised 33% of the total.

In the high risk category it is not possible to be definitive about the choice of postoperative therapy. Three investigators reported preliminary survival data at the 1981 meeting of the Society of Gynecologic Oncologists in carefully staged III and IV patients with tumor residua less than 2-3 cm. All used cisplatin containing regimens in 2-drug (cyclophosphamide-cisplatin), 3-drug (cyclophosphamide-cisplatin-adriamycin) or 4-drug combinations (cisplatin-adriamycin-cyclophosphamide-hexamethylmelamine) [12, 17, 22]. The long-term survival and relapse-free survival times quoted for the 'optimal' group of patients in these three studies were similar to the results obtained in the PMH series with pelvic plus abdominopelvic irradiation in the high risk group (Figure 7). Published studies of chemotherapy have not

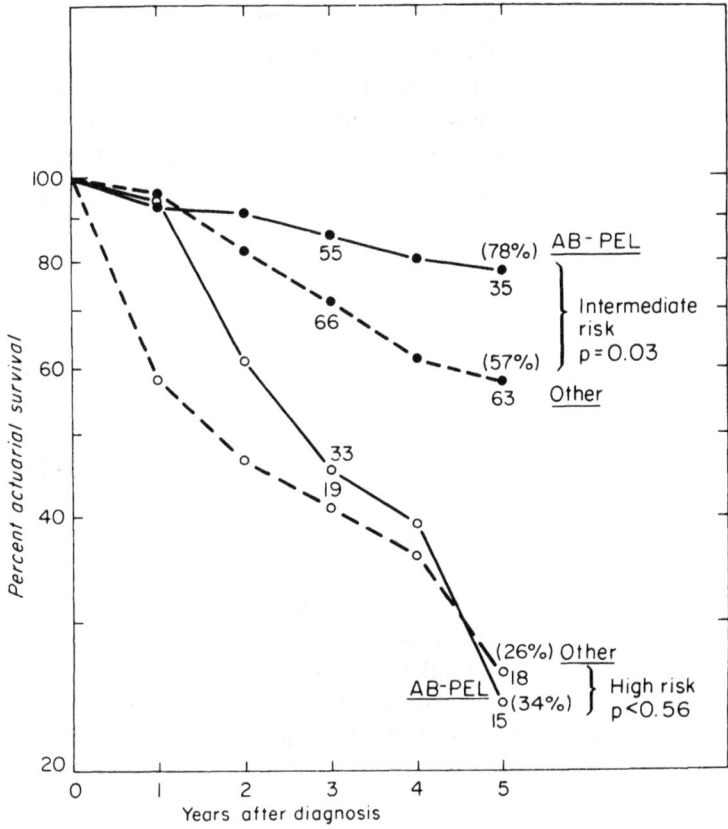

*Figure 7.* Survival by treatment in Stage II and III good-prognosis patients for the intermediate and high risk subgroups. (AB–PEL = all therapies which included pelvic plus abdominopelvic irradiation; other = pelvic irradiation alone or with chlorambucil.)

been analyzed in terms of high and intermediate risk as we have done: it is probable that the high risk factors for irradiation also apply to chemotherapy. Thus it is not immediately obvious that survival results will be improved if the PMH high risk, good prognosis patients were to be treated with chemotherapy instead of irradiation. This is a question requiring further study. Existing data suggest that this group of patients could probably be equally treated with irradiation or combination chemotherapy, but its prognosis is likely to be worse than the average 'good prognosis' or 'optimal surgery' patients.

In summary, we have tried to show in this section that multivariate analysis allows us to identify independent prognostic variables. These data can be used to classify patients into subgroups for purposes of choosing therapy or prognostication. The information derived from the use of several variables affords better characterization of patient subgroups than can be obtained by use of any one variable alone. Ovarian cancer is a complex disease and techniques of multivariate analysis allow us to take into account these complexities. The alternative path of univariate analysis is simpler, but this simplicity is acceptable only to the extent that the inaccuracies, distortions, and obstructions it presents to our understanding and to progress in this disease are acceptable.

## 3. CLINICAL TRIALS OF RADIATION THERAPY IN OVARIAN CANCER

Few large-scale randomized studies have been performed in patients with epithelial ovarian cancer. Those which have been published have sometimes yielded seemingly contradictory outcomes [14, 23]. The question as to whether chemotherapy or radiotherapy constitutes the most appropriate choice of therapy in good prognosis cases can not be resolved from published data. The answer awaits a carefully designed and executed comparative study in a well-characterized patient population. The intention in this section is to review selected clinical trials of external beam radiation therapy and chemotherapy, which illustrate current thinking and discuss the conclusions which may be derived from them. This is not a complete literature review.

### 3.1. Studies in Stage I

There are two questions of postoperative therapy in patients whose disease has not spread beyond the ovaries. The first is whether postoperative therapy is required for all patients. The second is what form postoperative therapy should take in patients for whom it is deemed indicated, i.e., what is effective therapy? It follows therefore that in both studies to be reviewed the designs included a control, no-treatment arm.

### 3.1.1. The Princess Margaret Hospital study in Stage IA.

Between 1971 and 1977, a period several months longer than the study period of the 430 cases described in Section 2, 54 patients with invasive Stage IA ovarian cancer were studied [5, 15]. After patient stratification by age, grade and pathology, treatment was randomized between observation (27 cases) and pelvic irradiation 4500 rads in 20 fractions (27 cases). A further 9 patients who originally entered on study were excluded because of incorrect staging (4 cases), borderline histology (1 case), refusal of treatment (2 cases), and protocol violation (2 cases).

This analysis (February, 1981) updates the previously reported re-

Table 3. Prognostic factors in 54 patients with Stage IA.

| | Proportion of tumor relapses | | | | |
|---|---|---|---|---|---|
| | Well differentiated[a] | Poorly/moderately differentiated | | All grades | |
| Factor | N | N | % | N | % |
| *Cyst rupture* | | | | | |
| yes | 0/9 | 4/14 | 29 | 4/23 | 17 |
| no | 0/14 | 5/17[b] | 29 | 5/31[b] | 16 |
| *Ascites* | | | | | |
| yes | 0/4 | 1/5 | (20) | 1/9 | 11 |
| no | 0/19 | 8/26[b] | 31 | 8/45[b] | 18 |
| *Capsular penetration* | | | | | |
| yes | 0/0 | 2/6 | (33) | 2/6 | (33) |
| no | 0/22 | 5/20 | 25 | 5/42 | 12 |
| unknown | 0/1 | 2/5 | (40) | 2/6 | 33 |
| *Adhesions* | | | | | |
| yes | 0/1 | 6/14[d] | 43 | 6/15 | 40 |
| no | 0/3 | 3/17[b,d] | 18 | 3/19 | 16 |
| not reviewed | 0/19 | — | | 0/20 | 0 |
| *Treatment* | | | | | |
| Pelvic irradiation | 0/11 | 5/16 | 27 | 5/27 | 19 |
| Observation | 0/12 | 4/15 | 31 | 4/27 | 15 |
| Total | 0/23[c] | 9/31[c] | (29) | 9/54 | 17 |

[a] Invasive only.
[b] One unknown, no relapse.
[c] $p = 0.008$, Fisher 2-tail.
[d] $p = 0.25$.

sults [5, 15]. The data have been analyzed to determine whether postoperative therapy is warranted for all Stage IA cases, or whether a subgroup could be recognized in whom the risk of relapse was so low that no postoperative therapy was indicated. As shown in Table 3, no relapses occurred in patients with well-differentiated carcinomas, even though cyst rupture had occurred in 9 patients (33%), and ascites was present in 4 patients (15%). All relapses occurred in patients with poorly and moderately differentiated tumors ($p = 0.008$, Fisher 2-tail). Even in these patients rupture, ascites and capsular penetration did not predict for relapse (Table 3). More relapses occurred in association with poorly differentiated lesions if adherence was present although the difference did not attain significance (43% *vs* 18%, $p = 0.25$).

Nine relapses have occurred (Table 3). These were evenly distributed between the two study arms, indicating no curative benefit for pelvic irradiation. The ratio of relapses in the abdomen alone *versus* those in the pelvis (with/without abdomen) was different in the two groups. In the pelvic irradiation arm, the ratio was 4 abdomen to 1 pelvis; in the observation arm it was 1 abdomen to 3 pelvis. These results indicate that the entire peritoneal cavity is at risk for relapse when relapse occurs. By reducing the frequency of pelvic recurrence, pelvic irradiation did not reduce the overall risk of relapse. The study was terminated when it was realized that control of pelvic disease was an inadequate objective of treatment. When treatment is indicated it should be directed at the whole peritoneal cavity. We currently recommend that pelvic plus abdominopelvic irradiation should be given. Some other investigators recommend chemotherapy, usually single agent therapy. This recommendation will be discussed below.

In summary this study demonstrated, (1) that tumor grade was the most important prognostic factor in Stage IA and treatment is not required if the tumor is well differentiated in its worst differentiated elements; (2) that other factors (rupture, ascites, capsule penetration) were of dubious prognostic value; (3) and that pelvic irradiation is inappropriate adjuvant therapy because the sites of relapse extend throughout the peritoneal cavity. In the series of over 800 cases treated by us between 1971 and 1978 and reviewed since this chapter was submitted, there were 56 patients in Stage I with well-differentiated invasive tumors [35]. Only 2 of these have experienced tumor relapse.

Our conclusions above, particularly regarding the weak prognostic effect of tumor adherence in Stage I are seemingly in contradiction to the Mayo Clinic results reported by Webb *et al.* [6] The difference may have occurred for several reasons. Some patients with densely adherent tumors in our series were upstaged and so do not appear in our Stage I results. However the proportion of adherent tumors in our series (15/54 = 28%), is higher than in the Mayo Series (28 of 219 evaluable cases = 13%). The negative prognostic effect of adherences, rupture and extracystic excrescences in their series is difficult to comment upon without knowing whether the majority of the deaths associated with these lesions were in poorly differentiated tumors.

It is noteworthy, too, that the proportion of Stage I cases in the Mayo Series was high (36.5% of the total) and 25% of these did not have BSOH performed. Because of the time period spanned by this study (1950–66) surgical staging may have been less thorough than it would be nowadays. Thus, many Stage I cases in the Mayo Series, particularly densely adherent and high grade lesions, might well have been in Stage III.

*3.1.2. The Gynecology Oncology Group (GOG) study of adjuvant therapy in Stage I.* This study was conducted between 1971 and 1978 by more than 20 institutions participating in the GOG. The study design and results are shown in Figure 8. The question asked are very important: Does postoperative therapy with melphalan or pelvic irradiation reduce the frequency of relapse compared with surgery alone, and if so, is one form of postoperative therapy superior to the other? Like the PMH study above, the failure analysis showed that most relapses were distributed throughout the peritoneal cavity when they occurred. Of the 86 evaluable patients studied 14 had tumor relapses: in only 3 was recurrent tumor confined to the pelvis while in 7 there was evidence of abdominal relapse as well [24]. It is justifiable to conclude from analyzing the sites of relapse that therapy directed towards the pelvis alone is not a rational strategy in these patients.

Comparative analysis of treatment results as presented by these authors should be interpreted with caution [25]. First, because 49% (82/168) entered on study were removed from the analysis, the three treatment arms were unequally matched with respect to patient numbers and with respect to the distribution of prognostic variables [24]. The comparison was, therefore, not of similar patient groups. Because the reasons for removing patients from study after randomization included physician preference for treatment, bias could have been introduced.

As seen in Figure 8, there was no significant difference in the proportion of relapses between the melphalan and control arms (2/34 $vs$ 5/29, $p = 0.30$, Fisher 2-tail) or between the pelvic radiation and control arm (7/23 $vs$ 5/29, $p = 0.43$). These data indicate that neither method of postoperative therapy

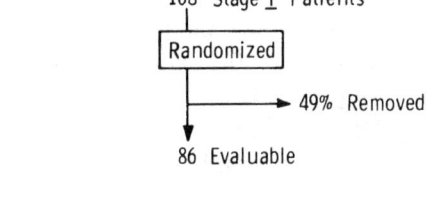

| Treatment | N | Recurrences N | % | p Values (Fisher) |
|---|---|---|---|---|
| Observation | 29 | 5 | 17 | }  0.43  } |
| Pelvic XRT | 23 | 7 | 30 | }  0.03  } 0.30 |
| Melphalan | 34 | 2 | 6 | |

*Figure 8.* Summary of the Gynecology Oncology Group Study. (Protocol #1; XRT = irradiation.)

prevented relapses to a significantly greater degree than occurred when no postoperative therapy was administered. Hence, the study yielded a null conclusion. However, there were significantly fewer relapses in the melphalan treated patients than among those who received pelvic irradiation (2/34 vs 7/23, $p = 0.03$). The most likely explanation for this difference is *not* attributable to the treatment these patients received, but to the dissimilarity of the patient groups with respect to prognostic variables resulting from the large numbers of patients withdrawn from study after randomization.

The Ovarian Cancer Study Group, more recently joined by the GOG, is attempting to study postoperative treatment methods (melphalan, observation, intraperitoneal $p^{32}$, pelvic irradiation plus melphalan) in thoroughly staged patients with Stages I and II who have been stratified by histology, grade and stage [7, 21]. No treatment results are available.

### 3.2. Studies of radiotherapy in patients with Stages I, II and III, having minimal tumor residuum

One decade ago the evidence supporting the contribution of radiation therapy to cure of ovarian cancer was derived from retrospective evidence of the use of postoperative pelvic irradiation in patients with Stage II presentations (for review see [26] and [27]). Although the generally held view was that postoperative radiotherapy improved survival in Stage II, there was no evidence for its benefit in Stages I, III and IV [26]. Interpretation of the older literature is difficult because radiation techniques were variable (energy, dose, field-size), studies were usually not randomized, and equivalence of patients treated by the modalities being compared cannot be evaluated with respect to prognostic variables. Frequently the radiation used for Stage II was pelvic irradiation and abdominal irradiation was the technique used for Stage III [27]. In most instances the abdominal irradiation did not cover the entire peritoneal surface and the patients often had large residual tumor masses in the abdomen [16, 27].

Much work was done by Delclos and co-workers at the M.D. Anderson Hospital (MDAH) to rationalize and standardize radiation techniques [28, 29]. These investigators developed a modification of the Manchester technique of moving-strip irradiation to treat the abdomen and characterized its tolerance and complications. They presented evidence to suggest that its application resulted in fewer relapses than obtained when smaller fields were used, and that for radiation therapy, tumor control rates decreased in relation to increasing amounts of residual disease [29]. Their data reaffirmed the observation that most patients who die of ovarian cancer do so with disease confined to the abdominal cavity.

During this same period Smith and co-workers at the same institution produced evidence suggesting that metastatic ovarian cancer could be cured by chemotherapy in a proportion of cases [30].

From these therapeutic advances of the 'sixties certain questions emerged concerning the postoperative treatment of patients with ovarian cancer that had spread to pelvic or abdominal structures. Among these were; (1) could total abdominal irradiation control upper abdominal metastasis and lead to higher cure rates than pelvic irradiation alone, and (2) what were the relative efficacies and toxicities of radiation and chemotherapy? Two studies directed towards answering these questions were undertaken at The Princess Margaret Hospital and the M.D. Anderson Hospital.

*3.2.1. The Princess Margaret Hospital study for patients with Stages IB, II and III-asymptomatic presentations.* In addition to the information outlined above, the following factors were considered in the design of The Princess Margaret Hospital study. A retrospective study of ovarian cancer patients with Stage IB and II conducted by Bush *et al.* showed two patterns of disease relapse after pelvic irradiation: recurrence of disease within the pelvis, and relapse in the abdomen not accompanied by pelvic recurrence [4]. It therefore seemed rational to study the ability of whole abdominal irradiation to control upper abdominal metastases not identified at operation but accounting for a large proportion of treatment failures and deaths. In this review the patterns of relapse and survival was similar in patients with Stages IB and II, so they were grouped together for treatment purposes in the prospective study.

Second, it had long been demonstrated that the drainage of fluid and cell-sized particulate matter from the peritoneal cavity was via the diaphragmatic lymphatics [31]. Lymphoscintigraphic studies undertaken at PMH in patients with advanced ovarian cancer suggested that a major mechanism leading to ascites formation in these patients was obstruction of diaphragmatic lymphatics, presumably by metastatic tumor [32]. It seemed critical, therefore, if radiation was to be used to treat the abdomen, that the entire diaphragm be included in the treatment portals. This meant that liver shielding should not be used. Accordingly the decision was made to use a radiation dose within liver tolerance rather than use a higher dose and reduce the treatment volume by shielding the liver and, of course, a portion of the diaphragm [16].

The PMH retrospective review further suggested that the survival times of patients with Stage III who had no disease-related symptoms postoperatively was longer than those who had disease-related symptoms [4]. This observation formed the basis for dividing Stage III patients into the asymptomatic and symptomatic categories in the prospective study. It was hypothesized that the potentially curable Stage III patients were likely to be derived from the asymptomatic subpopulation, who were hence suitable for inclusion with Stage IB and II patients for purposes of study of treatment methods.

The design of the study for 190 patients with Stages IB, II and asymptomatic-III presentations entered between 1971 and 1975 is shown in Figure 9 [4, 14]. Stratification was by age, stage, pathology, grade and whether or not BSOH had been completed, prior to randomization. For Stages IB and II, pelvic irradiation 4500 rads midplane in 20 fractions (PEL) was taken as the standard postoperative therapy. The objective was to determine if survival could be improved by adding to this either chlorambucil 6 mg/day for 2 years (P+CH) or irradiation of the upper abdomen (P+AB). Stage III patients were randomized only between P+AB and P+CH.

The essential features of the technique of abdominopelvic irradiation used were: (a) therapy commenced with pelvic irradiation 2250 rads midplane in 10 fractions followed immediately by a downward moving-strip that encompassed the entire abdomen and pelvis; (b) the dose to the moving-strip was 2250 rads midplane in 10 fractions; (c) the upper border was radiologically verified to be at least 1 cm above the diaphragm in expiration; (d) no liver shielding was used but posterior renal shielding (5 HVL) was used throughout; (e) patients were treated prone using two fields per day with an iso-centric technique [16].

At the time of publication in 1979, patients had been at risk a median of 52 months. The survival difference for the 76 patients treated with pelvic plus abdominopelvic irradiation was not significantly superior to that of the 71 patients treated with pelvic irradiation and chlorambucil (60% vs 45%, $p = 0.13$) [14]. At the present time, all patients have been at risk for a minimum of 4 years since diagnosis (median 6.4 years), and the difference has become significant (58% vs 40%, $p<0.05$). However, as noted in the

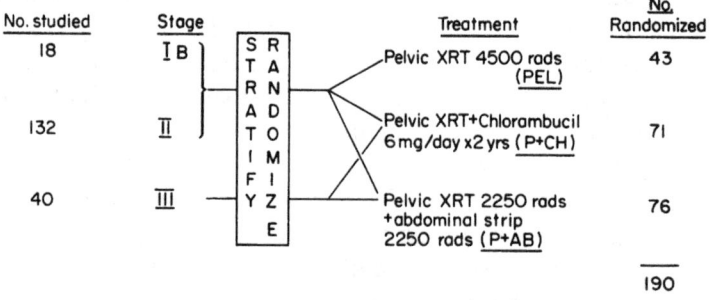

Figure 9. Design of The Princess Margaret Hospital Study for Stages IB, II and Asymptomatic III. (XRT = irradiation.)

original publication, the survival benefit applied only to patients in whom bilateral salpingo-oophorectomy and total abdominal hysterectomy (= BSOH) had been performed [14]. The following results are all updated.

When BSOH was completed (132 cases, or 69%) the 5-year actuarial survival was 62% compared with 21% when the operation was incomplete, usually due to disease ($p<0.0005$). None of the three treatment methods tested in the BSOH-incomplete group was superior to another. However, patients with no gross residuum in the BSOH-incomplete group had survival characteristics similar to the BSOH-complete group, indicating that it was the amount of residuum that determined prognosis rather than the procedure *per se*. Nevertheless the completeness of BSOH affords a sensitive index of whether or not the amount of gross tumor residuum was likely to be cured by postoperative therapy.

In contrast the outcome in the BSOH-completed group (i.e., small, or no, or uncertain residuum patients) was markedly dependent upon postoperative therapy. The following results refer only to the BSOH-completed group. For Stage II, relapse-free survival (and survival) was superior for abdominopelvic irradiation compared with pelvic irradiation alone: 73% *vs* 37%, $p = 0.005$. This advantage for abdominopelvic irradiation is seen in Stages IB and III as well as Stage II. The 5-year survival rates for abdominopelvic irradiation and pelvic irradiation plus chlorambucil were 78% *vs* 51%, $p = 0.004$ (Figure 10). The survival benefit correlated with a reduced risk of upper abdominal tumor relapse of 1/50 for abdominopelvic irradiation *vs* 14/51 for pelvic irradiation with chlorambucil ($p<0.001$), when pelvic disease was controlled. The proportion of patients with pelvic relapse was similar in all 3 treatment groups, approximately 25%. The patients treated by

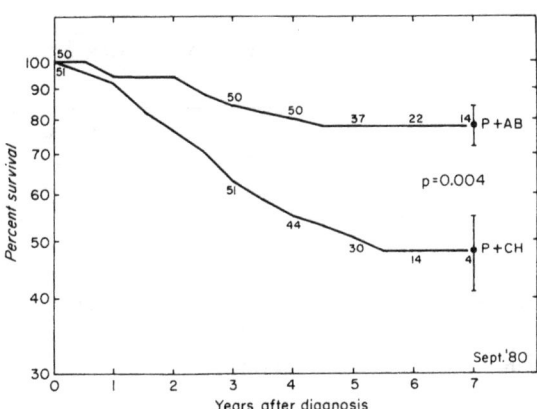

*Figure 10.* Survival by therapy in 101 patients with Stages IB, II, III, BSOH-completed.

*Table 4.* Proportion of relapses by residuum and treatment.

| Residuum | Treatment | |
|---|---|---|
| | P+AB | P+CH |
| None or uncertain | 4/32 [a] | 15/30 |
| Macroscopic | 10/18 | 12/21 |

[a] Lower than other 3 groups, $p<0.005$.

pelvic irradiation and chlorambucil and by abdominopelvic irradiation were comparable with respect to the variables age, stage, grade, histology and presence or absence of gross tumor residuum.

The prognostic effect of grade and stage seen with P+CH was largely overcome by P+AB therapy [14]. Residual disease, however, had an important influence on outcome of therapy (Table 4). The advantage of P+AB was found only in patients with all visible tumor removed (insofar as could be assessed from the operative reports), but was not evident where gross residuum was present. Disease relapse occurred mainly in the pelvis in patients who had gross tumor residuum postoperatively.

Treatment complications with the PMH technique of pelvic plus abdominopelvic irradiation were only rarely serious [14, 16]. Almost all patients experienced some degree of discomfort during the period of treatment. Cramping diarrhoea usually occurs during irradiation of the pelvis and fatigue, anorexia, nausea during upper abdominal irradiation. Significant myelosuppression can occur. The late complications are shown in Table 5 for 151 consecutive study patients treated by this technique. Symptomatic

*Table 5.* Late complications of pelvic plus abdominopelvic moving-strip irradiation in 151 consecutive study patients.

| | Number evaluable | Crude frequency | |
|---|---|---|---|
| | | No. | % |
| Basal lung fibrosis | 130 | 44 | 34 |
| Localized varicella zoster | 150 | 15 | 10 |
| Raised Alk Phos (>12 KAU) | 125 | 58 | 46 |
| Occasional diarrhoea | 149 | 15 | 10 |
| Mild sigmoid colon stenosis | 149 | 3 | 2 |
| Required operation | 149 | 4 | 3 |
| Fatal complication (?) | 151 | 2 | 1.5 |

late effects were infrequent. Only 4 patients required bowel surgery, and it is questionable whether radiation was really responsible for the 2 deaths attributed to therapy in Table 5 (one jaundice, one bowel obstruction). Serious complications were no more frequent with pelvic plus abdominopelvic irradiation than with pelvic irradiation alone [14]. However, if the abdominal portals are correctly applied, asymptomatic basilar pneumonitis or fibrosis and elevation of the serum alkaline phosphatase occur in a high proportion of patients. The most serious late complication occurring in the 76 patients treated with pelvic irradiation plus chlorambucil was fatal acute leukemia in two cases.

The conclusions from this study are summarized below. Cures were only rarely obtained with any of the three tested therapies in patients with Stages II and III who had residual disease and incomplete BSOH. As abdominopelvic irradiation is associated with significant acute upset, its use in this group of patients is not indicated. Abdominopelvic irradiation is curative in a significantly higher proportion of patients with Stage II BSOH-completed, than is pelvic irradiation alone. In complete-BSOH Stage IB, II and III patients, abdominopelvic irradiation controls occult upper abdominal metastasis in approximately 30% more cases than does pelvic irradiation plus chlorambucil, producing a similar increment in long-term survival. The benefit of abdominopelvic irradiation is greatest when visible disease has been removed. The survival gains with abdominopelvic irradiation in these patients considerably outweighs the risks of serious morbidity. The strategy of adding continuous single alkylating agent chemotherapy to pelvic irradiation did not increase survival rates, was difficult to administer, and was associated with a not inconsequential risk of leukemia.

The strong points of the PMH study of postoperative therapy are that it was conducted in a single institution, that the pathological material was all reviewed by a single pathologist, and that the stratified randomized design ensured comparability of therapy arms as far as can be ascertained with respect to the major prognostic variables. Nonetheless, the study has been criticized principally on two accounts. First, because meticulous surgical staging was not performed, some uncertainty exists as to comparability of the treatment arms with respect to stage. There are always unknown prognostic variables in clinical studies, but the purpose of randomization is to ensure as far as possible that these are evenly distributed between the treatment arms. Certainly the treatment groups were closely matched with respect to the known variables making the likelihood of imbalance small. The major problem arising out of the imprecise staging appears to be the difficulty in comparing these results with those obtained in other series which employed careful surgical staging. While it might be expected that approximately one third of cases in this study classed in Stages I and II would have been upstaged to Stage III if careful exploration had been performed, the true effectiveness of abdominopelvic irradiation in these 'meticulous' Stage III cases cannot be determined from the PMH data [14].

Another criticism, is that the results obtained with abdominopelvic irradiation seem as good as they do because results obtained with pelvic irradiation and chlorambucil are inferior to those obtainable with adequate chemotherapy. This concern seems to us to based more on theory than on observed results. The study was conducted in the pre-adriamycin and cisplatin era. As we have pointed out previously, the 3-year relapse-free survival rate of 54% reported for the 26 Stage II and III BSOH-completed no residuum cases treated with pelvic irradiation and chlorambucil in the PMH study, is not apparently inferior to the 39% result reported for similar patients treated with cyclophosphamide with or without adriamycin at the Mayo Clinic [1, 14, 18]. Of the 21 patients treated with pelvic irradiation and chlorambucil in Stages II and III BSOH-completed with macroscopic residual disease, 9 have not had tumor relapse having been at risk 4–9 years. Translating this into the terminology of responses, we have observed a complete response rate of over 35% which has lasted over 4 years from diagnosis. In patients with macroscopic residuum, this is not inferior to most results reported with chemotherapy. Our conclusions from these data are that the PMH results with pelvic irradiation and chlorambucil do not appear to be inferior to those obtainable with 'adequate' chemotherapy. Pelvic irradiation appears to have contributed to the result obtained rather than detracted from the ability to administer chemotherapy in adequate amounts. The results of trials employing cisplatin-containing combination have not been presented in a manner that permit comparison.

The apparent discrepancy between the results obtained at the PMH and MDAH for abdominal moving-strip irradiation will be discussed after the MDAH study is reviewed.

*3.2.2. The M.D. Anderson Hospital (MDAH) random trial between postoperative irradiation and chemotherapy.* Patients were entered onto this study between April 1969 and November 1975. However, detailed results have only been published of an interim analysis of 149 patients studied until May 1974 [23]. Postoperative patients with Stages I, II and III (and one Stage IV case) with epithelial ovarian cancer were randomized without prior stratification to receive moving-strip abdominal irradiation plus pelvic boost, or 12 cycles of melphalan 0.2 mg/kg/day for 5 days every 4 weeks, bloodcounts permitting. All had no gross residuum in areas which would be shielded from irradiation and had no gross residuum or residuum <2 cm elsewhere.

The technique of irradiation consisted of an upward moving-strip pelvi-

*Table 6.* Salient features of the M.D. Anderson study of radiation and chemotherapy.

|  | Treatment randomization | | | |
|---|---|---|---|---|
|  | Irradiation ($n = 70$) | | Melphalan ($n = 79$) | |
| Stage and residuum | N | (%) | N | (%) |
|---|---|---|---|---|
| No residuum (Stages I and IIA) | 19[b] | (27) | 35[b] | (44) |
| Residuum not stated (Stages IIB and III) | 51 | (73) | 44[a] | (57) |
| Actuarial 5-year survival rate | 71% | | 72% | |

[a] 1 Stage IV.
[b] $p = 0.044$, Fisher 2-tail.

abdominal field delivering a midplane dose of 2500 to 2800 rads in 8 fractions with liver and kidney shielding, followed or preceded by pelvic irradiation 2000 rads in 10 fractions.

Seventy patients were randomized to receive irradiation and 79 to receive chemotherapy (Table 6). Although patients were comparable with respect to pathology type there was a marked discrepancy by stage in favor of chemotherapy as shown in (Table 6). There were significantly more patients with Stages I and IIA in the chemotherapy arm. Information was not provided on comparability of the treatment arms with respect to tumor grade, or the presence or absence of macroscopic tumor residuum.

Overall 5-year survival rates were similar (71% vs 72%), and there was no significant difference in survival by stage between treatment arms. At the time of the report however, the authors were impressed by the difference in toxicity and monetary cost to patients between the two therapies. Seven (10%) of the irradiated patients required postirradiation surgery for small bowel injuries, often resulting in chronic malabsorption. There were no treatment related deaths in either arm. The expenses related to the radiation therapy (time, motel costs) were far greater than those related to chemotherapy. In view of these findings the authors concluded that chemotherapy was the preferred treatment method since it was as effective as irradiation, but less toxic and less costly.

A very brief updating of the study has been published [33]. Ninety-five patients received chemotherapy and 92 irradiation. The differences in survival between the two treatment methods remain nonsignificant for each stage. There were 2 deaths from radiation bowel injury out of a total of 7 who required surgery and 2 patients developed acute leukemia after chemotherapy.

The impression made by this study on the postoperative management of ovarian cancer in North America has been profound. Most physicians and institutions abandoned primary postoperative radiotherapy in favor of chemotherapy. It is important and interesting to scrutinize the data which led to this altered pattern of practice.

In contrast to the PMH study, patients in the MDAH study were subject to meticulous surgical staging. Yet the data in Table 6 indicate that the two treatment arms are unevenly weighted by stage significantly in favor of chemotherapy. Does this mean that the identical overall survival curves for the two reported treatment methods in fact signifies that irradiation is the superior treatment? Furthermore, no information is provided on the distribution of the even more important variables tumor grade and residuum. For example, if a greater proportion of irradiated patients in Stages IIB and III had macroscopic residuum than did the patients who received chemotherapy, then there would be an even greater survival advantage for patients treated by chemotherapy. Thus, the data are not sufficiently complete to justify the authors' conclusion that chemotherapy is as effective as radiotherapy.

A small number of patients treated by both methods have developed fatal treatment complications with further follow-up [33]. Although the period of maximum risk for development of radiation bowel damage may have passed, the same may not be true of chemotherapy-induced leukemia. This latter complication is particularly worrisome as the authors used melphalan as adjuvant therapy in patients with Stage I well-differentiated tumors.

It is hoped that a detailed follow-up report of the MDAH study will be published clarifying the issues of the distribution of all major prognostic variables between the two arms, with outcome corrected for imbalances by appropriate statistical means, and of the late toxicities of therapy.

A further reason for the disparity in efficacy between the PMH and MDAH radiation results relates to whether the whole peritoneal cavity was irradiated in all patients in the MDAH series. It is possible to calculate the length of treatment field used to treat the abdomen from the duration of treatment. This latter information was provided for 60 patients in the MDAH series [23]. For this calculation we have ignored treatment delays. In 16/60 (28%) the field length was 30 cm (12 strips) or less. In the PMH series the shortest field deemed adequate to cover the diaphragms was 37.5 cm (15 strips), but in 95% of patients a field length of 40 cm (16 strips) or longer was required. It appears, therefore, that in a appreciable proportion of patients in the MDAH series the *whole* abdomen was probably not irradiated. Even if it had been, the liver shielding provided a sanctuary site on the undersurface of the right hemidiaphragm. We believe inclusion of the diaphragm to be the explanation for the superior results reported with the use of the PMH technique. It is apparent that in most series where abdominal irradiation has been used in ovarian cancer, the fields employed unfortunately were not adequate to cover the whole peritoneal cavity [1, 16].

Comment is required on the different complication rates reported in the two series. The higher bowel complication rate in the MDAH series is most likely attributable to the higher radiation dose used (2800 rad/8 fractions vs 2250 rad/10 fractions). Patients in Houston were more likely to have had more numerous and extensive surgical procedures prior to their radiotherapy [33]. As well they were irradiated in both prone and supine treatment positions which, with altered flexion of the trunk in each position, might have produced high-dose regions. This would be less likely to occur with the isocentric radiation technique used in Toronto where patients are prone during the moving-strip therapy [16].

## 3.3. Summary

Irradiation of the whole abdomen, from above the diaphragm to below the obturator foramina, with no liver shielding, and with a boost-dose to the pelvis, appears to be effective postoperative therapy in ovarian cancer when all macroscopic tumor has been excised, or when there are small residual deposits. In situations where there are large residual deposits (BSOH-incomplete) there is no advantage to using this form of therapy.

Several issues require further clarification. It is not known whether the moving-strip technique which delivers a higher biologic dose (for normal tissues) to segments of the abdomen sequentially, is more effective than the open beam technique, which treats the entire peritoneal contents each day, but to a lower dose. One study which was undertaken to address this question produced inconclusive results [34].

The indications and limitations of abdominopelvic irradiation require better definition in terms of size, number, and site (pelvis vs abdomen) of residual deposits as well as the other factors discussed in Section 2. Optimal dosage schedules are not known for each of these situations.

The relative effectiveness of radiation and combination chemotherapy in patients who are at high and intermediate risk for relapse after radiation therapy needs to be compared. By combining information from several prognostic variables we have identified a group of patients who are at high risk for relapse after radiotherapy. We do not know whether cure rates can be improved in such cases by increasing radiation dose, or by using chemotherapy instead of, or in addition to irradiation. Methods of effectively combining chemotherapy with radiotherapy should be explored. Myelotoxicity appears to be the limiting factor.

## ACKNOWLEDGEMENTS

The authors appreciate the excellent secretarial assistance received from Mrs Isabelle Gamble. The Ovarian Cancer Project of The Princess Margaret Hospital is supported in part by a grant from The Ontario Cancer Treatment and Research Foundation. The invaluable collaboration of members of the Biostatistics Department, Mrs Joan Reid in particular, in this project is acknowledged.

## REFERENCES

1a. Griffiths CT: Surgical resection of tumor bulk in the primary treatment of ovarian carcinoma. Natl Cancer Inst Monogr 42:101-104, 1975.
1. Bush RS, Dembo AJ: Current status of treatment for patients with ovarian cancer. In: Ovarian Cancer, Advances in the Biosciences, Vol 26. Newman CE, Ford CHJ, Jordan JA (eds). Oxford: Pergamon Press, 1980, pp 115-135.
2. Easson EC, Russell MH: The cure of Hodgkin's disease. Br Med J 1: 1704-1707, 1963.
3. Smith JP: Surgery for ovarian cancer. In: Ovarian Cancer, Advances in the Biosciences, Vol 26. Newman CE, Ford CHJ, Jordan JA (eds). Oxford. Pergamon Press, 1980, pp 137-149.
4. Bush RS, Allt WEC, Beale FA, Bean H, Pringle JF, Sturgeon J: Treatment of epithelial carcinoma of the ovary: operation, irradiation and chemotherapy. Am J Obstet Gynecol 127:692-704, 1977.
5. Dembo AJ, Sturgeon JR, Bean HA, Beale FA, Pringle JF, Brown TC, Gospodarowicz M, Bush RS: The effectiveness of adjuvant abdominopelvic irradiation in ovarian cancer. In: Adjuvant Therapy of Cancer II. Jones SE, Salmon SE (eds). New York: Grune & Stratton, 1979, pp 467-474.
6. Webb MJ, Decker DG, Mussey E, Wiliams TJ: Factors influencing survival in Stage I ovarian cancer. Am J Obstet Gynecol 116:222-226, 1973.
7. Ovarian Cancer Study Group Protocol for all Stage Ic and II (A, B, C) and Selected Stage IAii and IBii Ovarian Cancer: NCI Protocol #7602, June 1976.
8. Peto R, Pike MC, Armitage P, Breslow NE, Cox DR, Howard SV, Mantel N, McPherson K, Peto J, Smith PG: Design and analysis of randomized clinical trials requiring prolonged observation of each patient. II. Analysis and examples. Br J Cancer 35:1-39, 1977.
9. Griffiths CT, Parker LM, Fuller AF: Role of cytoreductive surgical treatment in the management of advanced ovarian cancer. Cancer Treat Rep 63:235-240, 1979.
10. Smith JP, Day TG: Review of ovarian cancer at the University of Texas Systems Cancer Center, M.D. Anderson Hospital and Tumor Institute. Am J Obstet Gynecol 135:984-993, 1979.
11. Sturgeon JFG, Fine S, Gospodarowicz MK, Dembo AJ, Bean HA, Bush RS, Beale FA, Herman JG, Pringle JF, Thomas GM: A randomized trial of melphalan alone versus combination chemotherapy in advanced ovarian cancer. Gyn Oncol: Abstract 28, 268, 1980.
12. Ehrlich CE, Einhorn LH, Stehman FB, Roth LM, Blessing J: Responsive, 'second look' status and survival in Stage III-IV epithelial ovarian cancer treated with Cis-dichlorodiammine platinum II (Cis-platinum), adriamycin (ADR) and cytoxan (CTX). Gyn Oncol 10: Abstract 27, 367, 1980.

13. Young RC, Chabner BA, Hubbard SP, Fisher RI, Bender RA, Anderson T, Simon RM, Canellos GP, DeVita VT: Advanced ovarian adenocarcinoma. A prospective clinical trial of melphalan (L-PAM) versus combination chemotherapy. N Engl J Med 229:1261–1266, 1978.
14. Dembo AJ, Bush RS, Beale FA, Bean HA, Pringle JF, Sturgeon J, Reid JG: Ovarian carcinoma: Improved survival following abdominopelvic irradiation in patients with a completed pelvic operation. Am J Obstet Gynecol 134:793–800, 1979.
15. Dembo AJ, Bush RS, Beale FA, Bean HA, Pringle JF, Sturgeon J: The Princess Margaret Study of Ovarian Cancer: Stages I, II and Asymptomatic III Presentation. Cancer Treat Rep 63:249–254, 1979.
16. Dembo AJ, VanDijk J, Japp B, Bean HA, Beale FA, Pringle JF, Bush RS: Whole abdominal irradiation by a moving-strip technique for patients with ovarian cancer. Int J Radiat Oncol Biol Phys 5:1933–1942, 1979.
17. Vogl SE, Pagano M, Kaplan BH, Canalog A, Greenwald E, Arseneau J: Combination chemotherapy of advanced ovarian cancer with cyclophosphamide (C), hexamethylmelamine (H), adriamycin (A) and diamminedichloroplatinum (C) – The 'CHAD' regimen. Gyn Oncol 10: Abstract 30, 369, 1980.
18. Edmonson JH, Fleming TR, Decker DG, Malkasian GD, Jorgensen EO, Jefferies JA, Webb MJ, Kvols LK: Different chemotherapeutic sensitivities and host factors affecting prognosis in advanced ovarian carcinoma versus minimal residual disease. Cancer Treat Rep 63:241–247, 1979.
19. Rosenoff SH, Young RC, Anderson T, Bagley C, Chabner B, Schein PS, Hubbard S, DeVita VT: Peritoneoscopy: A valuable staging tool in ovarian carcinoma. Ann Int Med 83:37–41, 1975.
20. Piver MS, Barlow JJ, Lele SB: Incidence of subclinical metastasis in Stage I and II ovarian carcinoma. Obstet Gynecol 52:100–104, 1978.
21. Young RC: A strategy for effective management for early ovarian cancer. In: Adjuvant Therapy of Cancer II. Jones SE, Salmon SE (eds). New York: Grune & Stratton, 1979, pp 467–474.
22. Decker DG, Fleming TR, Malkasian GD, Webb MJ, Jefferies JA, Edmonson JH, Podratz KC, Gallenberg MM: A treatment program for Stage III and IV ovarian cancer. Cyclophosphamide versus cyclophosphamide and Cis-platinum. Gyn Oncol 10: Abstract 29, 368–369, 1980.
23. Smith JP, Rutledge FN, Delclos L: Postoperative treatment of early cancer of the ovary: A random trial between post-operative irradiation and chemotherapy. Natl Cancer Inst Monogr 42:149–153, 1975.
24. Hreshchyshyn MM, Park RC, Blessing JA, Norris HJ, Levy D, Lagasse LD, Creasman WT: The role of adjuvant therapy in Stage I ovarian cancer. Am J Obstet Gynecol 138:139–145, 1980.
25. Dembo AJ, Bush RS, DeBoer G. Letter to the Editor. Am J Obstet Gynecol 141:231, 1981.
26. Tobias JS, Griffiths CT: Management of ovarian carcinoma. Current concepts and future prospects. N Engl J Med 294:819–823, 1976 (Part I) and 294:877–882, 1976 (Part II).
27. Eltringham JR: Radiation therapy for ovarian carcinoma. Clin Obstet Gynecol 22:967–992, 1979.
28. Delclos L, Braun EJ, Herrera JR, Sampiere VA, Roosenbeek EV: Whole abdominal irradiation by Cobalt-60 moving-strip technique. Radiology 81:632–641, 1963.
29. Delclos L, Quinlan EJ: Malignant tumors of the ovary managed with postoperative megavoltage irradiation. Radiology 93:659–663, 1969.
30. Smith JP, Rutledge F: Chemotherapy in the treatment of cancer of the ovary. Am J Obstet Gynecol 107:691–703, 1970.

31. Courtice FC, Harding J, Steinbeck AW: The removal of free red blood cells from the peritoneal cavity of animals. Aust J Exp Biol Med Sci 31:215–225, 1953.
32. Coates G, Bush RS, Aspin N: A study of ascites using lymphoscintigraphy with $^{99m}$Tc-sulphur colloid. Radiology 107:577–583, 1973.
33. Delclos L, Dembo AJ: Ovaries. In: Textbook of Radiotherapy. Fletcher GH (ed). Philadelphia: Lea & Febiger, 1980, pp 834–851.
34. Fazekas JT, Maier JG: Irradiation of ovarian carcinomas: A prospective comparison of the open-field and moving-strip techniques. Am J Roentgenol 120:118–123, 1974.
35. Dembo AJ, Bush RS, Brown TC: Clinico-pathological correlates in ovarian cancer. Bulletin du Cancer (Paris), 69:292–297, 1982.
36. Dembo AJ, Brown TC, Bush RS, Sturgeon JFG: Prognostic significance of pathology subtype and differentiation in epithelial carcinoma of ovary (ECO). Proc Am Soc Clin Oncol, Abstract C408, 1982.

# 9. Heavy Particle Radiation Therapy in Gynecological Malignancies

ROBERT D. HILGERS, STEVEN E. BUSH and FRANCISCO AMPUERO

Microscopic populations of hypoxic tumor cells represent a major obstacle to the successful control of solid malignant neoplasms by radiation therapy. Hypoxic cells show a greater resistance to conventional radiation therapy (X-rays or gamma rays) than do oxygenated cells. Nearly every gynecologic malignancy is composed of poorly vascularized central zones with hypoxic cells. For successful therapy, treatment ports must encompass the geographic extent and volume of tumor, including both the target tissue and adjacent normally oxygenated tissues. Cancerocidal doses are often limited by normal tissue tolerance beyond which treatment doses may cause severe complications (Figure 1), and still leave behind a population of viable, although radioresistant, hypoxic cells which may serve as a nidus for future tumor relapse.

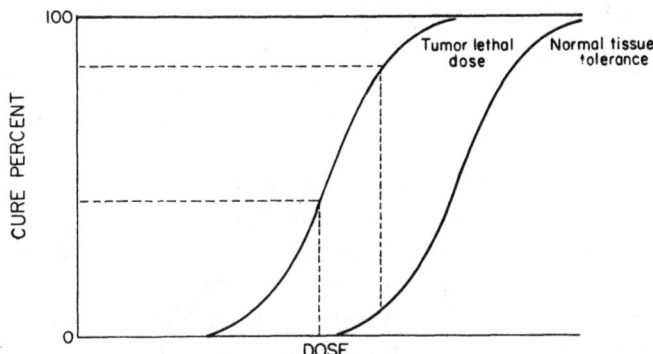

*Figure 1.* Therapeutic gain. Diagram shows parallel between tumor response and normal tissue tolerance curves and demonstrates the relationship between increasing dose, increasing cure rate and increasing morbidity. With conventional radiotherapy this diagram shows that an 80–90% cure rate can potentially be achieved with a 5–10% morbidity. Pushing the cure rate higher with a higher radiation dose increase morbidity.

*Griffiths, C. T. and Fuller, A. F. (eds.), Gynecologic Oncology.*
© *1983, Martinus Nijhoff Publishers, Boston. ISBN 0-89838-555-5.*
*Printed in The Netherlands.*

During the past decade innovative ideas have been explored with the objectives of both the antitumor effect of radiation therapy and reducing morbidity, thereby improving the therapeutic index in treatment of malignancies of the female pelvis. These innovations include the use of hyperbaric oxygen, chemical radiosensitizers, cell cycle synchronizers, hyperthermia, variable fractionation patterns, tumor localization through CT scanning and more penetrating beam therapy. Applied therapy, in some instances, depends upon achieving more sophisticated levels of development and interpreting the results of clinical studies.

Heavy particle and other high-LET radiation, the subjects of this review, offer an alternative for achieving local tumor control. The rationale for investigating high-LET radiation therapy as a therapeutic modality is based partly on the premise that hypoxic cells are the limiting factor in conventional radiotherapy and partly on their penetrating qualities which may minimize damage to normal tissues without reducing their ability to deliver curative doses to the tumor [1].

## 1. LINEAR ENERGY TRANSFER (LET)

Linear energy transfer (LET) is the amount of energy released (usually in keV) per micron of medium along the tissue track of any ionizing particle [3]. LET is not a constant or a static value but is different for the same ionizing particle over different portions of the radiated pathway. The rate of energy loss by ionizing particles depends upon particle charge ($Q$) and velocity ($V$). The quotient $Q^2/V$ indicates that a relatively slow moving, highly charged particle will have a high-LET. LET is an average quantity, as both track average, the mean of each quantum of energy deposited in a specified increment of length, and energy average, dividing the track into variable energy increments, occur.

Radiation can be subdivided by the density of the ionization formed within a submicroscopic volume of tissue [4]. A low density pattern of ionization (X-rays, gamma rays of cobalt, electrons, protons, and inflight pions) creates 'low linear energy transfer' (low-LET) radiation in tissue (Figure 2). A high density pattern of ionization (neutrons, heavy ions and stopping pions) is depicted as 'high-LET' radiation. A beam may be considered high-LET when it deposits more than 50 kilovolts per micron of tissue.

High-LET beams differ from conventional low-LET beams in their deposition of energy in tissue molecules. Figure 2 illustrates a high-LET beam passing through a DNA molecule, causing many densely concentrated points of ionization. The beam shown passing through the lower portion of

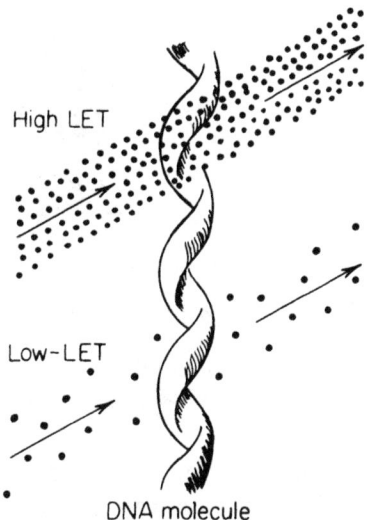

*Figure 2.* In the upper portion of the diagram, many ionization points proceed through the DNA molecule of the cell nucleus with high-LET radiation. Contrariwise, low-LET radiation is characterized by a relatively sparse distribution of ionization points.

the DNA molecule, causing only occasional impact by ionization, is a low-LET beam.

As an ionizing particle moves along its path through tissue, linear energy transfer increases. Such radiobiological interaction between the ionizing particle and the tissue in its path should reduce the damage to intervening normal tissue and increase the damage to a deep-seated tumor. Vital organs often restrict delivery of a tumor-determined dose to the treatment volume. Particles of high-LET are more likely to produce cytotoxic effects in a given volume of living matter because of their concentrated ionization points as they proceed through the tissue. Contrariwise, low-LET radiation is characterized by a relatively sparse distribution of ionization points and a critical molecule can potentially escape injury when low-LET radiation is used. As expected, with increasing LET there is greater biological damage to normal tissue as well.

Charged particles have an additional characteristic which makes them attractive for clinical investigation. While X-rays, gamma rays of cobalt, and neutrons (which have no electrical charge) deposit radiation exponentially as they pass through tissue, charged particles have a finite range in tissue. As these particles are slowed by the tissue they traverse, a greater density of ionizing events occurs, depositing a greater dose at the end of their range (the 'Bragg peak'). The rate of energy dissipated from a charged particle as it moves along its path in tissue exhibits a characteristic absorp-

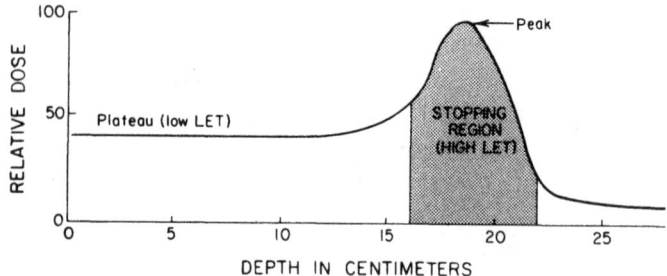

*Figure 3.* Hypothetical application of the 'Bragg peak' to therapeutic gain at the stopping region where high-LET ionization can be precisely localized at a specific tissue depth where the tumor target exists. Such precise localization makes high-LET radiation, such as pi mesons, especially attractive for therapeutic use because of theoretical protection of the interval normal tissue.

tion curve with a finite depth of penetration. The curve is composed of an initial, relatively low-LET, low dose plateau and a high dose terminal peak (Bragg peak) in the stopping region [1]. The distance the plateau extends inward from the body surface depends on the initial energy of the radiation beam. The charged particles lose energy, begin to slow down, and eventually stop when a proportionately greater amount of energy is absorbed per unit volume of tumor in the high dose peak range. The greater the dose at the peak stopping region in comparison to the plateau, the greater the probability that the beam will concentrate radiation in the tumor. This concept means that the heavy ions, i.e., neon and helium, the proton beam (even though it is low-LET), and the pion beam can be shaped to fit a specific tumor configuration (Figure 3), minimizing the amount of energy deposited in adjacent normal tissues. By superimposing a number of contiguous Bragg peaks within a defined tumor volume, the peak region can be spread to enhance effective dose deposition within the tumor volume, while largely sparing surrounding normal tissue (Figure 4) [5]. Heavy particles with broad

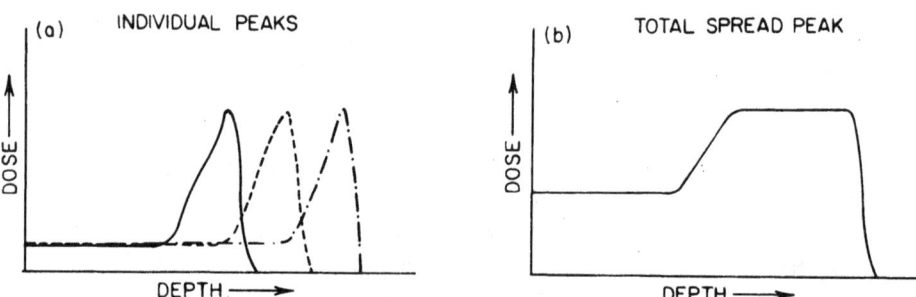

*Figure 4.* Schematic representation of change in depth dose distribution by range-modulation, i.e., movement of the Bragg peak at depth to assure a 'spread' peak of adequate width to encompass clinically relevant volumes.

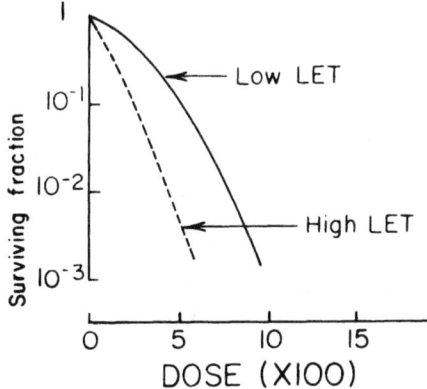

*Figure 5.* Schematic cell survival curves, characteristic of X-rays compared with that exhibited by high-LET radiation.

peaks are well suited for treating deep-seated tumor targets. A greater spread of the peak region of the ion beam, however, results in a lower differential in dose between the entrance and peak regions of the dose distribution. Thus the advantage of dose distribution with high-LET radiation includes sparing of superficial tissues, an adequate depth dose and maintenance of the sharply focused distribution at depth.

The radiobiological effect of high-LET radiation [6] results in (1) less repair of sublethal damage between radiation treatments; (2) less differential effect between oxygenated and hypoxic cells; and (3) a smaller difference between phases of the cell cycle when compared to low-LET radiation.

As LET increases, the shoulder characteristically observed with low-LET survival curves tends to disappear, resulting in a straight line, exponential curve (Figure 5). This exponential response suggests that critical molecular targets are not being repaired or replaced following injury by high-LET radiations. Each interaction is presumed lethal and little sublethal accumulation of damage occurs. Thus there is essentially no recovery between fractionated doses in high-LET radiation. One can expect that the cell survival curve will change from a sigmoid to an exponential curve between 165–220 keV/$\mu$m. The shoulder of the cell survival curve decreases with increasing LET and finally disappears at a critical transition point to higher LET energy levels. Furthermore, sublethal damage produced by low-LET radiation does not seem to enhance the sensitivity of cells to high-LET radiation. Damage produced by high-LET ionized particles also does not prevent the surviving cells from recovering from sublethal damage due to low-LET radiation. High-LET radiation acts independently of the damage induced by low-LET radiation.

The biological effects of high-LET radiation are nearly independent of any oxygen enhancement; high-LET radiation is more effective against hypoxic cells than are low-LET radiation. This means that for the same cytotoxic effect produced in healthy cells, high-LET radiation has high probability (1.5–3.0 times that of X-rays) of killing hypoxic tumor cells. When LET increases, OER* decreases, approaching unity as 150–200 keV/$\mu$m is approached. Low-LET energy tends to spare hypoxic, radioresistant proliferating tumor cells. This radioresistance may be more effectively overcome by combining high-LET radiation (low OER) with chemical radiosensitizers, i.e., metronidazole and misonisazole, than by treatment with either radiation modality alone.

High-LET radiation has greater relative biological effectiveness (RBE) than low-LET radiation, due to the greater number of ionizing events per microgram of tissue. The RBE of high-LET radiation for hypoxic cells is greater than that for oxygenated cells. Likewise, the RBE increases at the peak whereas it is less in the plateau region of the Bragg curve. Such differences in RBE enhance the dose localization advantage of high-LET radiation.

Relative radiosensitivity within the cell cycle to low-LET radiation is greatest at M phase and during late S phase. Multifractionated radiation therapy increases the likelihood of tumor cell damage in radiosensitive phases of the cell cycle. Likewise, low-LET radiation is less effective in breaking chromosomes than is high-LET radiation. The higher density of ionization by high-LET radiation increases the probability of inducing double strand breaks in DNA molecules, which are often difficult to repair, as compared to the more limited injury caused by low-LET radiation. Similarly the inhibition of repair by high-LET particles overcomes the protective effects of hypoxia and variations in cell cycle sensitivity which ordinarily inhibit the effectiveness of low-LET radiation. The greater the LET, the more efficient is the radiation at bringing about mutations or chromosomal alterations and the less likely that variations in killing effect within the cell cycle will occur.

## 2. FORMS OF IONIZING RADIATION

High-LET beams differ from low-LET beams in their deposition of energy in tissue molecules. Low-LET radiation is characteristic of conventional radiation therapy, i.e., X-rays or gamma rays from a cobalt source. High-LET radiation results in a spatial rate of energy loss significantly higher than that for low-LET radiation.

---

* See Glossary on p. 310.

*2.1. Low-LET radiations*

X-rays and gamma rays are forms of electromagnetic radiation which have no mass or charge (photons). They do not differ in nature or properties but rather in the manner in which they are produced. X-rays are the kinetic energy resulting from the impact of accelerated electrons on a tungsten or gold target and are therefore extranuclear in origin. Contrariwise, gamma rays are emitted intranuclearly by the decay of radioactive isotopes such as $Co^{60}$. They represent excess energy given off as an unstable nucleus breaks up and decays to reach a stable form. The energy released by electromagnetic radiation may be thought of as a stream of 'photons' or packets of energy. These individual packets of energy are quantified into large packets of energy, each of which is big enough to break a chemical bond and initiate a change of events which culminates in biological change. The potency of X-rays or gamma rays in matter is a function not so much of the total energy absorbed as it is of the size of the individual energy packet. In their interactions with matter, the energy of photons is transferred by collision, usually with an orbiting electron in an atom of the absorbing medium. Thus the damaging actions of X-rays and gamma rays are exerted almost entirely through secondary fast electrons ejected from the atoms. Since the interaction of X-rays and gamma ray photons with matter depend upon chance collision with electrons, they are capable of penetrating deeply and passing though vast distances in tissue without interacting with any of its molecules. Conventional radiotherapy deposits energy into tissue via ionized or excitated electrons that lose their energy slowly, resulting in a low linear energy density along the electron track (low linear transfer, or low-LET).

*2.2. High-LET radiation*

High-LET radiation results from particulate or heavy particle radiation. Particulate radiation may have both mass and charge. These properties make interactions with matter possible both by direct collision with electrons in the orbits of atoms and also by the interactions between their charge and that of the orbital electrons. The final result of both, i.e., electromagnetic or particulate radiation, is the same, ionization, the production of high speed electrons in matter. The difference in biological response to high-LET radiation results from dense ionization in critical molecules, so that cells are not able to repair molecular injuries in a manner similar to the repair after low–LET radiation. Common forms of high-LET radiations include neutrons as well as heavy ions and stopping pions. A special characteristic of pion radiation involves low-LET radiation expended during the plateau phase of energy loss and a combination of high- and low-LET energy lost at the stopping region of Bragg's peak (Figure 3).

## 3. PHYSICAL AND CLINICAL FEATURES OF PARTICULATE RADIATION

### 3.1. Neutrons

Neutrons [6] are electrically neutral particles with a mass similar to that of a proton. Because they are electrically neutral they cannot be accelerated in an electrical device.

Neutrons are emitted as a byproduct of U-235 or Cf-252 undergoing fission or they are produced when a charged particle such as deuteron is accelerated to a high energy level and then made to impinge upon a suitable target material. Six MeV neutrons result from impingement of a deuteron of suitable energy on a target of beryllium; the proton is 'stripped' from the deuteron leaving a neutron which carries much of the kinetic energy of the original deuteron. Neutrons generated at 14 million electron volts (MeV) exhibit essentially the same dose distribution as gamma rays from a cobalt-60 source.

Neutron beams cannot be localized to the tumor target in the same manner as high-LET radiations exhibiting a Bragg peak. The radiation dose of neutron radiation therapy falls off exponentially as it passes through the tissue and depth dose localization cannot be designed to fit the actual geographic limits of the tumor in the depth dimension, although collimation of lateral borders of a tumor volume is possible.

In 1974 the first results of neutron therapy from Hammersmith Hospital were reported by Catterall [7]. She believed that undesirable late effects of fast neutron therapy could be prevented by careful attention to dose and by careful treatment planning. In those early studies, necrosis appeared to be an occasionally serious side effect. She pointed out that when normal tissue necrosis occurred, a serious predisposing event acted as a co-factor. She also observed that the margin between the optimal dose and dose causing undesirable after-effects (the therapeutic index) appeared to be narrower for high-LET than for low-LET radiation.

In 1977, Parker and co-workers [8] reviewed the results of over 700 patients with diverse malignancies treated with fast neutron beam therapy in three United States programs since 1972. The normal tissue tolerance was considered to be good. Beam doses ranged between 2000 rads (total neutron and gamma doses) with 2, 3 or 5 increments per week for 6 to 8 weeks to a maximum of 2240 rads with 2 or 4 increments per week for 6 to 8 weeks. Fifty-seven patients with Stage IIB, III and IVA carcinoma of the uterine cervix have been treated by one of the following treatment arms: photons only, combined neutron and photon therapy, photons followed by neutron boost, and neutrons only. Seventeen of 22 (77%) patients, treated with a mixed beam pattern of 2 increments of fast neutrons and 3 increments of photons weekly, and 6 of 17 patients (35%), treated by fast neutron beam only in 2 increments weekly, showed good local control. Stratification in both of these arms was inadequate; a greater percentage of patients treated by mixed beam exhibited earlier stage disease and were associated with fewer instances of pre-radiation pelvic surgery.

Morita and co-workers [9] reported 24 cases of gynecologic malignancy treated by fast neutron therapy without detailed follow-up analysis. Five patients treated for Stage III squamous cell carcinoma of the cervix with a mixed beam approach combining 2550 rads in 15 fractions over 5 weeks with 800 neutron rads (generated from a deuteron beam on a beryllium target) in 10 fractions over the same period resulted in complete tumor regression in all cases.

Recently, Dutriex and Tubiana [10] cautioned that dose distribution and energy absorption in the target tissues may be contributing to the marginal success of these patients. Conclusions from neutron therapy may not be extended to high-LET radiations, e.g. pions and heavy ions, which can be localized in a finite range and offer a superior dose distribution with sparing of normal tissues and potential prevention of unacceptable late normal tissue reactions. Halan [11] evaluated normal tissue response to neutron irradiation and concluded that adjustment of dosage seems essential in view of the undesirable incidence of apparent normal tissue damage at high doses.

In 1980 Maruyama [12] reported the use of intracavitary Cf-252 followed by high dose whole pelvis radiotherapy in advanced cervical and vaginal carcinoma. The results support a prospective clinical trial for this modality of cancer therapy.

More recently, Morales *et al.* [13] have published preliminary results of a randomized trial comparing conventional irradiation with or without intracavity radium with mixed beam neutron therapy for advanced cervical carcinoma. Analysis of 75 patients with stages IIB–IVA or locally recurrent cancer following surgery when followed for an average of 25 months showed no statistically significant differences in local control, survival or complications between the 2 groups. The authors emphasized the technical inadequacies of the neutron equipment available for the trial.

*3.2. Pions*

Pions (pi meson) represent the binding energy which holds neutrons and protons together in the nuclei of atoms [6]. They are negatively charged particles with a mass 273 times as great as the electron and approximately 1/7th the mass of a proton. Pions are currently produced from highly energetic proton beams generated by synchrocyclotrons or linear accelerators. They are unstable and have a mean life of $2.54 \times 10^{-8}$ seconds. Negative pions with energies of 60–90 MeV (range 12–23 centimeters in tissue) are of interest in clinical radiotherapy. (Figure 6).

Pions distribute their dose with a Bragg peak, a region of intense radiation which can be readily localized at the level of the tumor target. In contrast, neutrons, which have no charge, deposit their dose in tissue exponentially, similar to the dose absorption of gamma rays. Pions have the advantage of both high-LET and low-LET radiation because they deposit low-LET radiation as they pass through normal tissue (plateau region) and produce a predominantly high-LET component in the tumor (peak region) (Figure 3). Due to their negative charge, the stopping pions are absorbed by the positively charged nuclei of oxygen, carbon, and nitrogen. This excess energy makes the nuclei unstable and they disintegrate, releasing large, densely ionizing subnuclear fragments of short energy range. These events increase the total dose in the pion stopping region, and alter the biological effectiveness (RBE) because of the dense ionization produced by the alpha particles, neutrons, and heavy ions.

The rationale for pion radiotherapy is primarily related to two factors: (1) a different biological response in the stopping region of the pion beam from that seen in conventional photon radiation therapy, and (2) the capability for localization of this response within the limits of the target volume,

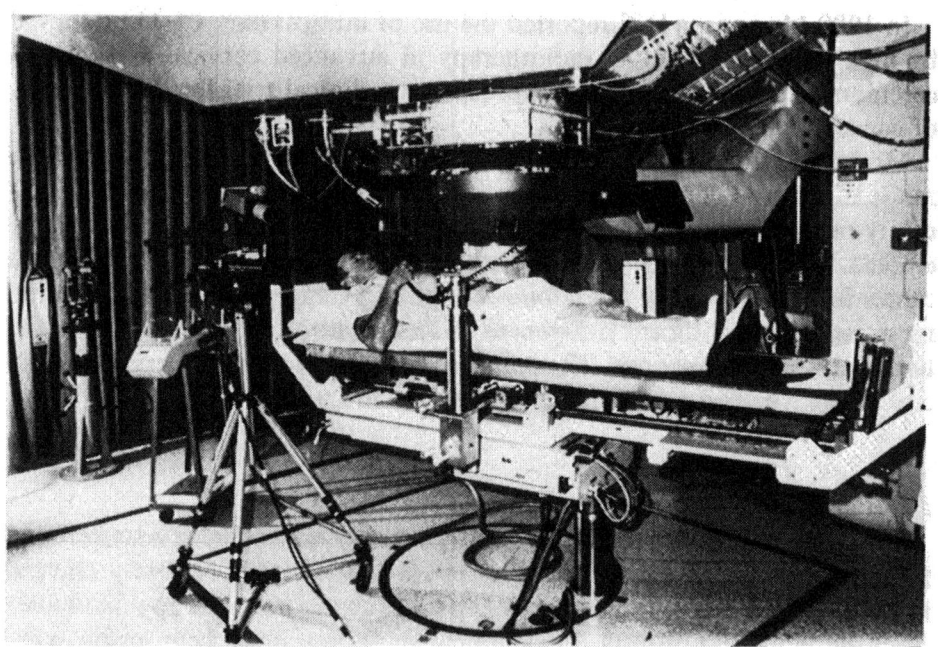

*Figure 6.* Biomedical facility at the Los Alamos Medical Facility. The patient is positioned under the collimated shaped pion beam and is monitored through closed circuit television screen.

largely sparing surrounding normal tissues. There is an increased chance of irreparable damage of critical molecules which overcomes the protective effect of hypoxia and reduces differences in cellular sensitivity due to cell cycle variations. Depth dose localization is a special advantage of pion radiotherapy because pions exhibit an unusually advantageous peak to plateau ratio and a concentreated high-LET fraction in the peak.

In gynecology, studies have been initiated to study the effect of pi mesons on metastatic lesions as well as Stage IIIA, IIIB and IVA squamous cell carcinoma of the uterine cervix. The authors were involved in the latter studies. To date nine patients with advanced previously untreated squamous cell carcinoma of the uterine cervix have been treated with pi meson

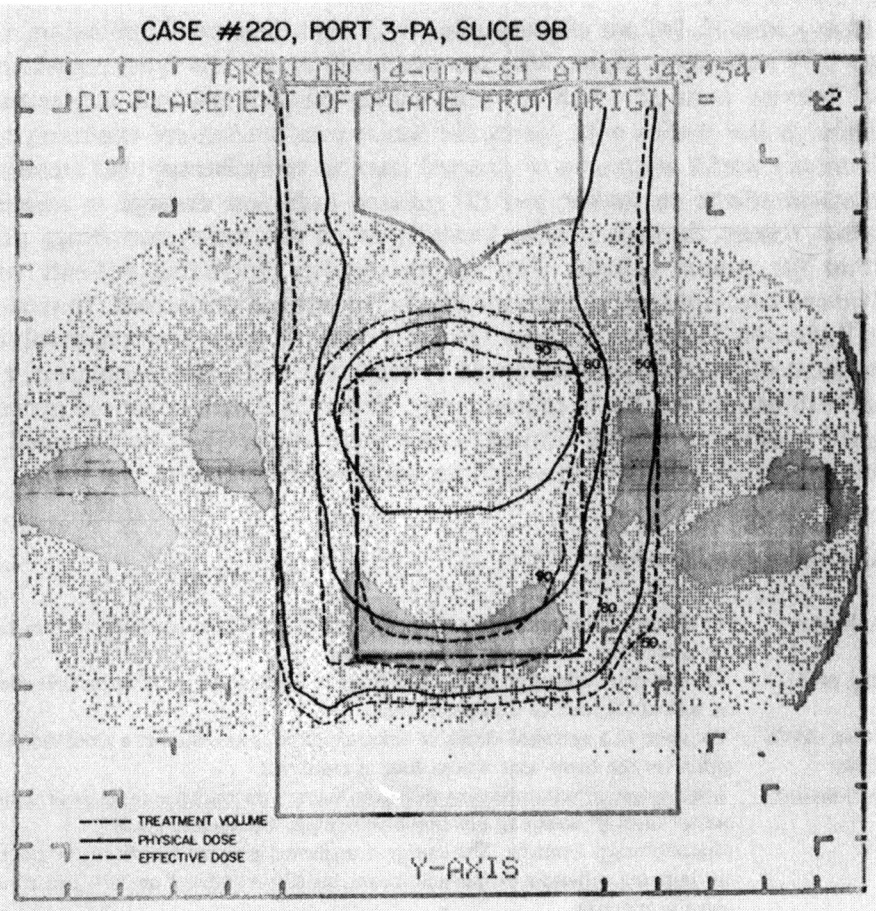

*Figure 7.* Dose distribution for pion radiotherapy by a posterior port (top of figure) of a conedown volume of the central pelvis at the level of the pubis for advanced cervix carcinoma with bladder invasion. Isodose lines are indicated for the measured physical dose and for the effective biological dose taking account of the variability in cell killing across the pion peak region.

radiation therapy alone or in combination with conventional X-ray therapy and have been followed for a minimum of 8 months. The complication rates are tolerable and in 6 of 9 patients, local tumor control has occurred. One patient received 4500 pion rads followed by an interstitial template implant, giving an additional 2400 rads, developed small bowel changes consistent with radiation enteritis and expired of metastatic disease 1 year following treatment. One patient has died of metastatic disease present at the time pion radiation therapy was initiated and two have died with local recurrence and metastases. An example of dose localization by particle irradiation is exhibited in Figure 7.

### 3.3. Heavy ions

Heavy ions [6, 14] are characterized by a high density of ionization, i.e., high-LET radiations. Heavy ions are produced by the 184 Synchrocyclotron and Belevac, both of which are high energy physics research accelerators. Similar to the studies with pions, the heavy ions studies are exploring two potentially useful attributes of charged particle radiotherapy: (1) increased biological effects on tumor, and (2) reduced radiation damage to adjacent normal tissues through precise localization of the heavy ion Bragg peak within the tumor volume. Few clinical studies, including patients with advanced carcinoma of the uterine cervix, have been performed. Currently, the Radiation Therapy Oncology Group is carrying out a protocol involving treatment of patients with advanced or recurrent malignant neoplasms, any site, with helium ion beam radiotherapy. Experience with advanced gynecological neoplasms is very limited. Later these studies will be extended to pilot studies of beams of heavier ions such as carbon, neon and argon.

### RADIOBIOLOGICAL TERMS

Accelerator: An electronic channel which imparts energy to charged particles, such as electrons, protons, deuterons and helium ions.

Bragg peak: The dramatic release of energy just prior to the time an ionizing particle comes to rest at the end of a particle track.

Percent depth dose: The dose at a specified depth in tissue relative to the dose at a fixed reference point on the beam axis where dose is maximal.

Fractionation: A technique of administering radiation therapy in multiple doses over a number of days or weeks to achieve a maximum therapeutic ratio.

LET: Linear Energy Transfer. The energy transferred per unit length of the track of an ionizing radiation or particle beam, usually expressed as keV/$\mu$m of unit density material.

OER: Oxygen Enhancement Ratio. The ratio of radiation dose required to produce an effect under hypoxic conditions to the dose required to produce the same effect under oxygenated conditions. For conventional radiation therapy, this quantity ranges between 2.5–3.0.

| | |
|---|---|
| RBE: | Relative Biological Effectiveness. This term defines the ratio of two different forms of radiation required to produce a biological effect. The RBE of a test radiation ($D_t$) is compared to a standard radiation ($D_{std}$) defined by the ratio $D_t/D_{std}$. $D_t$ and $D_{std}$ are the doses required to achieve an equal biological effect. |
| Sublethal damage: | A cell radiated by conventional X-rays exhibits reversible damage in some, but not all, of the critical target molecules, in a cell. Although cell damage occurs, lethality does not occur and cellular repair takes place in the interval between fractionated doses. When a critical number of damaged target sites accumulate, lethality finally occurs. |
| Therapeutic gain: | Increasing the tumor dose without exceeding the normal tissue tolerance (Figure 1). Beyond a critical point small increases in radiation dose may lead to large increases in the percentage of postradiation complications. |

## REFERENCES

1. Kilgerman MM, Knapp EA, Petersen DF: Biomedical program leading to therapeutic trials of pion radiation at Los Alamos. Cancer 36:1675–1680, 1975.
2. Hall EJ: Radiobiology for the Radiologist. Hagerstown: Harper & Row, 1973.
3. Pizzarello DJ, Witcofski RL: Medical Radiation Biology. Philadelphia: Lea & Febiger, 1972.
4. Kilgerman MM, Sternhagen CJ: Radiation oncology. In: The Physiopathology of Cancer, Vol 2. Homburger F (ed). Basel: S Karger, 1976, pp 135–181.
5. Yuhas JM, Li AP, Kilgerman MM: Present status of the proposed use of negative pi mesons in radiotherapy. Adv Radiation Biol 8:51–53, 1979.
6. Raju MR: Heavy Particle Radiotherapy. New York: Harcourt Brace Jovanovich, 1980.
7. Catterall M: The treatment of advanced cancer by fast neutrons from the Medical Research Council's cyclotron at Hammersmith Hospital, London. Eur J Cancer 10:343–347, 1974.
8. Parker RG, Berry HC, Caderao JB, et al.: Preliminary clinical results from US Fast Neutron Teletherapy Studies. Cancer 40:1434–1438, 1977.
9. Morita S, Tsunemoto H, Umegaki Y: Preliminary clinical results of Fast Neutron Therapy with NIRS Medical Cyclotron. Int J Radiation Oncology Biol Phys 3:281–282, 1977.
10. Dutriex J, Tubiana M: Evaluation of clinical experience concerning tumor response to high-LET radiation. In: Proceedings of the Third Meeting on Fundamental and Practical Aspects of the Application of Fast Neutrons and Other High-LET Particles in Clinical Radiotherapy. Oxford: Pergamon Press, 1978.
11. Halan K: Evaluation of normal tissue responses to high-LET radiations. In: Proceedings of the Third Meeting on Fundamental and Practical Aspects of the Application of Fast Neutrons and other High-LET Particles in Clinical Radiotherapy. Oxford: Pergamon Press, 1978.
12. Maruyama Y, Beach JL, Feola J, et al.: Low dose rate fast neutron therapy of advanced cervical cancers. In: Second International Symposium on Biological Bases and Clinical Implications of Tumor Radioresistance (in press).
13. Morales P, Hussey DH, Maor MH, et al.: Preliminary report of the M.D. Anderson Hospital Randomized Trial of Neutron and Photon Irradiation for locally advanced carcinoma of the uterine cervix. Int J Radiation Oncology Biol Phys 7:1533–1540, 1981.
14. Sala JM, Kilgerman MM: Clinical experience with negative pi mesons and other high-LET radiations. In: Advances in Medical Oncology, Research & Education, Vol 6, Basis for Cancer Therapy 2. Moore M (ed). New York: Pergamon Press, 1979, pp 215–221.

# 10. Growth of Gynecologic Neoplasms in Tissue Culture and as Heterografts

CHARLES E. WELANDER and JOHN L. LEWIS Jr.

## 1. INTRODUCTION

A major challenge to investigators studying human tumors is the development of a laboratory model in which the behavior and response of the tumor is the same or similar to that of the patient. Since the early part of this century [1, 2], tissue culture of human cells, both benign and malignant, has been one of the approaches used to understand tumor behavior. The difficulties inherent in tissue culture techniques, particularly in the days before antibiotics were available, prompted investigators to look further, to the study of animal tumor model systems. Recognition of immunologically privileged sites in laboratory animals permitted the first successful growth of human tumors in another species ('heterografts') [37–41]. In addition to the use of such immunoprivileged sites for tumor transplantation, methods resulting in total body immunosuppression could be added to enhance the probability of tumor growth in a foreign host [42–45]. It was not until the discovery of the athymic nude mouse, however, that a widespread use of animal heterografts for the study of human cancers was possible [50, 51].

The technique of *in vitro* growth of tumor cells in tissue culture flasks or *in vivo* growth in animal transplants developed over several decades. Credit for specific developments belongs to many investigators. The subsequent use of these techniques to answer specific questions concerning the biology and pathophysiology of tumor cells presently occupies our interests.

Two broad areas will be considered in this chapter: the development of techniques necessary to grow human cancers in the laboratory, and the application of these new techniques to the study of clinical cancer treatment. Included in the section on clinical applications of new techniques are the serologic approach to cell surface antigen identification, hybridoma studies, and descriptive analyses of chromosomal changes in human tumors. The other area to be considered within this same section will be therapeutically

*Griffiths, C. T. and Fuller, A. F. (eds.), Gynecologic Oncology.*
© *1983, Martinus Nijhoff Publishers, Boston. ISBN 0-89838-555-5.*
*Printed in The Netherlands.*

important information concerning chemotherapy response that can be obtained from *in vitro* studies. The human tumor stem cell assay is a recent technical innovation used for chemotherapy sensitivity testing. Drug testing using heterograft model systems will also be presented.

## 2. TISSUE CULTURE

During the first decade of the twentieth century Alexis Carrel developed techniques for growth of human tissues *in vitro* [1]. As a result of the work in his laboratory at the Rockefeller Institute, Carrel became a leading figure and proponent of this new field of cell culture, and was responsible for many of the early technical innovations. His interests in *in vitro* cell growth extended to many types of cells, both normal and malignant [2]. The popularity of tissue culture developed slowly because of difficulties encountered in achieving sustained growth of human cells. It was not until 1923 that Carrel introduced the culture flask, which greatly facilitated the maintenance of aseptic growth conditions. One recent biographer described Carrel's efforts as primarily directed at popularizing his new technique, without adequate emphasis on practical application of it [3].

After the discovery of antibiotics and the development of defined culture media, tissue culture began growing rapidly as a research tool. At the American Association of Cancer Research meeting in 1952, Dr George Gey of Johns Hopkins University presented a paper describing the establishment of a human cervical adenocarcinoma in cell culture, which had at that time been grown more than one year in serial subcultures [4]. This cell line, designated HeLa, continues to be propagated to the present time. This success introduced a new era in the advancement of tissue culture techniques.

In the years since the establishment of the HeLa cell line, widespread efforts have been made to establish other gynecologic malignancies in continuous culture. Established cell lines are often started using solid tumors from surgical specimens; selection of a sterile tumor fragment with the greatest proportion of tumor cells to stroma (or fat) is important. Tumor cells must be viable and free of necrosis when placed into culture in order to achieve successful growth. Viability may be enhanced by shortening the elapsed time from removal of the specimen by the surgeon in the operating room to its arrival in the culture laboratory [5, 6] sterile handling throughout transport is mandatory.

Laboratory preparation begins with washing the tumor in saline containing antibiotics. Fat and fibrous tissue are trimmed away prior to mincing the tumor into chunks as small as possible. Mincing the tissue automatically releases free cells into the medium [7]. An unusual amount of fibrous stroma may require additional enzymatic digestion using collagenase and deoxyribonuclease to liberate more single cells [6]. It is necessary to disaggregate the specimen as completely as possible to facilitate attachment of tumor cells to the culture flask. Few primary cultures of human tumor cells will proliferate initially in suspension; attachment to the flask is essential in order to maintain continued cell viability.

Occasionally gynecologic cancer patients have large volumes of ascites and pleural fluid which contain viable tumor cells. Preparation of cultures from this material is simplified; it is not necessary to disaggregete a solid mass prior to primary cell culture. An excessive number of erythrocytes can by lysed with a hypotonic solution in order to count the number of tumor cells to be plated in culture.

A major set of problems with the growth of human cancer *in vitro* relates to the limited understanding of the nutritional requirements of tumor cells. The basic medium contains glucose, electrolytes, amino acids, trace elements, and vitamins in known quantities. The addition of various types of serum to the medium has resulted in increased chance of successful growth. Presumably, there are growth-promoting substances in the sera [8], for efforts to grow cells in chemically defined medium free of serum have only recently become successful. Hormonal additives to the medium vary with

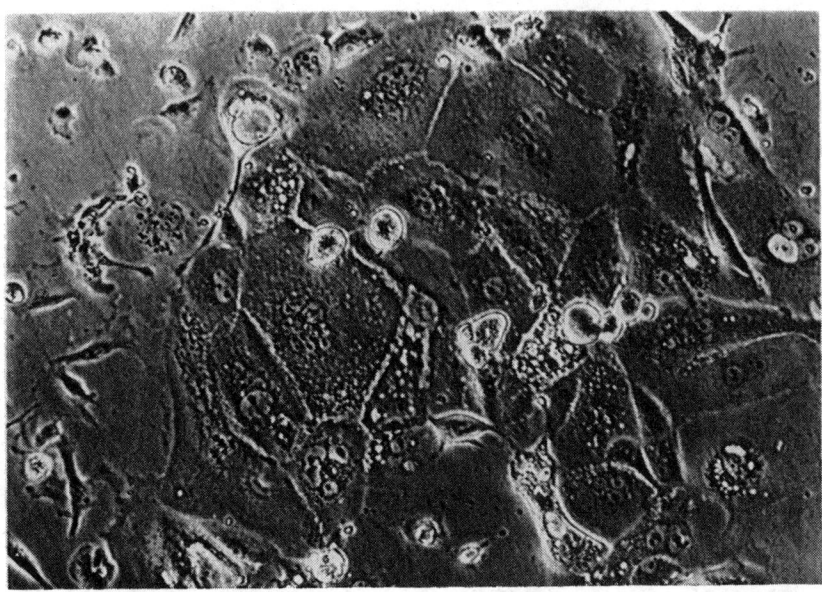

*Figure 1.* Ovarian carcinoma cells after 28 days in primary culture. Cells become large, flat, vacuolated, and rarely divide any longer; ×96.

the type of cell being cultured; gynecologic tumors often require insulin, growth hormone, progesterone, estrogen and glucocorticoids [8-11]. Great efforts have been made in the past ten years to identify additional growth factors that will make dormant cells divide again. These include the somatomedins and multiple growth factors: epidermal, fibroblast, macrophage, and nerve growth factors. In the presence of an optimally enriched culture medium, cells attach quickly to the flask and begin a sequence of rapid cell divisions. The process of cell division, however, often slows, and within a few weeks mitotic activity ceases completely. With this slowed metabolic rate, the cells change shape and often acquire large intracytoplasmic vacuoles (Figure 1). We might conclude that initial vigorous growth followed by gradual reduction in cell division is related to the absence of some factor in the medium essential for continued viability. The perfect medium containing the exact nutritional requirements of culture tumor cells is not known.

An additional problem precluding the establishment of successful tumor cell cultures is the overwhelming presence of fibroblasts in some primary cultures. The single cell suspension prepared from the tumor specimen includes both tumor cells and the adjacent stroma; as a result the culture is often heavily plated with fibroblasts from the beginning (Figure 2). There is no simple way to exclude fibroblasts. Since differential growth rates usually favor the fibroblast, the tumor cells may be completely overgrown. Small

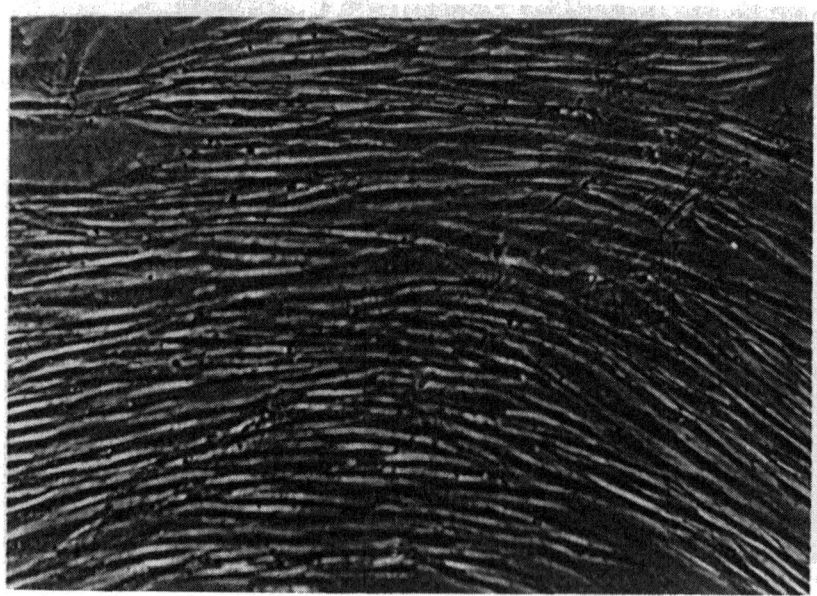

*Figure 2.* Fibroblasts growing in a primary monolayer culture; ×96.

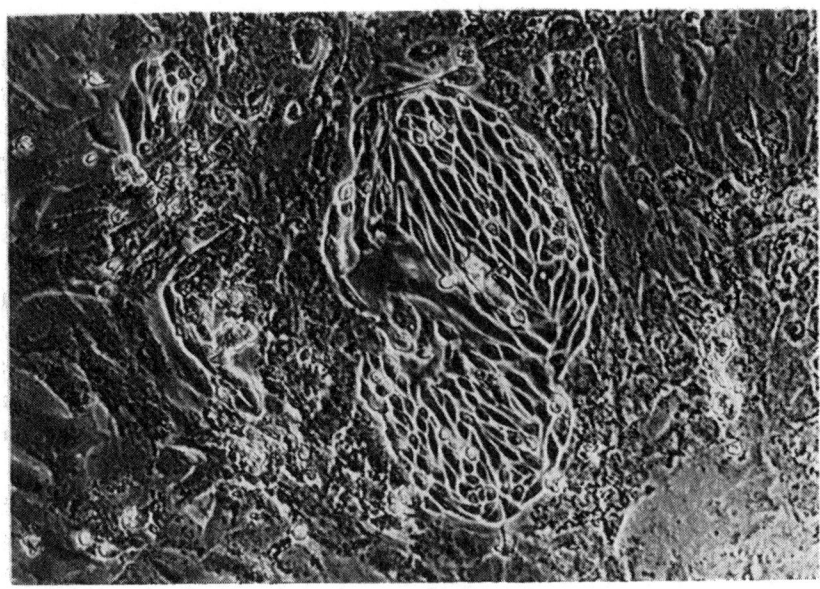

*Figure 3.* Small islands of epithelial cells in the center of the field become surrounded by more rapidly dividing fibroblasts; ×60.

islands of epithelial cells then disappear when subcultured as they are overtaken by the rapidly dividing population of fibroblasts (Figure 3).

Ascitic or pleural fluids which contain tumor cells usually also have mesothelial cells from peritoneal surfaces mixed together. These mesothelial cells are as difficult to separate from tumor cell population as are the stromal fibroblasts in a solid tumor [12].

For these reasons, the establishment of gynecologic cancers in long-term culture has been rare. A review published in 1975 described only 11 cervical carcinoma lines, including the original HeLa line [13]. There are few reports of cell lines derived from endometrial cancer [14–18], vulvar carcinomas [19, 20], or choriocarcinomas [21].

Probably the most extensive efforts to grow gynecologic carcinomas in the tissue culture in the past decade have been carried out with ovarian carcinomas. During the years 1974 to 1979 fifteen established lines of epithelial ovarian cancers were reported [22–27]. The reason for improved success rate is not clear from these published studies. One observation was the growth-enhancing effect of macrophages on cell cultures of ovarian carcinomas. Removal of the macrophages from the cultures decreased the growth of tumor cells; growth could be restored by replacing the macrophages or, to a lesser degree, by substituting conditioned medium prepared from supernatant of cultures of peritoneal macrophages or adherent spleen cells [28, 29]. Using a modification of the conditioned medium technique, irradiated peritoneal macrophages can be incorporated into the culture flasks as a feeder layer, over which the primary tumor cell suspension is plated. This technical modification is based on the presumption that the macrophages produce some soluble substance which diffuses through the medium of the culture and enhances epithelial tumor cell growth. Use of this feeder layer has increased the initial attachment of epithelial tumor cells during the first twenty-four to forty-eight hours, in culture. The feeder layer promoted persistence of epithelial cells in serial subcultures, in contrast to frequent overgrowth of fibroblast. Using this technique in 64 primary cultures we have successfully grown 25 cell lines (39%) beyond the fifth passage from both solid and ascitic ovarian tumor specimens over the past 3 years [30]. The macrophage growth-promoting effect noted in ovarian carcinomas has not yet been investigated in other types of cancer.

Assurance that the tumor cells grown in long-term cultures and serial passages have retained their original identity deserves further consideration. The epithelial tumor cells can be overgrown and ultimately replaced by fibroblasts, yielding a culture devoid of malignant cells. Morphology alone is not a safe criterion of malignancy [12].

Commonly accepted criteria for malignancy in cell lines include long-term growth in tissue culture, karyotypic analysis, growth in soft agar, expression of specific tumor cell markers, and growth in nude mice [20, 31-33]. Additional information such as analysis of glucose-6-phosphate dehydrogenase isozymes may be valuable in insuring that cell lines are not contaminated by animal or even other human cells (such as HeLa cells) [34-36]. Most of the criteria listed above must be met in order to be certain that the cell line actually represent tumor material from the original donor.

## 3. HETEROGRAFT EXPERIMENTS

Coincident with the development of *in vitro* tissue culture techniques in the early 1950s, an *in vivo* means of studying human tumors became popular. Heterografts of human cancers were found to grow in various animal systems under carefully defined conditions. The growth of a human tumor in a laboratory animal not only provided a reservoir of tumor for serial experimental studies, but also different animals bearing the same human tumor could be treated simultaneously with differing therapies. Early heterograft experiments generally followed two courses: selection of an immunologically privileged site, or systemic immunosuppression.

The anterior chamber of the eye [37], the brain [38, 39], and the cheek pouch of the hamster [40, 41], were initially identified as immunologically privileged sites. Technical difficulties in the anterior chamber of the eye limited the volume of tumor that could be grown. While the brain remained suitably protected from tumor rejection, particularly in young animals, serial measurement of tumor growth was difficult prior to autopsy. Choriocarcinoma was grown in each of 10 attempts in the brain of adult rhesus monkeys, without the requirement for systemic immunosuppression with antilymphocyte serum [39]. Viable choriocarcinoma was recovered from the brains of all ten monkeys and was transplanted into hamster cheek pouches. Of all the putatively privileged sites, the hamster cheek pouch has been the most frequently used. Tumors can be implanted easily, growth measured, and results of therapy evaluated. Of the human gynecologic neoplasms, one tumor successfully grown in hamsters was choriocarcinoma. Hertz was able to transplant seven different choriocarcinomas in 30 attempts. Serial transplantation has been possible in each of the seven tumors described [40]. In those that failed, the tumor graft grew for 10 to 12 days, and then spontaneously regressed. In the face of a spontaneous tumor regression without additional immunosuppression of the hamster, antitumor therapy could not be evaluated. The tumor rejection was the result of species-specific antigenicity of the heterograft that precluded evaluation of rejection based on tumor-specific antigens [41].

Systemic immunosuppression was another method designed to enhance heterograft acceptance. Early experiments were carried out with subcutaneous tumor transplants in mice, rats and hamsters treated with whole body irradiation in doses up to 600 rads [42–44]. Tumor growth was sustained for an average of only 8 days, followed by regression of the implanted nodule. Corticosteroid administration to the irradiated animals extended the tumor growth to 12 to 20 days [45]. Some of these tumors could be grown successfully when they were subsequently implanted in other immunosuppressed animals. Systemic administration of corticosteroids was also beneficial in hamster cheek pouch experiments [46]. However, it was not until heterologous anti-lymphocyte serum (ALS) was used that graft rejection could be forestalled long enough to evaluate cytotoxic drug therapy. ALS treatment of hamsters resulted in a greater proportion of successful tumor transplants, larger tumor volumes, prolonged tumor survival and occasional distant metastases.

Surgical ablation of the thymus carried out in neonatal or adult rats and mice has achieved increased immunological tolerance [47, 48]. However, within studies of gynecologic tumors, the hamster has been the animal commonly used. Thymectomy in the adult hamster delayed immunologic recovery following ALS treatment [49]. Compared to either modality alone or to untreated controls, growth of human choriocarcinomas in the hamster cheek pouch is enhanced significantly when combined with ALS treatment.

Because of difficulties and side effects involved in producing systemic immunosuppression required for successful human tumor growth in animals, none of these systems found widespread acceptance. In the late 1960s the discovery of a strain of mice that were congenitally athymic and thus immunologically hyporesponsive greatly facilitated investigation of human tumor heterografts [50, 51]. This association of the athymic state with the absence of body hair led to the naming of this strain of mouse, *nude,* (given the symbol nu/nu) for the homozygous state. The primary immunologic deficiency is in cell-mediated immunity, which is related to T lymphocyte function. The mice are not deficient in tumor immunity, which is primarily a B lymphocyte function. These nude mice accept transplants to xenogeneic tumors without requiring additional immunosuppression. Since the first report of a successful human colon carcinoma heterograft in a nude mouse in 1969 [52] numerous investigators have grown a variety of human gynecologic tumors, including cervix, endometrium, uterine stromal sarcomas, ovary, vulva and choriocarcinoma [53–57]. A registry listing laboratories around the world which have successfully transplanted human tumors into nude mice has been established in Copenhagen and has reported a large number of generally successful heterotransplants [58].

Subcutaneous implantation of a small piece of human tumor [59] is the technique commonly used for heterotransplantation of solid tumor specimens into nude mice. The tumor grows in the subcutaneous space and is

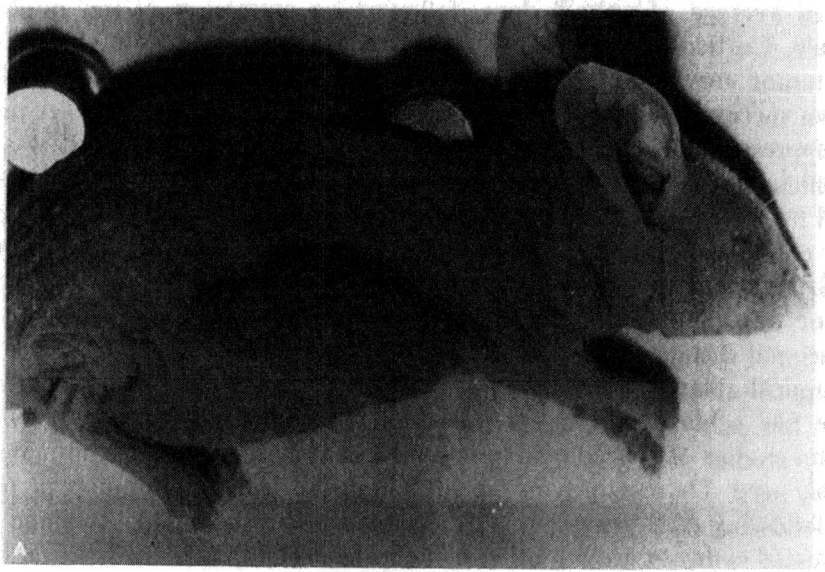

*Figure 4a*

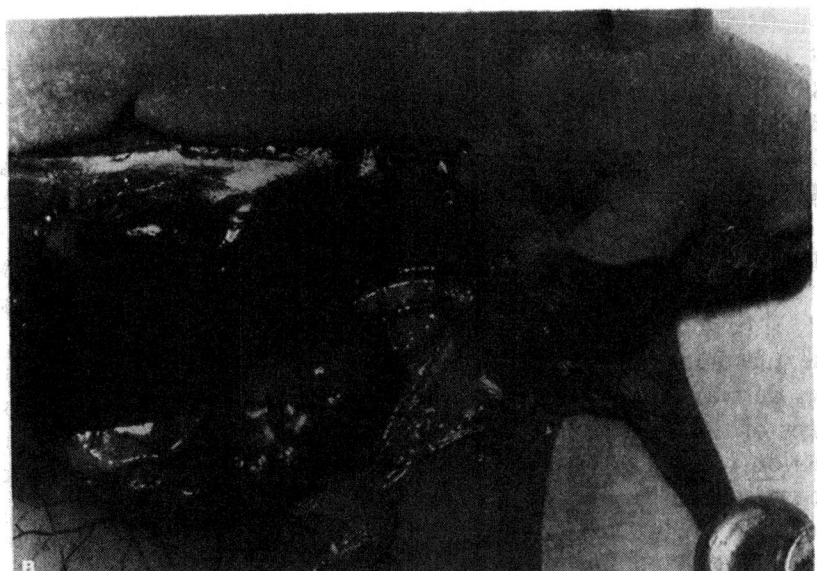

*Figure 4b*

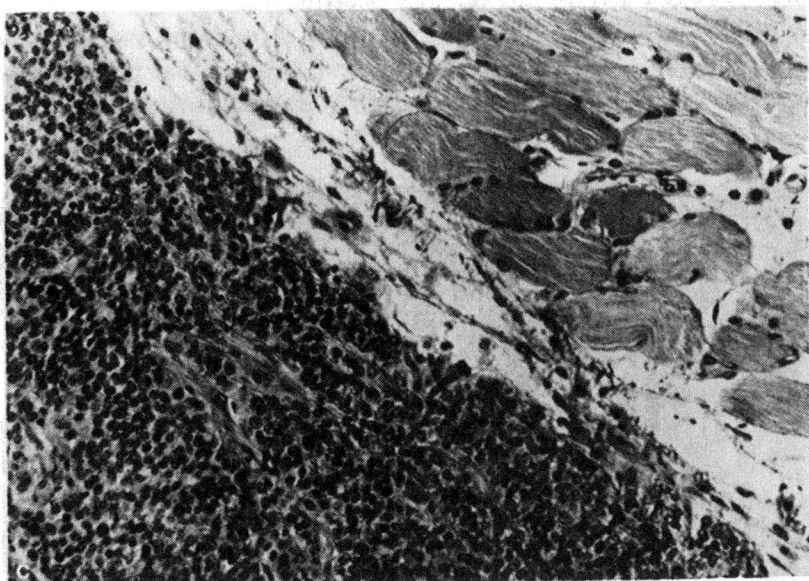

*Figure 4c*

*Figure 4.* (a) Nude mouse with human tumor implanted subcutaneously. (b) Human tumor dissected free from body wall of nude mouse. Note the vascular supply to the tumor from the mouse. (c) Microscopic section of nude mouse tumor. Note the plane between the human carcinoma and the mouse striated muscle, with no invasion of the mouse tissue by the carcinoma; ×96.

vascularized from the periphery (Figure 4). Human connective tissue and other benign stromal elements, transplanted together with the malignant tumor cells, will not grow in the nude mouse; only the malignant portion of the human tumor will grow [31]. Despite the disappearance of human stromal tissue, proliferation of mouse stroma restored the histopathologic architecture of the original tumor [60]. Cell lines of human tumors in tissue culture may also be grown subcutaneously in the nude mouse [32]. The solid tumor nodule which forms after injection of tissue-cultured cells also develops the same architecture as that of the initial primary surgical specimen [33] (Figure 5).

The question of contamination of heterotransplanted human tumors with tissues derived from the nude mouse host has been raised. Chromosomal analysis of tissue-cultured tumor cells before and after nude mouse transplantation reveals an identical karyotype [61]. Glucose-6-phosphate dehydrogenase phenotypes of human tumors following nude mouse transplantation remain the same as those of the patient from which the tumor was obtained [62]. Although the possibility exists of contaminating the human tumor cells with murine xenotropic virus, gynecologic tumors in nude mice have not yet been scrutinized for this possibility.

In addition to the use of the nude mouse as a reservoir for human tumor growth in the laboratory, it has been observed that initial tumor growth in the nude mouse facilitates the subsequent establishment of that tumor in

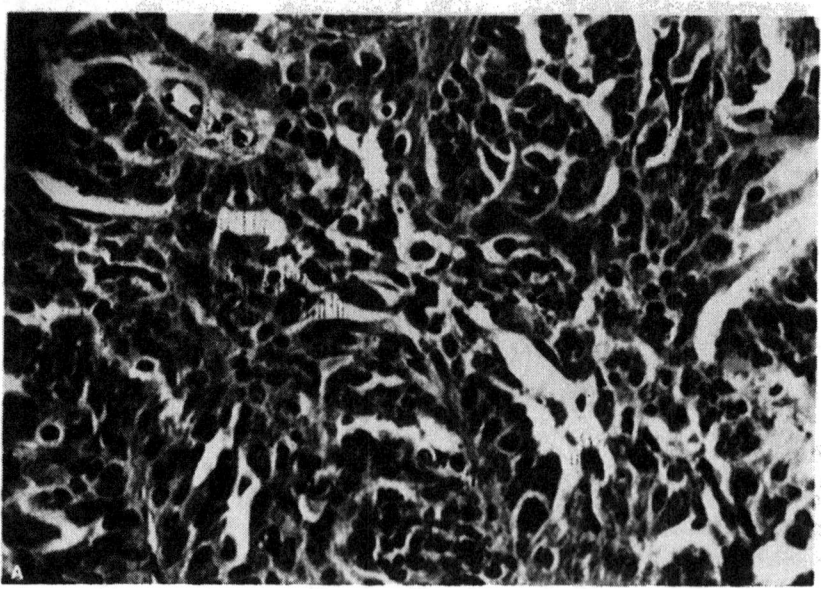

*Figure 5a*

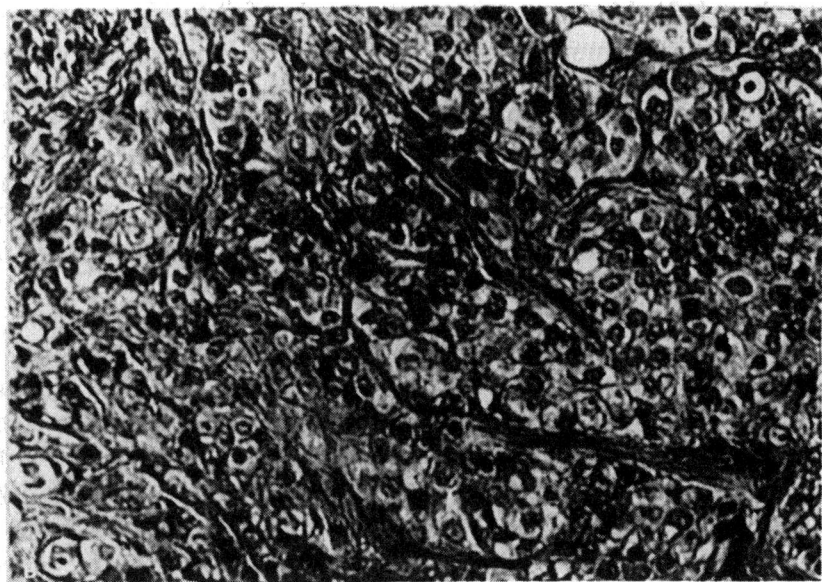

*Figure 5b*

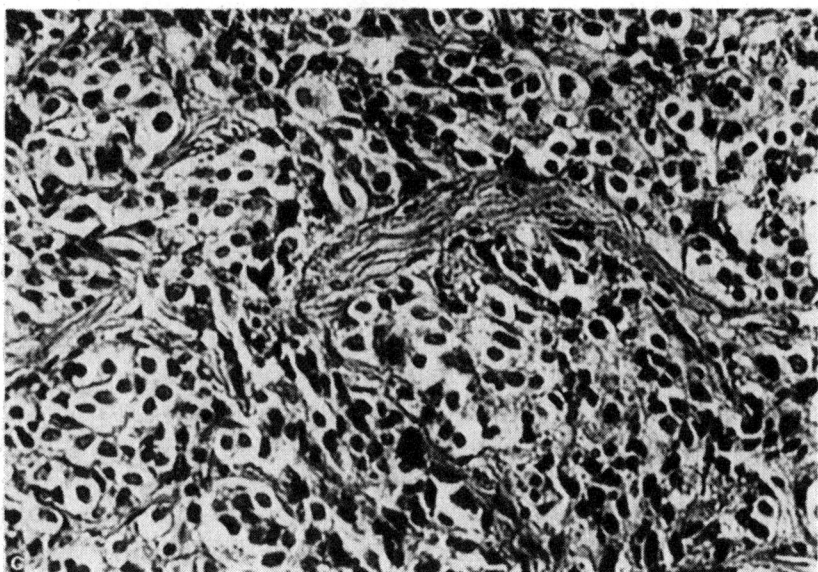

*Figure 5c*

*Figure 5.* (a) Section of original surgical specimen of ovarian carcinoma removed from a patient; ×96. (b) Section of the same human tumor growing subcutaneously in the nude mouse; ×96. (c) Section of tumor prepared by injecting tissue cultured cells of the original surgical specimen into the nude mouse; ×96.

tissue culture [63]. Many surgical specimens that fail to grow in tissue culture will grow in the nude mouse. Once established in the nude mouse, the tumor explant can then be dissected from surrounding mouse tissues and mechanically minced for tissue culture, where it often grows successfully *in vitro*. Growth in the nude mouse may have encouraged the selective overgrowth of the most aggressive fraction of the human tumor cell population. In addition, there is little stroma in the nude mouse tumor, rendering fibroblast overgrowth less likely, thus minimizing the common problem of fibroblast predominance in primary cultures [31].

Cross breeding of a mutant mouse strain having congenital asplenia with nude mouse strains resulted in a hybrid strain of mice with agenesis of both spleen and thymus that could facilitate heterotransplantation of human tumors. Impairment of both humoral immunity and cell-mediated immunity in this animal would theoretically provide an ideal recipient for all types of heterografts. Such a mouse has been developed by B. Lozzio, and given the designation of LASAT mouse (Lozzio A-Splenic A-Thymic) [64]. Significant problems exist, however, with the breeding and maintenance of these animals because of extreme susceptibility to infection. These difficulties have temporarily relegated the LASAT mouse to laboratory curiosity.

## 4. SEROLOGIC APPROACH TO CELL SURFACE ANTIGEN IDENTIFICATION

One of the most important applications of tissue culture is the search for tumor-specific antigens. Whether such antigens exist has not yet been clearly answered for human cancer. Because of the formidable problems of growing gynecologic cancers *in vitro*, most immunologic studies have used heterologous antisera rather than tissue culture as a means for identifying putative tumor antigens. Heterologous antisera have been prepared by injecting tumor homogenates as antigenic material into rabbits. Serum is later collected and purification of specific antibodies attempted by sequential absorption. Numerous studies of ovarian cancers have been published which have identified substances proposed as tumor-associated antigens [65–75]. Exhaustive analyses, however, have frequently found that these substances are differentiation antigens which appear on normal cells at some stage during the process of differentiation. None of the antigens identified so far have been sufficiently tested so that they can be considered tumor specific; yet they may have clinical merit as tumor markers.

Dr Lloyd Old and his group have applied several serologic tests to the search for cell surface antigens, in a variety of human cancers [76–81]. This serologic approach termed as *autologous typing*, has four features: (1) use of established cell lines in tissue culture for serologic testing. (Primary cultures often contain too many fibroblasts to be useful in serologic assays.) Established cell lines, essentially free of fibroblasts, are required for optimal results; (2) direct serologic tests using tumor cells and serum from the same patient. Such an autologous immune response eliminated the confusion of allo-antibody reactivity. It can also detect unique surface antigens present only on that one patient's tumor cells and not shared with any other tumors; (3) absorption tests that can classify the presence and quantity of antigens on cells; (4) the use of multiple serologic techniques simultaneously, reducing the possibility that autologous antibody of a particular class might not be identified. The four serologic procedures used have been the mixed hemadsorption assay, immune adherence assay, anti-C3 mixed hemadsorption assay, and protein A assay [76-81]. Cell surface antigens identified by these procedures have been divided into three classes. Class I antigens are those restricted to autologous combinations of serum and tumor cells. There is no sharing of these antigens with other similar cancers or with normal cells. Class II antigens are shared with allogeneic tumors of the same cell type, but not with normal cells. Class III antigens are ubiquitous and are found on both normal and malignant allogeneic cells, even on heterogeneic cells. Background contamination with antigens derived from the heterologous sera used in cell culture (principally fetal calf serum) can complicate these studies [82]. Work to date includes studies of melanomas, renal cell carcinomas, astrocytomas, and leukemias. A variety of class I and class II antigens have been identified in these tumor types. It appears that the technique of *autologous typing* to detect cell surface tumor-specific antigens could be applied to the evaluation of gynecologic tumor antigens.

The objective subsequent to the identification of human tumor-specific antigens is the determination of the immunological response evoked in the host by these antigens. Based on the presumed existence of such host responses, pilot studies of therapeutic vaccine programs for melanoma and renal cell carcinoma have been established at Memorial Sloan-Kettering Cancer Center, as an outgrowth of the serologic identification of these cell surface antigens. Changes in patients' antibody titers can be recorded using irradiated autologous or allogeneic cells as the immunogenic stimulus and correlating such changes in titers with clinical tumor responses [83].

Viral oncolysates further enhance the immunogeneicity of a tumor cell vaccine [84, 85]. A viral oncolysate can be prepared from a tumor cell culture infected with either vesicular stomatitis virus or vaccinia virus. Following viral infection of the cell cultures, the cells are mechanically disrupted, leaving antigenic fragments of cell membrane intact in the absence of whole viable cells. The material is then irradiated with ultraviolet light to inactivate any remaining active virus. A predetermined amount of oncolysate is then injected intradermally into the tumor-bearing patient.

No gynecologic cancer has yet been studied serologically in depth in order to identify either unique or shared tumor-specific cell surface antigens. Nevertheless, the idea of tumor vaccine remains intriguing to investigators. Patients with advanced cancers in a number of institutions have been injected with irradiated autologous or allogeneic tumor cells [86-88]. In addition to tumor cell vaccines, nonspecific immunopotentiation with Bacillus Calmette-Guerin (BCG) or *Corynebacterium parvum* has also been investigated [89]. The end-points used in such historical studies have been measurement of tumor volume as well as overall survival. Experimental groups have been small, often without randomized controls. Results have not been conclusive and consist mainly of anecdotal cases of tumor response.

## 5. HYBRIDOMAS

The classic work of Kohler and Milstein in 1975 opened a new technology for the preparation of antibodies [90]. Previously antisera was prepared by heteroimmunization, injecting antigenic material into animals and attempting to isolate antisera of desired specificity. Since the immunizing substance was not pure, antibodies were made to all the antigens contained in the substance. It was subsequently necessary to remove (by absorption) the undesired antibodies, many of which were present in higher titers than the desired ones. The new hybridoma technology now permits the production of monoclonal antibodies with defined specificity. Immunogens used to create monoclonal antibodies have included whole tumor cells, preparations of viral material, and purified tumor markers [91, 92]. Six distinct monoclonal antibodies have been identified by Dippold *et al.* using cultured melanoma cells as the immunogen [93], thereby extending the serologic identification of cell surface antigens. None of those six distinct antigenic systems identified are clearly tumor specific. One of the problems noted is that expression of tumor-specific antigens may be of a low level and difficult to detect within the range of sensitivity possible with direct serologic tests. Nonetheless the search for purified antibody continues using the hybridoma technology [94].

## 6. GENETIC STUDIES

Tissue culture has provided material for some of the early investigations of chromosomal abnormalities in tumor cells. Karyotypic analysis of tumor cells in culture has demonstrated several points: (1) the deviation from normal chromosomal complements of primary tumor cells, (2) the changes in karyotype which become evident in long-term tumor cell cultures, and (3) the cytogenetic detection of contaminating cells in established malignant cell lines [34, 95].

Prior to the development of chromosome banding techniques, it was not possible to precisely describe marker chromosomes. Many of the chromosomes previously described as *normal* might have been abnormal if stained by newer banding procedures [96, 97]. A paper from Roswell Park Memorial Institute reported the cytogenetic studies of fresh ovarian tumor specimens prepared in short-term tissue cultures. Cells were grown only 2 to 3 days in culture, avoiding karyotypic changes observed in long-term cell cultures. Chromosomes were stained with Giemsa followed by quinacrine mustard. The most frequent abnormality which was seen in eight of twelve ovarian cancer cases studied was 6q− and 14q+. This appeared to be a characteristic of papillary serous adenocarcinoma of the ovary [98].

Chromosomal analyses of tumors can also be performed using the stem cell clonogenic assay technique in agar. It is possible to study mitotic cells at the periphery of tumor cell clusters in a high percentage of tumors. Trent has published a report of successful chromosomal preparation in 15 of 22 ovarian tumors and in 2 of 3 uterine tumors cultured in agar [99]. With the ability to study many different tumors *in vitro*, it is now possible to correlate karyotypic heterogeneity with clinical tumor behavior. Increasingly mutant karyotypes within subpopulations of tumor cells may be found in those cases with poor clinical prognosis [100]. Further investigation of this hypothesis will be possible using the clonogenic assay technique. The karyotypes of drug-resistant tumor cell clones can be identified, testing the association of drug resistance with a particular cytogenetic abnormality [101, 102]. At this time these promising studies have only begun.

## 7. CLONOGENIC STEM CELL ASSAY

The successful growth of human cancers in tissue culture and the concurrent development of many effective cytotoxic chemotherapeutic agents in the 1950s and 1960s led to attempts at *in vitro* drug sensitivity testing of tumors. It was hoped that tissue culture would facilitate testing the effectiveness of established drugs on specific tumors and screening new compounds for tumor cytotoxicity.

Successful testing of bacterial sensitivity to antibiotics provided the hope that the same principle of *in vitro* testing would be applicable to the determination of tumor sensitivity to anticancer drugs. As a result, major laboratory efforts were directed toward drug screening. Various end-points were selected for measurement of drug effects on tumor cells. Some investigators observed only morphologic effects in cultured cells after incubation with dilutions of drugs [103–106], whereas others measured drug effects on cell growth [107, 108], counting attached cells in the culture flask or by measuring total protein content of the culture flask. A biochemical means of measuring dehydrogenase activity was also promoted as a method of determining tumor cell sensitivity to specific drugs [109–111]. In recent years, more sophisticated techniques have measured drug-induced inhibition of cellular DNA synthesis by recording changes in uptake of radiolabeled nucleic acid precursors as a measure of cell division [112, 113]. Common to all these tests is the measurement of a morphologic, metabolic or reproductive change in the target cell. Each technique utilized tissue culture in testing established cell lines as well as fresh solid tumor specimens.

There are two fundamental flaws in these *in vitro* techniques. First, the methods assume morphologic changes and metabolic dysfunction as equivalent to loss of the potential for cell division. Drug effects on tumor cells are important only if they render cells incapable of dividing. Second, in a culture of tumor cells, none of the methods can distinguish between damage to normal fibroblasts and damage to the tumor cells themselves. What may appear to be effective cell-kill might only represent destruction of the fibroblast matrix in the tumor stroma without affecting tumor cell viability. Because of these limitations, efforts to find more suitable techniques of *in vitro* sensitivity testing have continued.

The stem cell assay in agar is presently the most reliable method to identify loss of clonogenicity in the tumor cell population. The problem of drug-induced damage to fibroblasts in the culture is not encountered in the soft agar stem cell inhibition assay, as benign stromal elements will not grow in an unanchored state [114, 115]. Moreover, colonies will not arise from single cells which have incurred lethal damage as a result of exposure to a chemotherapeutic agent. The effects of cytotoxic drugs on the integrity of tumor cell membranes in soft agar cultures more closely resemble the observed *in vivo* effects than when they are grown in monolayer cultures [116].

The fundamental theory supporting use of the clonogenic assay is based upon tumor cell kinetics. Human solid tumors are composed of many elements, including tumor cells and stromal components. Three types of cells are present within the tumor cell compartment: (1) stem cells, capable of both self-renewal and production of tumor-specific progeny, (2) progenitor cells, capable of extensive proliferative growth, and (3) differentiated progeny with only limited potential for future cell division [117]. The largest masses of a human tumor specimen is made up of differentiated cells, which have only limited or absent ability to divide. This contrasts to the progenitor compartment, in which cells can undergo extensive cell division. Cells in this compartment are usually considered to constitute less than 1% of the nucleated cells in the tumor [118]. In the context of earlier work with hematopoietic tumors, single cell suspensions of clonogenic cells could be plated in soft agar and develop into colonies in the agar matrix [119, 120]. Because cells from nonmalignant stromal tissue are anchorage dependent, they will not grow in a suspended state, as in agar. Likewise, differentiated progeny which have limited capabilities for cell division will not grow from a single cell to a colony (by definition, size greater than 50 cells) [117].

Application of the clonogenic stem cell assay to clinical problems has included testing of tumor sensitivity to chemotherapeutic drugs. Because drug sensitivity of the cells in the stem cell compartment may predict clinical response, the soft agar assay can, in theory, identify stem cell susceptibility to chemotherapeutic agents.

Before attempting quantitative stem cell drug assays for a given tumor type, one must first show that such tumors grow predictably in soft agar cultures. The utility of the assay is greater in those tumors which have a high rate of successful *in vitro* growth and also in those for which there are several clinically effective drugs. It is important to demonstrate the linear relationship between the number of cells plated in the agar culture and the number of colonies formed. Without demonstration of linearity, it is not possible to reliably interpret a reduction in colony formation as an effect of drug toxicity [121].

Application of the agar technique has been successful in many human solid tumors, including carcinomas of the ovary [121], bladder [122], colon [123], and in melanomas [124], neuroblastomas [125], and brain tumors [126]. Although results from these initial studies have been promising, these technical problems remain: (1) preparation of single cell suspensions from a solid tumor biopsy specimen [6], (2) definition of nutritional requirements of the cells, and (3) determination of the best method of cell exposure to the varied chemotherapeutic agents being tested [127].

The use of this technique in the study of human gynecologic cancers has thus far been mainly limited to ovarian cancer. Fortunately, successful growth of a majority of solid ovarian tumor specimens or malignant ovarian effusions has been accomplished. Hamburger and Salmon reported successful colony growth in 85% of specimens obtained from 31 patients with ovarian cancer. In addition to predictable growth in agar cultures, linearity of plating efficiency has been shown in a range of $10^4$ to $10^6$ cell per 35 mm plate [121]. This high rate of successful growth and linear relationship between cells cultured and colonies formed permits the system to be used to predict clinical responsiveness of a given tumor to the drugs tested.

Specimens are collected under sterile conditions and prepared in a man-

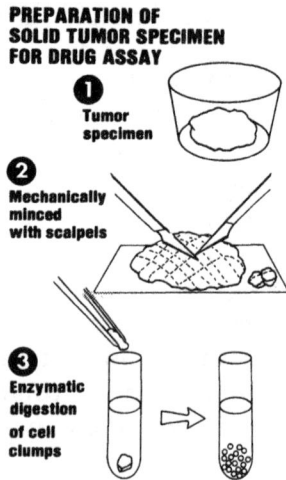

*Figure 6.* Method of preparation of solid tumor specimens for culture.

ner similar to that described for primary tissue cultures [29] (Figure 6). Because mechanical mincing of a tumor specimen will usually not release the number of single cells necessary for extensive drug assays, enzymatic digestion with 0.5% collagenase is used to further disaggregate clumps of cells [6].

The method of exposure of the tumor cells to chemotherapeutic drugs prior to culturing in agar has been studied empirically [127]. The drug concentrations used in *in vitro* assays have been based on pharmacologic studies in humans. Peak plasma levels can be measured in patients following intravenous injection of a given dose of drug; for the *in vitro* drug exposure one utilizes this maximal plasma concentration with additional drug concentrations one log above and one below this concentration (Figure 7). Since the tissue concentrations within a bulky tumor mass are probably lower than the measured peak plasma concentration, at least three drug dilutions over a two-log range are used for each assay in order to cover the range of tissue levels likely to be encountered in a patient's tumor.

The appropriate length of time for exposing cells to the drug prior to culture in agar is also unclear. Times empirically tried have varied from one hour to 24 hours of incubation prior to plating the cells in agar. While there is some variation in optimal exposure time for different drugs, one hour has been chosen as standard. The alternative method has been to test continuous exposure of the tumor cells to the chemotherapeutic agent by incorporation of the drug into the agar. However, there is uncertainty about the stability of some drugs in agar at 37 °C over a long period of time. Therefore, this method of continuous exposure has not been chosen, but the one-

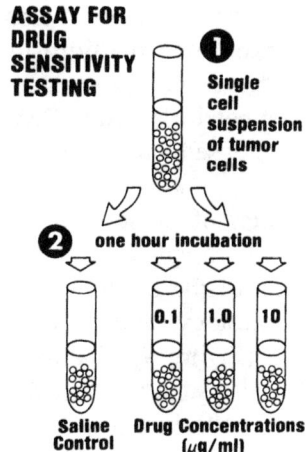

*Figure 7.* Method of exposing tumor cell suspension to drug dilutions in vitro.

hour incubation at 37 °C has instead been accepted as routine [125]. Following drug incubation, the chemotherapeutic agent is washed from the cell suspension. The tumor cells are then mixed with molten agar (0.3%) and plated over the agar underlayer (Figure 8).

Prior to plating the tumor cell suspension in agar, the underlying layer of agar for each culture dish is prepared. Earlier in this chapter, we discussed the use of conditioned medium, prepared from supernatant of adherent spleen cell cultures. Some soluble substance produced by these adherent cells has an apparent growth enhancing property for certain types of tumor cells. Although conditioned medium has been shown to be beneficial for

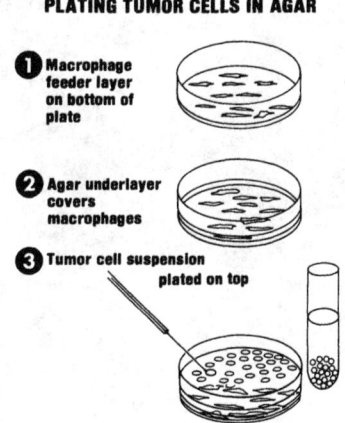

*Figure 8.* Method of preparing the feeder layer, agar underlayer, and tumor cell plating layer.

increasing colony growth in ovarian cancer, we have modified that protocol slightly. Instead of using conditioned medium in the manner described by Hamburger *et al.* [121] we have incorporated a macrophage feeder layer attached to the bottom of the petri dish and covered by the agar underlayer. In our experience this has increased the colony formation of ovarian tumor specimens [30] (Figure 8).

The malignant characteristics of those clonogenic cells in soft agar have been evaluated by the use of morphologic and biologic studies. Staining techniques have been applied to the study of cellular and nuclear detail of the colonies [128]. The morphology of these cells is similar to that seen in the original tumor specimen (Figure 9). Comparison of markers produced by the original tumor with those identified in the agar culture provide further evidence that the tumor cells in culture are the same as those in the original tumor. These markers have included acid phosphatase, melanin, vanillylmandelic acid, and catecholamines [129]. Techniques of cytogenetic analysis developed by Trent *et al.* [99] describe varying degrees of aneuploidy, with some marker chromosomes, as noted previously, and provide further evidence of malignancy.

The ultimate utility of this assay will be measured by comparison of the results in the agar assay with chemotherapeutic response in patients. A patient's tumor is arbitrarily considered to be responsive to a drug *in vitro* if there has been at least a 70% reduction in colony formation when compared

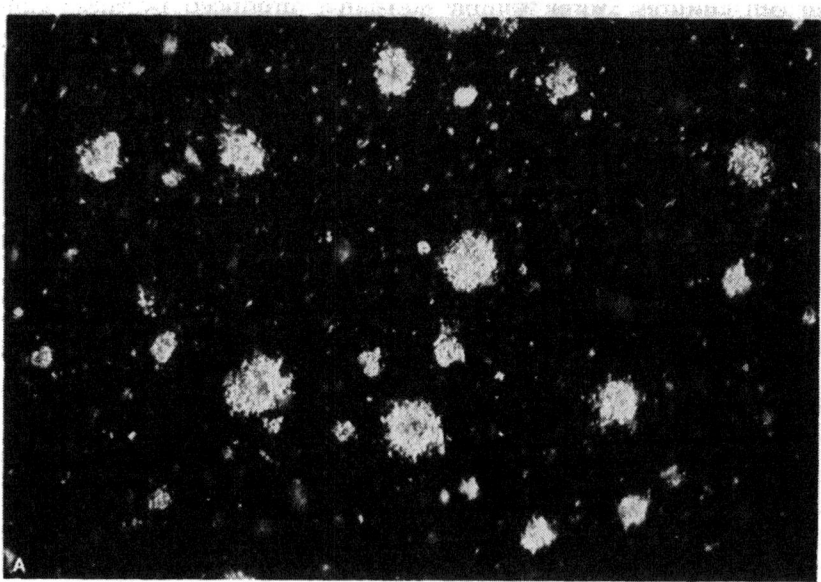

*Figure 9a*

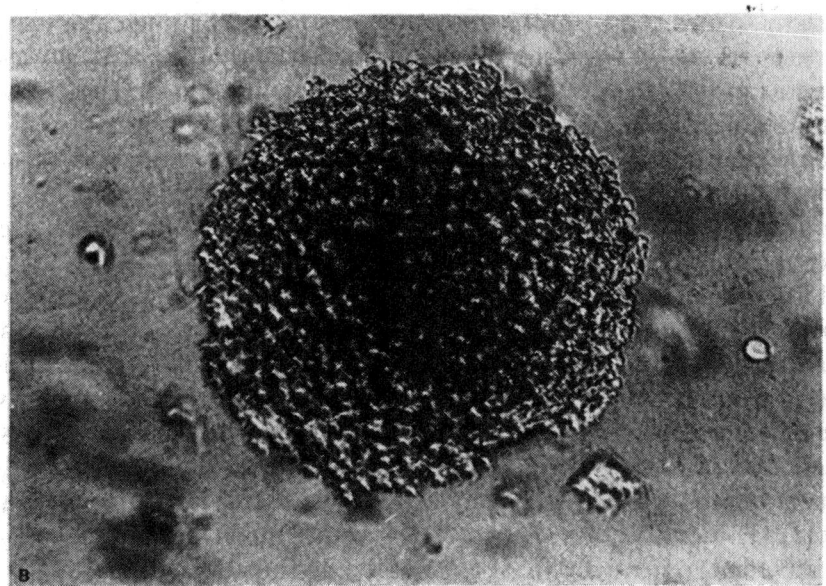

*Figure 9b*

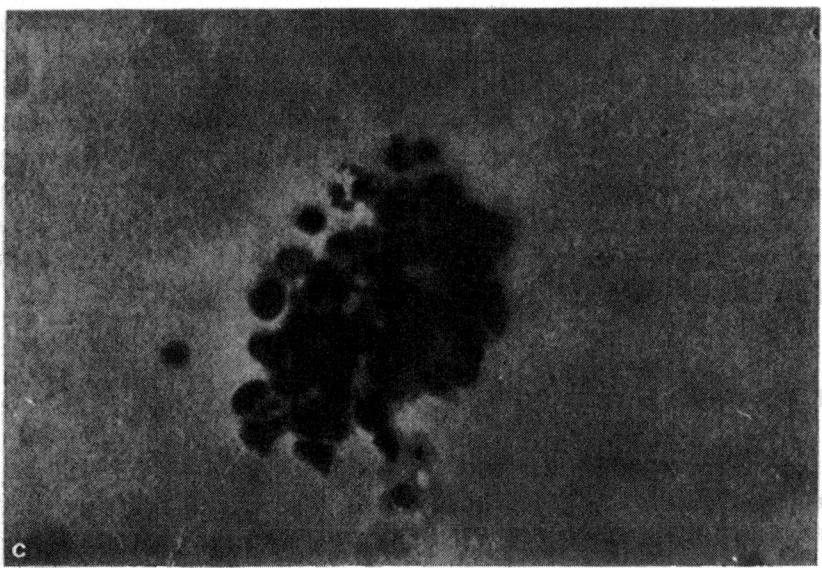

*Figure 9c*

*Figure 9.* (a) Ovarian colony growth in agar at 14 days; ×15. (b) Single ovarian colony in agar at 14 days; ×96. (c) Portion of stained ovarian colony in agar at 14 days; ×240.

to control plates. Less inhibition of colony formation indicates relative unresponsiveness. *In vivo* drug responsiveness is determined clinically and is defined as greater than 50% reduction of tumor mass for longer than one month. Stable disease or tumor shrinkage less than 50% has not been considered a clinical response. Results obtained in patients with ovarian cancer demonstrate a high degree of correlation between the *in vitro* clonogenic assay results and patient responses to specific chemotherapeutic agents. Alberts *et al.* have reported results in 40 patients with ovarian carcinoma [130]: when the *in vitro* assay predicted responsiveness, clinical response occurred in 62% of the patients; when the *in vitro* assay predicted nonresponsiveness, 99% of the patients failed to respond. The prevalence of drug-sensitive ovarian tumors is directly related to previous therapy, either with single or multiple agent chemotherapy. Although drug sensitivity assays are far less likely to identify active agents in patients who have already received the most effective drugs, the assay can still be useful in selecting Phase II drugs [131]. Identification of such drugs which might be useful can avoid ineffective and potentially toxic chemotherapy in patients with progressive cancer.

An additional application of the stem cell assay could be screening new compounds for activity against a variety of tumor cell lines. The commonly accepted assay for screening the potential value of a new chemotherapeutic agent tests its activity against L-1210 and P-388 murine leukemias, transplanted in syngeneic mice. Further studies are subsequently carried out with those drugs which show any activity in the mouse systems [132]. In parallel or as an alternative to the mouse screening program, it would seem logical to screen active compounds against a variety of human tumors using the stem cell assay. Significant reduction in cost and time could be achieved with this *in vitro* test as well as decreasing the risk of overlooking valuable drugs for human cancers.

## 8. HETEROTRANSPLANTATION EXPERIMENTS

Earlier in this chapter heterograft experiments were discussed as part of the historical development of human tumor transplantation into a variety of recipient animals. Prior to the availability of nude mice in the late 1960s, earlier attempts to test for sensitivity to chemotherapy by using either immunologically privileged sites or immunosuppressed animals were beset with serious problems. Ultimate tumor rejection rendered data on drug-induced tumor shrinkage difficult to interpret. The discovery of the athymic nude mouse provided a convenient heterograft recipient for human tumors. Advantages of the nude mouse include convenient measurement of subcutaneously implanted tumors and serial transplantation of such tumors. The histology and differentiation of the original human tumor specimen is retained when the tumor is heterotransplanted into nude mice [60].

There are several disadvantages to the nude mouse model, however. A prolonged time, often more than three months, is required to establish growth in the mouse. The biologic variations in success and rate of tumor growth among various nude mice require many animals for any drug sensitivity experiment, increasing the costs of a large-scale project. Breeding and maintenance costs of a nude mouse colony are significantly higher than are the costs for conventional laboratory animals. The nude mouse sensitivity to airborne bacteria and viruses requires elaborate facilities and care to ensure disease-free life span sufficiently long to perform experiments such as drug sensitivity testing. At this time the correlation of *in vitro* responses in nude mouse heterografts with clinical responses is uncertain.

Among gynecologic tumors tested for drug sensitivity in the nude mouse, mixed results were reported for two patients with gestational trophoblastic disease [133]. Davy and co-workers observed the response of one ovarian carcinoma transplanted to nude mice, treated with either 5-fluorouracil or thio-TEPA® (Triethylene thiophosphoramide) [55]. A positive correlation with thio-TEPA® was noted; as both the patient and the nude mouse had a partial clinical response. Nongynecologic tumors have also been studied, measuring tumor regression as an index of drug sensitivity. Giovanella has reported some correlation between the nude mouse and the patient responses in breast cancer [134]. Helson has also demonstrated the same correlation with chemotherapy of neuroblastomas [135]. A colon cancer model has been used to test a wide variety of drugs for activity against human colon tumors, without clinical correlation [136]. Modifying the standard subcutaneous tumor transplantation technique, Bogden *et al.* developed an assay for human tumors implanting blocks of tumor tissue beneath the kidney capsule of a nude mouse. This *subrenal capsule assay* is capable of yielding drug sensitivity data within 11 days for human colon, breast, and lung cancers [137].

The use of nude mouse heterografts for determining chemotherapeutic sensitivity appears to be a valid concept. The ultimate value of this assay depends upon its accuracy in predicting clinical response. These clinical correlations await further investigation.

REFERENCES

1. Carrel A, Burrows MT: Cultivation of tissues *in vitro* and its technique. J Exp Med 13:387–396, 1911.
2. Carrel A, Burrows MT: Cultivation *in vitro* of malignant tumors. J Exp Med 13:571–575, 1911.

3. Witkowski JA: Alexis Carrel and the mysticism of tissue culture. Med Hist 23:279–296, 1979.
4. Gey G: Tissue culture studies of the proliferative capacity of cervical carcinoma and normal epithelium. Cancer Res 12:264, 1952.
5. Povlsen CO, Rygaard J: Heterotransplantation of human adenocarcinomas of the colon and rectum to the mouse mutant nude. A study of nine consecutive transplantations. Acta Pathol Microbiol Scand 79:159–169, 1971.
6. Pavelic ZP, Slocum HK, Rustum YM, Creaven PJ, Karakousis C, Takita H: Colony growth in soft agar of human melanoma, sarcoma, and lung carcinoma cells disaggregated by mechanical and enzymatic methods. Cancer Res 40:2160–2164, 1980.
7. Liebovitz A: Development of media for isolation and cultivation of human cancer cells. In: Human Tumor Cells in Vitro. Fogh J (ed). New York and London: Plenum Press, 1975, pp 23–50.
8. Hayashi I, Larner J, Sato G: Hormonal growth control of cells in culture. In Vitro 14:23–30, 1978.
9. Gospodarowicz D, Greenburg G, Bialecki H, Zetter BR: Factors involved in the modulation of cell proliferation in vivo and in vitro: The role of fibroblast and epidermal growth factors in the proliferative response of mammalian cells. In Vitro 14:85–118, 1978.
10. Stanley MA, Parkinson EK: Growth requirements of human cervical epithelial cells in culture. Int J Cancer 24:407–414, 1979.
11. Ioachim L, Sabbath M, Andersson B, Barber HRK: Tissue culture of ovarian carcinomas. Lab Invest 31:381–390, 1974.
12. Cailleau RM: Old and new problems in human tumor cell cultivation. In: Human Tumor Cells In Vitro. Fogh J (ed). New York and London: Plenum Press, 1975, pp 79–114.
13. Fogh J, Trempe G: New human tumor cell lines. In: Human Tumor Cells In Vitro. Fogh J (ed). New York and London: Plenum Press, 1975, pp 115–159.
14. Kuramoto H, Tamura S, Notake Y: Establishment of a cell line of human endometrial adenocarcinoma in vitro. Am J Obstet Gynecol 114:1012–1019, 1972.
15. Kuramoto H, Hamano M: Establishment and characterization of the cell line of a human endometrial adenoacanthoma. Eur J Cancer 13:253–259, 1977.
16. Gorodecki J, Mortel R, Ladda RL, Ward SP, Geder L, Rapp F: Establishment and characterization of a new endometrial cancer cell line (SCRC-1). Am J Obstet Gynecol 135:671–679, 1979.
17. Ishiwata I, Nozawa S, Inoue T, Okumura H: Development and characterization of established cell lines from primary and metastatic regions of human endometrial adenocarcinoma. Cancer Res 37:1777–1785, 1977.
18. Merenda C, Sordat B, Mach JP, Carrel S: Human endometrial carcinomas serially transplanted in nude mice and established in continuous cell lines. Int J Cancer 16:559–570, 1975.
19. Giard DJ, Aaronson SA, Todaro GJ, Arnstein P, Kersey JH, Dosik H, Parks WP: In vitro cultivation of human tumors: Establishment of cell lines derived from a series of solid tumors. J Natl Cancer Inst 51:1417–1423, 1973.
20. Dodson MG, Klegerman ME, Menon M, Kerman RH, Lange CF, O'Leary JA: Establishment and characterization of a squamous cell carcinoma of the vulva in tissue culture and immunologic evaluation of the host. Am J Obstet Gynecol 131:606–619, 1978.
21. Patillo RA, Gey GO: The establishment of human hormone-synthesizing trophoblastic cells in vitro. Cancer Res 28:1231–1236, 1968.
22. DiSaia PJ, Morrow M, Kanabus J, Piechal W, Townsend DE: Two new tissue culture lines from ovarian cancer. Gynecol Oncol 3:215–219, 1975.
23. Sinna GA, Beckman G, Lundgren E, Nordenson I, Roos G: Characterization of two new human ovarian carcinoma cell lines. Gynecol Oncol 7:267–280, 1979.

24. Kimoto T, Ueki A, Nishitani K: A human malignant cell line established from ascites of patient with embryonal carcinoma of ovarium. Acta Pathol Jpn 25:89–98, 1975.
25. Freedman RS, Pihl E, Kusyk C, Gallager HS, Rutledge F: Characterization of an ovarian carcinoma cell line. Cancer 42:2352–2359, 1978.
26. Yamada T: The cellular biology of a newly established cell line of human ovarian adenocarcinoma *in vitro*. Keio J Med 23:53–70, 1974.
27. Woods LK, Morgan RT, Quinn LA, Moore GE: Comparison of four new cell lines from patients with adenocarcinoma of the ovary. Cancer Res 39:4449–4459, 1979.
28. Buick RN, Fry SE, Salmon SE: Effect of host cell interactions on clonogenic carcinoma cells in human malignant effusions. Br J Cancer 41:695–704, 1980.
29. Hamburger AW, Salmon SE: Primary bioassay of human tumor stem cells. Science 197:461–463, 1977.
30. Welander CE, Natale RB, Lewis JL, Jr.: *In vitro* stimulation of human ovarian cancer cells by xenogeneic peritoneal macrophages. J Natl. Cancer Inst 69 (november) 1982.
31. Giovanella BC, Stehlin JS, Williams LJ Jr: Heterotransplantation of human malignant tumors induced by injection of cell cultures derived from human solid tumors. J Natl Cancer Inst 52:921–927, 1974.
32. Fogh J, Fogh JM, Orfeo T: One hundred and twenty-seven cultured human tumor cell lines producing tumors in nude mice. J Natl Cancer Inst 59:221–226, 1977.
33. Hajdu SI, Fogh J: The nude mouse as a diagnostic tool in human tumor cell research. In: The Nude Mouse in experimental and Clinical Research. Fogh J, Giovanella BC (eds). New York, San Francisco, London: Academic Press, 1978, pp 235–266.
34. Herrick PR, Baumann GW, Merchant DJ, Shearer MC, Shipman C Jr, Brackett RG: Serologic and karyologic evidence of incorrect identity of an animal cell line (guinea pig spleen). *In Vitro* 6:143–147, 1970.
35. Gartler SM: Genetic markers as tracers in cell culture. Natl Cancer Inst Monogr No 26:167–178, 1967.
36. Fogh J, Wright WC, Loveless JD: Absence of HeLa cell contamination in 169 cell lines derived from human tumors. J Natl Cancer Inst 58:209–214, 1977.
37. Greene HSN: The significance of the heterologous transplantability of human cancer. Cancer 5:24–44, 1952.
38. Greene HSN: The transplantation of tumors to the brain of heterologous species. Cancer Res 11:529–534, 1951.
39. Lewis JL Jr, Brown WE, Hertz R, Davis RC, Johnson RH Jr: Heterotransplantation of human choriocarcinoma in monkeys. Cancer Res 28:2032–2038, 1968.
40. Hertz R: Serial passage of choriocarcinoma of women in the hamster cheek-pouch. In: Choriocarcinoma. Holland JF, Hreshchyshyn MM (eds). Berlin, Heidelberg, New York: Springer-Verlag, 1967, pp 26–32.
41. Lewis JL Jr, Davis RC, Ross GT: Hormonal, immunologic, and chemotherapeutic studies of transplantable human choriocarcinoma. Am J Obstet Gynecol 104:472–478, 1969.
42. Sommers SC, Chute RN, Warren S: Heterotransplantation of human cancer. I. Irradiated rats. Cancer Res 12:909–911, 1952.
43. Toolan HW: Successful subcutaneous growth and transplantation of human tumors in X-irradiated laboratory animals. Proc Soc Exp Biol Med 77:572–578, 1951.
44. Friedman M, Fogh J: Evaluation of malignancy in tumors produced in X-radiated and cortisone treated rats injected with human cells in continuous culture. Cancer Res 18:879–886, 1958.
45. Toolan HW: Growth of human tumors in cortisone-treated laboratory animals: The possibility of obtaining permanently transplantable human tumors. Cancer Res 13:389–394, 1953.

46. Lewis JL Jr, Davis RC, Parker JT: Modification of the immunologic response to human choriocarcinoma in the hamster cheek pouch by heterologous antilymphocyte serum. Cancer Res 29:1988–1994, 1969.
47. Jeejeebhoy HF: Effects of rabbit anti-rat-lymphocyte plasma on immune response of rats thymectomised in adult life. Lancet 2:106–107, 1965.
48. Monaco AP, Wood ML, Russell PS: Studies on heterologous anti-lymphocyte serum in mice. III. Immunologic tolerance and chimerism produced across the H-2 locus with adult thymectomy and anti-lymphocyte serum. Ann NY Acad Sci 129:190–209, 1966.
49. Davis RC, Lewis JL Jr: The effect of adult thymectomy on the immunosuppression obtained by treatment with anti-lymphocyte serum. Transplantation 6:879–884, 1968.
50. Flanagan SP: 'Nude', a new hairless gene with pleiotropic effects in the mouse. Genet Res 8:295–309, 1966.
51. Pantelouris EM: Absence of thymus in a mouse mutant. Nature 217:370–371, 1968.
52. Rygaard J, Povlsen CO: Heterotransplantation of a human malignant tumor to nude mice. Acta Pathol Microbiol Scand 77:758–760, 1969.
53. Sharkey FE, Fogh JM, Hajdu SI, Fitzgerald PJ, Fogh J: Experience in surgical pathology with human tumor growth in the nude mouse. In: The Nude Mouse in Experimental and Clinical Research. Fogh J, Giovanella BC (eds). New York, San Francisco, London: Academic Press, 1978, pp 187–214.
54. Giovanella BC, Stehlin JS, Williams LJ, Lee SS, Shepard RC: Heterotransplantation of human cancers into nude mice. Cancer 42:2269–2281, 1978.
55. Davy M, Mossige J, Johannessen JV: Heterologous growth of human ovarian cancer. Acta Obstet Gynecol Scand 56:55–59, 1977.
56. Kullander S, Rausing A, Trope C: Human ovarian tumors heterotransplanted to 'nude' mice. Acta Obstet Gynecol Scand 57:149–159, 1978.
57. Kim WS, Takahashi T, Nisselbaum JS, Lewis JL Jr: Heterotransplantation of human choriocarcinoma in nude mice. I. Morphologic and biologic characteristics. Gynecol Oncol 6:165–182, 1978.
58. Sordat B, Tamaoki N, Povlsen CO: List of human tumors transplanted to nude mice. In: Proceedings of the Second International Workshop on Nude Mice. Nomura T, Ohsawa N, Tamaoki N, Fujiwara K (eds). Stuttgart, New York: Gustav Fischer Verlag, 1977, pp 587–595.
59. Kyriazis A, Kyriazis AP: Preferential sites of growth of human tumors in nude mice following subcutaneous transplantation. Cancer Res 40:4509–4511, 1980.
60. Hattler BG, Soehnlen B, Seaver NA, Satoh P: Heterotransplantation of human malignant neoplasms to the mouse mutant nude. Surg Forum 25:127–129, 1974.
61. Visfeldt J, Povlsen CO, Rygaard J: Chromosome analysis of human tumors following heterotransplantation to the mouse mutant nude. Acata Pathol Microbiol Scand 80:169–176, 1972.
62. Fogh J, Bean MA, Bruggen J, Fogh H, Fogh JM, Hammar SP, Kodera Y, Loveless JD, Sorg C, Wright WC: Comparison of a human tumor cell line before and after growth in the nude mouse. In: The Nude Mouse in Experimental and Clinical Research. Fogh J, Giovanella BC (eds). New York, San Francisco, London: Academic Press, 1978, pp 215–234.
63. Giovanella BC, Fogh J: Present and future trends in investigations with the nude mouse as a recipient of human tumor transplants. In: The Nude Mouse in Experimental and Clinical Research. Fogh J, Giovanella BC (eds). New York, San Francisco, London: Academic Press, 1978, pp 281–312.
64. Lozzio BB: The LASAT mouse: A new model for transplantation of human tissues. Biomedicine 24:144–147, 1976.
65. Levi MM, Keller S, Mandl I: Antigenicity of a papillary serous cystadenocarcinoma tissue homogenate and its fractions. Am J Obstet Gynecol 105:856–861, 1969.

66. DiSaia PJ, Sinkovics JG, Rutledge FN, Smith JP: Cell-mediated immunity to human malignant cells. Am J Obstet Gynecol 114:979–989, 1972.
67. Gall SA, Walling J, Pearl J: Demonstration of tumor-associated antigens in human gynecologic malignancies. Am J Obstet Gynecol 115:387–393, 1973.
68. Chen SY, Koffler D, Cohen CJ: Cell-mediated immunity in patients with ovarian carcinoma. Am J Obstet Gynecol 115:467–470, 1973.
69. Bhattacharya M, Barlow JJ: Immunologic studies of human serous cystadenocarcinoma of ovary. Cancer 31:588–595, 1973.
70. Dorsett BH, Ioachim HL: Common antigenic component in ovarian carcinomas: Demonstration by double diffusion and immunofluorescence techniques. Immunol Commun 2:173–184, 1973.
71. Knauf S, Urbach GI: Ovarian tumor specific antigens. Am J Obstet Gynecol 119:966–970, 1974.
72. Knauf S, Urbach GI: Purification of human ovarian tumor-associated antigen and demonstration of circulating tumor antigen in patients with advanced ovarian malignancy. Am J Obstet Gynecol 127:705–710, 1977.
73. Burton RM, Hope NJ, Lubbers LM: A thermostable antigen associated with ovarian cancer. Am J Obstet Gynecol 125:472–477, 1976.
74. Pant KD, Dahlman HL, Goldenberg DM: A putatively new antigen (CSAp) associated with gastrointestinal and ovarian neoplasia. Immunol Commun 6:411–421, 1977.
75. Imamura N, Takahashi T, Lloyd KO, Lewis JL Jr, Old LJ: Analysis of human ovarian tumor antigens using heterologous antisera: Detection of new antigenic systems. Int J Cancer 21:570–577, 1978.
76. Carey TE, Takahashi T, Resnick LA, Oettgen HF, Old LJ: Cell surface antigens of human malignant melanoma: Mixed hemadsorption assays for humoral immunity to cultured autologous melanoma cells. Proc Natl Acad Sci USA 73:3278–3282, 1976.
77. Shiku H, Takahashi T, Oettgen HF, Old LJ: Cell surface antigens of human malignant melanoma. II. Serological typing with immune adherence assays and definition of two new surface antigens. J Exp Med 144:873–881, 1976.
78. Shiku H, Takahashi T, Resnick LA, Oettgen HF, Old LJ: Cell surface antigens of human malignant melanoma. III. Recognition of autoantibodies with unusual characteristics. J Exp Med 145:784–789, 1977.
79. Ueda R, Shiku H, Pfreundschuh M, Takahashi T, Li LTC, Whitmore WF, Oettgen HF, Old LJ: Cell surface antigens of human renal cancer defined by autologous typing. J Exp Med 150:564–579, 1979.
80. Garrett TJ, Takahashi T, Clarkson BD, Old LJ: Detection of antibody to autologous human leukemia cells by immune adherence assays. Proc Natl Acad Sci USA 74:4587–4590, 1977.
81. Pfreundschuh M, Shiku H, Takahashi T, Ueda R, Ransohoff J, Oettgen HF, Old LJ: Serological analysis of cell surface antigens of malignant human brain tumors. Proc Natl Acad Sci USA 75:5122–5126, 1978.
82. Old LJ: Cancer immunology: The search for specificity – GHA Clowes memorial lecture. Cancer Res 41:361–375, 1981.
83. Livingston PO, Oettgen HF, Old LJ: Specific active immunotherapy in cancer therapy. In: Immunological Aspects of Cancer Therapeutics. Mihich E (ed) (in press).
84. Wallack MK, Steplewski Z, Koprowski H, Rosato E, George J, Hulihan B, Johnson J: A new approach in specific active immunotherapy. Cancer 39:560–564, 1977.
85. Boone CW, Austin FC, Gail M, Case R, Klein E: Melanoma skin test antigens of improved sensitivity prepared from vesicular stomatitis virus infected tumor cells. Cancer 41:1781–1787, 1978.

86. Currie GA: Effect of active immunization with irradiated tumor cells on specific serum inhibitors of cell-mediated immunity in patients with disseminated cancer. Br J Cancer 28:25-35, 1973.
87. Krementz ET, Samuels MS, Wallace JH, Benes EN: Clinical experiences in immunotherapy of cancer. Surg Gynecol Obstet 133:209-217, 1971.
88. Hudson CN, Levin L, McHardy JE, Poulton TA, Curling OM, Crowther M, English PE, Leighton M: Active specific immunotherapy for ovarian cancer. Lancet 877-879, 1976.
89. Rao B, Wanebo HJ, Ochoa M, Lewis JL Jr, Oettgen HF: Intravenous *Corynebacterium parvum*. An adjunct to chemotherapy for resistant advanced ovarian carcinoma. Cancer 39:514-526, 1977.
90. Kohler G, Milstein C: Continuous cultures of fused cells secreting antibody of predefined specificity. Nature 256:495-497, 1975.
91. Koprowski H, Gerhard W, Croce CM: Production of antibodies against influenza virus by somatic cell hybrids between mouse myeloma and primed spleen cells. Proc Natl Acad Sci USA 74:2985-2988, 1977.
92. Kohler G, Milstein C: Derivation of specific antibody-producing tissue culture and tumor lines by cell fusion. Eur J Immunol 6:511-519, 1976.
93. Dippold WG, Lloyd KO, Li LTC, Ikeda H, Oettgen HF, Old LJ: Cell surface antigens of human malignant melanoma: Definition of six antigenic systems with mouse monoclonal antibodies. Proc Natl Acad Sci USA 77:6114-6118, 1980.
94. Monoclonal antibodies and cancer. Lancet, 421-423, 21 Feb 81 (unsigned editorial).
95. Yamada K, Takagi N, Sandberg AA: Chromosomes and causation of human cancer and leukemia. II. Karyotypes of human solid tumors. Cancer 19:1879-1890, 1966.
96. Tiepolo L, Zuffardi O: Identification of normal and abnormal chromosomes in tumor cells. Cytogenet Cell Genet 12:8-16, 1973.
97. Kakati S, Hayata I, Oshimura M, Sandberg AA: Chromosomes and causation of human cancer and leukemia. X. Banding patterns in cancerous effusions. Cancer 36:1729-1738, 1975.
98. Wake N, Hreshchyshyn MM, Piver SM, Matsui SI, Sandberg AA: Specific cytogenetic changes in ovarian cancer involving chromosomes 6 and 14. Cancer Res 40:4512-4518, 1980.
99. Trent JM, Salmon SE: Human tumor karyology: Marked analytic improvement by short-term agar culture. Br J Cancer 41:867-847, 1980.
100. Nowell PC: Tumors as clonal proliferation. Virchows Arch (Cell Pathol) 29:145-150, 1978.
101. Trent JM, Salmon SE: Potential applications of a human tumor stem cell bioassay to the cytogenetic assessment of human cancer. Cancer Genet Cytogenet 1:291-296, 1980.
102. Biedler JL, Spengler BA: Metaphase chromosome anomaly: Association with drug resistance and cell-specific products. Science 191:185-187, 1976.
103. Biesele JJ: Some negative screening results with miscellaneous compounds in tissue culture of several tumors. Cancer Res Suppl 1:1-5, 1953.
104. Eichorn PA, Huffman KV, Oleson JJ, Haliday SL, Williams JH: A comparison of *in vivo* and *in vitro* tests for antineoplastic activity of eight compounds. Ann NY Acad Sci 58:1172-1182, 1953-1954.
105. Wright JC, Walker D: A predictive test for the selection of cancer chemotherapeutic agents for the treatment of human cancer. J Surg Oncol 7:381-392, 1975.
106. Wright JC, Cobb JP, Gumport SL, Golomb FM, Safadi D: Investigation of the relation between clinical and tissue-culture response to chemotherapeutic agents on human cancer. New Eng J Med 257:1207-1211, 1957.
107. Berry RJ, Laing AH, Wells J: Fresh explant culture of human tumors *in vitro* and the assessment of sensitivity to cytotoxic chemotherapy. Br J Cancer 31:218-227, 1975.

108. Eagle H, Foley GE: The cytotoxic action of carcinolytic agents in tissue culture. Am J Med 21:739–749, 1956.
109. Kondo T: Prediction of response of tumor and host cancer chemotherapy. Natl Cancer Inst Monogr No 34:251–256, 1970.
110. DiPaolo JA, Dowd JE: Evaluation of inhibition of human tumor tissue by cancer chemotherapeutic drugs with an *in vitro* test. J Natl Cancer Inst 27:807–815, 1961.
111. Knock FE: Qualitative and quantitative *in vitro* sensitivity tests for cancer chemotherapy. Natl Cancer Inst Monogr No 34:247–249, 1970.
112. Roper PR, Drewinko B: Comparison of *in vitro* methods to determine drug-induced cell lethality. Cancer Res 36:2182–2188, 1976.
113. Shrivastav S, Bonar RA, Stone KR, Paulson DF: An *in vitro* assay procedure to test chemotherapeutic drugs on cells from human solid tumors. Cancer Res 40:4438–4442, 1980.
114. Shin SI, Freedman VH, Risser R, Pollack R: Tumorigenicity of virus-transformed cells in nude mice is correlated specifically with anchorage independent growth *in vitro*. Proc Natl Acad Sci USA 72:4435–4439, 1975.
115. Freedman V, Shin SI: Use of nude mice for studies on the tumorigenicity of animal cells. In: The Nude Mouse in Experimental and Clinical Research. Fogh J, Giovanella BC (eds). New York, San Francisco, London: Academic Press, 1978, pp 353–384.
116. Good M, Lavin M, Chen P, Kidson C: Dependence on cloning method of survival of human melanoma cells after ultraviolet and ionizing radiation. Cancer Res 38:4671–4675, 1978.
117. Steel GG: Growth Kinetics of Tumors. Oxford: Clarendon Press, 1977, pp 217–267.
118. Steel GG: Cytokinetics of neoplasia. In: Cancer Medicine. Holland JF, Frei E (eds). Philadelphia: Lea and Febiger, 1973, pp 125–140.
119. Moore MAS, Spitzer G, Williams N, Metcalf D, Buckley J: Agar culture studies in 127 cases of untreated acute leukemia: The prognostic value of reclassification of leukemia according to *in vitro* growth characteristics. Blood 44:1–18, 1974.
120. Buick RN, Till JE, McCulloch EA: Colony assay for proliferative blast cells circulating in myeloblastic leukemia. Lancet 1:862–863, 1977.
121. Hamburger AW, Salmon SE, Kim KB, Trent JM, Soehnlen BJ, Alberts DS, Schmidt HJ: Direct cloning of human ovarian carcinoma cells in agar. Cancer Res 38:3438–3444, 1978.
122. Buick RN, Stanisic TH, Fry SE, Salmon SE, Trent JM, Krasovich P: Development of an agar methylcellulose clonogenic assay for cells in transitional cell carcinoma of the human bladder. Cancer Res 39:5051–5056, 1979.
123. Buick RN, Fry SE, Salmon SE: Application of *in vitro* soft agar techniques for growth of tumor cells to the study of colon cancer. Cancer 45:1238–1242, 1980.
124. Meyskens FL, Salmon SE: Inhibition of human melanoma colony formation by retinoids. Cancer Res 39:4055–4057, 1979.
125. Von Hoff DD, Casper J, Bradley E, Trent JM, Hodach A, Reichert C, Makuch R, Altman A: Direct cloning of human neuroblastoma cells in soft agar culture. Cancer Res 40:3591–3597, 1980.
126. Rosenblum ML, Vasquez DA, Hoshino T, Wilson CB: Development of a clonogenic cell assay for human brain tumors. Cancer 41:2305–2314, 1978.
127. Alberts DS, Chen HSG, Salmon SE: *In vitro* drug assay: Pharmacologic considerations. In: Cloning of Human Tumor Cells. Salmon SE (ed) New York: Alan R Liss Inc, 1980, pp 197–207.
128. Salmon SE, Buick RN: Preparation of permanent slides of intact soft-agar colony cultures of hematopoietic and tumor stem cells. Cancer Res 39:1133–1136, 1979.

129. Von Hoff DD, Johnson GE: Secretion of tumor markers in the human tumor stem cell system. Proc Am Assoc Cancer Res 20:51, 1979.
130. Alberts DS, Salmon SE, Chen HSG, Surwit EA, Moon TE: Correlative and predictive assay of the human tumor stem cell assay (HTSCA) for anticancer drug activity in ovarian cancer patients. Proc Am Soc Clin Oncol 21:431, 1980.
131. Salmon S, Alberts D, Meyskens F, Durie B, Jones S, Soehnlen B, Young L: A new concept: *In vitro* phase II trial with the human tumor stem cell assay. Proc Am Soc Clin Oncol 21:329, 1980.
132. DeVita VT, Oliverio VT, Muggia FM, Wiernik PW, Ziegler J, Goldin A, Rubin D, Henney J, Schepartz S: The drug development and clinical trials programs of the Division of Cancer Treatment, National Cancer Institute. Cancer Clin Trials 2:195–216, 1979.
133. Hayashi H, Kameya T, Shimosato Y, Mukojima T: Chemotherapy of human choriocarcinoma transplanted to nude mice. Am J Obstet Gynecol 131:548–554, 1978.
134. Giovanella BC, Stehlin JS, Randall CS: Experimental chemotherapy of human breast carcinoma heterotransplanted in nude mice. In: Proceedings of the Second International Workshop on Nude Mice. Nomura T, Ohsawa N, Tamaoki N, Fujiwara (eds). Stuttgart, New York: Gustav Fischer Verlag, 1977, pp 475–481.
135. Helson L, Helson C, Rubenstein R, Hajdu SI: Human neuroblastomas in nude mice. In: Proceedings of the Second International Workshop on Nude Mice. Nomura T, Ohsawa N, Tamaoki N, Fujiware K (eds). Stuttgart, New York: Gustav Fischer Verlag, 1977, pp 291–303.
136. Osieka R, Johnson RK: Evaluation of chemical agents in phase I clinical trial and earlier stages of development against xenografts of human colon carcinoma. In: Proceedings of the Symposium on the Use of Athymic (Nude) Mice in Cancer Research. Houchens DP, Ovejera AA (eds). Stuttgart, New York: Gustav Fischer Verlag, 1978, pp 217–223.
137. Bogden AE, Kelton DE, Cobb WR, Esber HJ: A rapid screening method for testing chemotherapeutic agents against human tumor xenografts. In: Proceedings of the Symposium of the Use of Athymic (Nude) Mice in Cancer Research. Houchens DP, Ovejera AA (eds). Stuttgart, New York: Gustav Fischer Verlag, 1978, pp 231–250.

# 11. Clinical Trials in Gynecologic Oncology: Cooperative Group Research

GEORGE C. LEWIS Jr., JOHN BLESSING and JOHN R. KELLNER

1. INTRODUCTION

The appearance of anticancer drugs that were effective in animal tumor systems and also showed promise in human malignancies set the stage for development of a new specialty of medical oncology. At the same time, it was realized that clinical trials required to establish the effectiveness of drugs would not keep up with the anticipated flood of new agents unless investigators from several institutions collaborated. Since such cooperative endeavors required the expenditure of money, physicians sought funding to develop cooperative groups not restricted to a single system or disease. The original two purposes for which groups were developed were development of therapeutic concepts and the testing of chemical agents. Over the years the second purpose broadened to cover every method of dealing with cancer and later with precancerous lesions.

The establishment of three multi-institutional groups in 1955, the Acute Leukemia Group A, the Acute Leukemia Group B, and the Eastern Group for Solid Tumor Chemotherapy marked the onset of cooperative group research. In 1956, two additional groups, the Southeastern Cancer Study Group and the Southwestern Oncology Group were formed. Simultaneously, the veterans hospitals developed five groups [1]. Over the ensuing years, 37 groups were formed and 15 are presently active. The initial decade of cooperative group research was almost entirely restricted to advanced solid tumors and to hematologic malignancies.

Participation by cooperative groups in gynecologic cancer research came relatively late in the course of group development. Higher priorities were given to those malignancies least controlled by radiation and surgery. Both modalities had been reasonably successful in treating gynecologic cancer thereby further reducing the need for immediate inclusion of gynecologic cancers in cooperative clinical trials. Over the decades, much of the progress made in gynecologic cancer has been through clinical research by gynecologic surgeons, pathologists, and radiation therapists as individuals or in small teams within single institutions. Beginning in the late 1950s gynecologic cancers were included incidentally in new drug screening programs by cooperative groups. An initial gynecologic group, the Surgical Ovarian Adjuvant Group formed in the late 1950s, terminated in 1964 after conducting only limited trials in this one area. From 1963 until 1968 another gynecologic group, the Surgical Endometrial Adjuvant Group, represented one of the earliest multidisciplinary efforts among gynecologists, pathologists, biostatisticians, and radiation therapists [2]. The Gynecologic Oncology Group formed in 1970 grew out of the Endometrial Study Group. The Gynecologic Oncology Group was designed to deal with all forms of gynecologic cancer with every available therapy which would be applied by representatives of the appropriate specialties, gynecologic oncology, pathology, radiation oncology and medical oncology.

The original cooperative groups did not have a multidisciplinary organization but, rather, they were dominated by medical oncologists. Multidisciplinary research was initiated in 1966 by nongynecologic groups for Stage II Hodgkin's disease and Wilms tumor [1]. Multidisciplinary participation in groups expanded in the late 1960s with the formation of a variety of disease committees in many of the groups. By 1978, 11 groups had developed gynecologic protocols or Phase II–III studies of several diseases including gynecologic malignancies.

In just over twenty-three years, 8,520 patients with gynecologic cancer were entered into 177 protocols; 5,879 patients were considered evaluable

Table 1. Cooperative group protocols and patient entries by site of malignancy, 1958–1978.

| Site | # protocols | # patients entered by nongynecologic groups | # patients entered by nongynecologic groups | Total # patients entered |
|---|---|---|---|---|
| Cervix | 49 | 683 | 1944 | 2627 |
| Ovary | 74 | 1513 | 1788 | 3301 |
| Tube | 1 | 3 | 0 | 3 |
| Uterus | 35 | 221 | 2288[b] | 2509 |
| Vagina | 2 | 2 | 0 | 2 |
| Vulva | 5 | 1 | 65 | 66 |
| Gynecologic site not specified | 11 | 1 | 11 | 12 |
| Total | 177[a] | 2424 | 6096 | 8520 |

[a] Number larger than true total because of multi-site protocols.

[b] 700 from endometrial adjuvant group.

Table 2. Number of gynecologic protocols and patients entered by cooperative groups, 1958–1978.

| Group | # Protocols | # Patients entered | # Patients evaluated |
|---|---|---|---|
| *Nongynecologic specialty groups* | | | |
| CALGB | 7 | 92 | 92 |
| ECSG | 1 | 5 | 5 |
| COG | 3 | 58 | 41 |
| ECOG | 19[a] | 1 078 | 857 |
| NCOG | 2 | 6 | – |
| RTOG | 4[a] | 220 | 170 |
| SECSG | 10 | 109 | 109 |
| SWOG | 24 | 817 | 663 |
| WOG | 5 | 39 | 38 |
| *Gynecologic specialty groups* | | | |
| EAG[b] | 1 | 700 | 525 |
| GOG | 59[a] | 5 396 | 3 379 |
| Total | 135 | 8 520 | 5 879 |

[a] Total includes one study shared; patients counted under group entered.
[b] Endometrial adjuvant group.

(Tables 1–3). Currently, there are seven multisystem groups conducting gynecologic studies. One additional group, the Gynecologic Oncologic Group, GOG, is devoted entirely to gynecologic oncology. The seven multisystem groups are: Cancer and Acute Leukemia Group B (CALGB), the Eastern Cooperative Oncology Group (ECOG), the Northern California Oncology Group (NCOG), the Radiation Therapy Oncology Group (RTOG), the Southeastern Cancer Study Group (SECSG), the Southwestern

Table 3. Cooperative group treatment protocols involving pelvic cancer according to site of tumor origin and agent, 1958–1980.

| Agent/procedure | Total # of protocols | Cervix | Uterus | Ovary | Others |
|---|---|---|---|---|---|
| Placebo | 4 | 0 | 1 | 3 | 0 |
| Radiation | 16 | 5 | 4 | 7 | 0 |
| Bleomycin | 13 | 12 | 0 | 1 | 0 |
| Vincristine | 8 | 4 | 1 | 3 | 0 |
| Methotrexate | 4 | 1 | 1 | 2 | 0 |
| Adriamycin | 30 | 10 | 8 | 12 | 0 |
| Cis-platinum | 27 | 9 | 2 | 14 | 2 |
| Surgery | 8 | 2 | 5 | 0 | 1 |

*Table 3.* (continued).

| Agent/procedure | Total # of protocols | Cervix | Uterus | Ovary | Others |
|---|---|---|---|---|---|
| Progestins | 7 | 0 | 6 | 1 | 0 |
| Melphalan | 19 | 1 | 3 | 15 | 0 |
| 5-fluoromacil | 9 | 0 | 3 | 6 | 0 |
| Dactinomycin | 5 | 0 | 0 | 5 | 0 |
| Cytoxan | 20 | 2 | 4 | 14 | 0 |
| Hexamethylmelamine | 9 | 0 | 0 | 9 | 0 |
| Chlorambucil | 2 | 0 | 0 | 2 | 0 |
| CCNU | 9 | 5 | 1 | 2 | 1 |
| MeCCNU | 6 | 2 | 1 | 2 | 1 |
| Pathlology cytology surgery | 10 | 3 | 3 | 3 | 1 |
| Hydroxyurea | 1 | 1 | 0 | 0 | 0 |
| C. Parvum | 2 | 1 | 0 | 1 | 0 |
| DTIC | 1 | 0 | 1 | 0 | 0 |
| Piperazinedione | 4 | 1 | 1 | 1 | 1 |
| VP-16 | 8 | 2 | 2 | 3 | 1 |
| DAG | 5 | 1 | 1 | 1 | 2 |
| Baker's antifol | 2 | 1 | 0 | 1 | 0 |
| ICRF-159 | 2 | 1 | 0 | 1 | 0 |
| Maytansine | 2 | 1 | 0 | 1 | 0 |
| Prednisone | 2 | 0 | 1 | 1 | 0 |
| ThioTEPA | 1 | 0 | 0 | 1 | 0 |
| YOSHI 864 | 3 | 1 | 1 | 1 | 0 |
| BCG | 4 | 1 | 1 | 2 | 0 |
| Porfiromycin | 4 | 1 | 1 | 1 | 1 |
| Cryotherapy | 2 | 2 | 0 | 0 | 0 |
| Mitomycin | 1 | 1 | 0 | 0 | 0 |
| Hyperbaric $O_2$ | 1 | 1 | 0 | 0 | 0 |
| Phenestrim | 1 | 0 | 0 | 1 | 0 |
| Levamisole | 2 | 0 | 0 | 2 | 0 |
| MGBG | 1 | 0 | 0 | 1 | 0 |
| Vinblastine | 2 | 0 | 0 | 2 | 0 |
| BCNU | 1 | 0 | 0 | 1 | 0 |
| Total (40 agents/procedures) | 258 | 72 | 52 | 123 | 11 |

16 other agents/procedures etc. were included in protocols that accumulated 20 or less patients. Most in broad Phase II multi-disease – with 1–5 GYN cases.

Oncology Group (SWOG), and the North Central Cancer Treatment Group (NCCTG). Approximately 9% of the budget of the NCI's Division of Cancer Treatment is devoted to support of investigations designated as gynecologic in all groups. Justification of this financial support can be obtained by appreciating the fact that 19% of all cancers in women arise from the genitalia.

In light of the overall development of cancer management, the turn to gynecologic cancer by multidiscipline groups and the birth of the GOG should have been expected. Fifty years of successful progress in surgical treatment and radiation therapy had reached such a point of excellence in gynecology in comparison to nongynecologic sites that results were essentially reaching a plateau. Cytologic screening introduced at mid-century increased overall success primarily through earlier discovery. The ovarian cancer picture remained dismal as did the situation for tubal and vaginal cancer. Success in gynecologic oncology prior to the entry of cooperative groups on the scene could be attributed to the large number of individual clinical investigators who varied from single individuals in nonacademic hospitals to complex teams in recognized cancer centers. The Study Populations varied widely from retrospective analyses of pitifully small clusters of patients to random assignment of treatment in select patient populations. Too often results were of little or borderline importance. Claims for improvements in treatments were based at times on historical controls and at times on the intuition of the individual investigator. Undoubtedly, there were times when treatment results depended more upon the varied characteristics of patient populations or variations in the disease process than on the therapeutic approach. Some retrospective studies extend so far back in time that the management and supportive care changed considerably during the long period of accrual. Variables within patient populations were not initially recognized including differing histologic interpretation, variations in calculations of drug dosage and variations in extent of surgical procedures or radiation treatment. Too frequently, specifications for these factors were neither detailed nor accounted for in conducting studies. As a result of all variables and problems cited, many claims and counterclaims were advanced in support of a host of therapeutic approaches. It became difficult for the clinician to judge what was really best for a given situation. At this point in the late 1960s, investigators began to advocate a large-scale multidisciplinary approach to gynecologic cancer research supported by adequate quality control.

In the decade ending in 1970, the subspecialty of gynecologic oncology came of age: board certification developed, a society of gynecologic oncologists was organized and a multi-institutional cooperative group for therapeutic trials in gynecologic oncology was initiated. The same factors stimulated multisystem cooperative groups to initiate or expand their work in gynecologic oncology. Clinical investigation in gynecologic oncology was stimulated by the appearance of fellowship programs, many of which were in cancer centers where clinical research was common place. The graduates of fellowships tended to seek staff positions in teaching institutions and particularly the graduates from cancer centers looked for the opportunity to continue research through cooperative group programs.

Full development of cooperative clinical trials in gynecologic oncology by the mid-1970s resulted from many interacting factors: the appearance of many new drugs to be tested, the recognized limitations of the individual investigator, the accomplishments of multidisciplinary groups in other specialty areas, subspecialty development in gynecologic oncology, expansion of fellowships, and the need for larger numbers of patients to be entered into sequentially interrelated studies. As experience has been gained in the application of cooperative effort, groups have come to serve as intermediaries between the scientific laboratory and the Phase I clinical level and the community practitioner. Because of their wide geographic spread and contacts with affiliate hospitals, cooperative group members can play a very active role in translating research into effective clinical practice.

Rapid patient accrual, organizational network and sequential study building are three major aspects that groups offer in research that are unmatched by individuals. Twenty-five years of patient accrual by an individual might be matched by a center in ten years and by a group in one year. Funding of multiple institutions because they mutually have passed peer review for the same shared task cannot be matched by individual researchers. Study building can be done by any investigator, but the first two attributes of groups, accrual and organizational network, make the third, sequential study building, more likely to be accomplished by a group.

## 2. ORGANIZATION - GOG

It is apparent that a group comprised of many institutions must have preconceived guidelines as to membership, administrative organization, protocol design, data flow, quality control, data analysis and publication. The Gynecologic Oncology Group has its primary guidelines embodied in a Constitution and Bylaws. Institutions are the members of the Gynecologic Oncology Group. Membership in the group is obtained after formal application and review. Membership requirements must be filled to gain entry and must be maintained to continue membership. Funds to carry out the Gynecologic Oncology Group's activities are not obtained from the group but from the federal government, Division of Cancer Treatment, National Cancer Institute. Grants are sought by application from member institutions to support the various portions of the Gynecologic Oncology Group activities. Investigators from each of the institutions or their representatives, serve on committees and carry out the business.

## 2.1. The operations office, the statistical office and committee functions

The operations office is responsible for administrative and financial correspondence and the origination and coordination of most committee activities. It is responsible for the arrangement of all interim and regular meetings. The office staff coordinates the quality control including patient records, pathology reports, operative reports, microscopic slides, X-ray films and special study material. It controls patient entry procedures and it is the primary collection agency for forms. The office monitors adverse effects by a phone notification system which it turns over to a Data and Safety Monitoring Committee.

The statistical office, under the direct supervision of the group biostatistician is responsible for the statistical design of studies, preparation of randomization schemes for each study, incorporation of the results of quality control review into the data files and the review of patient data with protocol chairmen, who periodically visit the statistical office for this purpose. Data is entered into a computer directly via video terminals. Analysis is performed and the results are disseminated in biannual statistical reports, abstracts and manuscripts. At the semiannual meetings of investigators, communications between committees, communications between statistical and operational offices, and individual investigators are coordinated through the operations office.

The overall direction of the group is under a chairman who is elected by the membership. The chairman, in turn, nominates the group biostatistician and the associate group chairman, who must be approved by the executive committee and the membership of the group.

The Gynecologic Oncology Group has stressed interdisciplinary operation and structure. An institutional membership requirement is to have at least three treatment modalities represented. The Executive Committee has specialists representing Gynecologic Oncology, Pathology, Radiation Oncology, and Medical Oncology. Chairpersons of standing committees are appointed by the Group Chairman after approval by the Executive Committee. Committee members are appointed by Committee Chairmen with approval of the Group Chairman. The most important committee, aside from the executive committee, is the Protocol Committee which directs studies of the group. It consists of the chairmen of Site and Modality committees. All committee actions require approval by a majority of the full members. Full members vote in the general session and their representative may be elected to the executive committee or the chairmanship. There are two other categories of membership. Provisional status applies to a new institution to provide a period of observation while it tries to meet specifications for full membership. Probationary status is the label given to the institution that does not continue to meet membership requirements. Both provisional and probationary members may hold appointed positions on committees but are not elected to office.

*2.2. The patient*

The basic elements of cooperative clinical trials in terms of organization are the patient, the investigator and the institution. Up until just a decade ago, the patient was incidental to research. A pharmaceutical company providing samples of new drugs to select practitioners accomplished inexpensive collection of physician's impressions. Frequently reports derived from such informal trials were cursory, retrospective and testimonial in nature. Today, the patient must receive primary consideration in all human research projects. Committees for human research look at the balance between possible gain to the patient and possible detriment. Investigations for the Gynecologic Oncology Group and for other clinical investigators must prepare a statement of informed consent for the patient describing this risk-benefit balance. There must also be assurance as to the confidentiality of patient information, the responsiveness to questions, the compensation for injury, the ability to withdraw, alternative therapy, etc. Gradually the various rules governing informed consent that must be signed with research procedures have been expanded by the Food and Drug Administration in agreement with the National Cancer Institute to the point where very detailed and frightening explanations are presented to patients. These detailed statements are disturbing both to the patients and to the attending physician. Thus, there is a tendency to avoid presentation of such projects and consent forms to patients with relatively treatable disease. Instead the patient tends to be an individual who has run the gamut of all the therapies and has only two options – no additional treatment or the treatment under investigation. Hopefully, as the cooperative groups, such as the Gynecologic Oncology Group, expand studies and include more early disease patients, the process of informed consent will not provide the obstacle that it has in the past.

During the early years of cooperative group research, patients were essentially selected because of the terminal nature of the disease. Palliation was a more practical goal than cure. Chemotherapy has now progressed to the point where it can be offered as primary definitive treatment with a reasonable potential for cure rather than as a terminal care effort. Improvements in radiation therapy and surgery now permit the Gynecologic Oncology Group to offer to patients protocols that examine in detail the factors that may define prognosis and help establish a risk score which will guide treatment. This approach is leading to protocols for patients with early as well as late disease. Evaluation of patients with limited malignancy indicates that all are not cured and current methods of therapy are not innocuous. Generally accepted management of every patient does not segregate the less fortunate patients for investigation of why their treatment failed. Thus, as 'standard' therapy is applied to all regardless of the potential for failure high risk patients are lost to research procedures aimed at improving their prognosis. The Gynecologic Oncology Group is making a special effort, through presurgical staging procedures as well as surgical staging, to identify and include in study programs patients with a wide range of disease conditions. Because of financial limitations, patients included in the Gynecologic Oncology Group protocols have been for the most part those at academic institutions. Efforts are now underway to extend these protocols to affiliated institutions so that patients in these institutions may benefit from studies designed for early and late disease and so that physicians in the affiliated institutions may be able to offer their patients possibly more effective treatments with less risk than they are currently offering.

*2.3. The investigator*

It is impossible to assign a financial value to contributions from investigators in terms of time, services and materials given outright to cooperative group studies. In individual institutions, pathologists, radiation oncologists and gynecologic oncologists all assist without compensation in studies not primarily based in their own specialty. Recognition of this fact is needed as well as recognition of the personal contributions and sacrifices of individual investigators within the specialty covered by the protocol. The major role provided by the group mechanism is the coordination of clinical investigation which when properly conducted takes advantage of the interaction of knowledge of numerous investigators in the development of the conceptual phase of the protocol. A properly functioning group will efficiently guide research projects through progressive steps, taking a concept from preliminary pharmacologic (dose seeking) programs through tumor screening to final randomized clinical trials. With well coordinated investigators, the group should be in a position to define and conduct appropriate data flow systems and quality control regulations. By utilizing nationally distributed experienced specialists in various modalities, there should emerge from group activities the feeling of assurance as to dependability of such things as tumor grading, specification of cell type and tumor origin, definition of operative procedures, details for appropriate radiotherapy and chemotherapy, etc.

Within the Gynecologic Oncology Group, each participating institution names one individual as the principal investigator. He is directly responsible within his own institution for the supervision and direction of the group's protocols. He carries out all the administrative responsibilities within his own institution and at group meetings he is responsible for coordinating the other representatives from his institution. He is responsible within his own institution for collaboration with representatives of other specialties. Within the group the principal investigator will be contributing to protocol design, reviews of studies, and decisions to activate or terminate particular programs. The principal investigator needs to organize a grant application and seek funding for his institution. When his institution first enters into a cooperative group, such as the Gynecologic Oncology Group, an individual investigator in gynecologic oncology can join with a representative from medical oncology, radiation therapy, and pathology to form the representative team. Up to a dozen patients can be entered into group protocols annually on behalf of the institution by the investigators without having to go to great expense in terms of paperwork, patient enlistment, therapy coordination and other aspects of clinical research. Group requirements for membership, however, in the Gynecologic Oncology Group have now gone beyond this limited number of entries and impose an obligation upon the investigators at a new institution to produce relatively large numbers of patients with the assistance of data clerks, secretaries, nurses and others. The team of investigators at an institution new to the group must demonstrate to the group their ability to enroll patients who will become evaluable. Pending full approval by the group, the investigators must initially conduct this program at their own expense, getting support from their own departmental chairman, psychologically as well as monetarily.

Success for investigators in the Gynecologic Oncology Group comes in two ways. The first is in inducing other specialists and nononcologic obstetrician-gynecologists to support GOG studies and refer patients or participate in the studies themselves, encouraging local patient enrollment and participation, and using continued education to interest fellow staff physicians in strengthening the position of the participating institution within the Gynecologic Oncology Group. It also lays the groundwork for successful application for funds from the National Cancer Institute. The Gynecologic Oncology Group has a point system whereby it gives from 6 to 12 points for each patient entered into a high priority protocol and as low as 1 or 2 points for patients entered into pilot studies and staging studies. When enough patients are entered into studies from an institution to acquire at least 100 points from high priority patients and a total of 150 points minimum from all varieties of patients, an institution with investigators in at least three specialty areas has a good chance of full membership. Full membership is required by the NCI before an application for funding will be considered. The second way for investigators to succeed in the Gynecologic Oncology Group is for the representatives to participate in activities of the group such as committee membership, preparation of protocols, and publication of results.

## 2.4. *The institution*

Contributions are expected from the institution as they are from the individual investigator. In the Gynecologic Oncology Group, nineteen institutions have received funding averaging 50% of the requested amount although recently budgets have been trimmed further. A year's waiting period is required for new institutions before any funding is available. Therefore, during the waiting period an institution must support its own research costs. Funding comes to the individual institutions from the National Cancer Institute and not from the GOG headquarters. In some groups, discretionary funds from headquarters provide minimal temporary support to new members for a secretary, data clerk or possibly travel. Recent budget restrictions have prevented the GOG from continuing this practice. When an institution applies for funding to the NCI, its application is reviewed by a peer review committee, the Clinical Cancer Investigation Review Committee (CCIRC). If approval is granted priority scores are given according to the relative merit of the application. With limited funding the priority score level required to receive funding becomes very strict and limiting. When funds are awarded, and the priority score is adequate, the grants are usually for four years unless there is some question raised by the CCIRC. In such cases, the grant may be for two years. When a member is dropped from a group funding ceases immediately.

When the Gynecologic Oncology Group was initiated, contributing institutions entered 15 to 20 patients per year per institution. This figure rapidly increased so that the average patient entry currently is 54 patients per year. Some contributors enter over 100 patients each year. The largest contributor has arranged a network of regional hospitals to be coordinated with the medical school. It has set up a centralized system for human research clearance that saves a lot of administrative effort. Another large contributor is made up of a number of hospitals associated with medical schools in a large urban area. These institutions function under the sponsorship of a cancer center so that the net effect is a regional system. It is very likely in the future that more regional arrangements will be developed and small individual institutions will either join regional networks or be dropped from group membership.

Over the past few years, the National Cancer Institute has developed a policy restricting membership of institutions in groups to one national group with the exception that groups representing limited interest such as radiation therapy, gynecology and pediatrics may co-exist in the same institution as a multisystem group. This action by the National Cancer Institute permits the Gynecologic Oncology Group to reach a wide distribution of institutions and gather together much needed material especially for the more rare pelvic malignancies. The tying together of institutions in regions across the nation helps encourage multimodal management of patients and will, in the long run, be beneficial to the medical profession and the patients they serve.

Approximately five years ago, the Cancer Control Program of the National Cancer Institute recognized that cooperative group institutions were generally hospitals that were very closely related to medical schools. To a large extent institutions which were off-campus were not included. Patients might be referred from the off-campus hospitals to the medical school hospitals, but not routinely. It was felt that a large percentage of patients with cancer in this country are still treated in off-campus hospitals, with or without official ties to the medical schools. A program was initiated for affiliate hospitals to encourage participation of physicians, nurses and other supportive personnel in protocols of cooperative groups. The Cancer Control Program has recently re-issued a request for proposals which is intended to assist cooperative groups in extending their protocols to all hospitals affiliated with and/or collaborating with medical schools. The teaching hospitals associated with groups have had the advantage of funding for handling data, quality control, staff education and other activities. Academic institutions with gynecologic service and a division of gynecologic oncology, tend to have a more vigorously supervised program for the conduct of research. The patients are usually admitted with advanced or recurrent disease. Very early lesions such as Stage I endometrial carcinoma and Stage I ovarian carcinoma would be less frequently encountered than in the services of an off-campus institution. When an academic institution is participating in a clinical trial, the quality of records, the standards of therapy and quality of care will be better than would be expected in the absence of the peer review system of a cooperative group. In a single institution not tied to a cooperative group network there is likely to be a higher incidence of early malignancy and stress upon the individual physician's conduct of practice. The performance of tests, the extent of therapy, the follow-up all will be less regulated and supervised than they would be for similar activities carried out in an institution associated with a cooperative group.

*2.5. Research costs*

Over 2,000 gynecologic patients are entered yearly into cooperative group studies. On the basis of data provided in grant awards, the cost per entry ranges widely from less than $ 900 to over $ 2,000 in direct costs from federal sources. This is a bargain when it is realized that the very same money must cover the cost of follow-up for over 4,000 patients being followed currently from a few months to five years. The research funds are almost entirely spent for administrative and statistical costs, including meetings, travel, communications, purchase of study materials, analysis and preparation of reports, etc. In the Gynecologic Oncology Group the total indirect and direct costs per year are just under $ 3.2 million. Thirty percent of this cost is the headquarters with the majority going to the Operations Office. Headquarters covers all the travel costs except for travel of individual investigators to the twice yearly business meeting. In institutions, costs largely revolve about the secretary and nurse who are responsible for protocol procedures, data and material handling, and the reporting of cases to the headquarters. In institutions, partial salary support may be provided for administrative activities, not for patient care, which is paid for by the patient or third party. Phase II research drugs not available to pharmacies are provided by the National Cancer Institute. All considered, the total cost incurred in the course of investigation in the Gynecologic Oncology Group of one patient dwarfs the $ 1,500 direct cost per patient derived from federal funding of the Gynecologic Oncology Group.

Without exaggeration it can be shown that the federal dollar spent per patient is a good investment in many ways. For every patient entered into a protocol three to four patients not eligible or willing to participate and cared for by the same investigator will be treated by a program identical to one of the arms of a cooperative protocol. Physicians in the same hospitals or other regional hospitals in the area of a group member, may apply protocol-type therapies to patients outside of the research setting even though the physician who gives the treatment is not a group participant. In addition, all of the member hospitals of the Gynecologic Oncology Group have residency and student programs. Under these clinical trial programs, the students, residents, nurses and others associated with patient care are exposed to the concepts and procedures of top-quality clinical management. Thus, the research dollar is also an educational dollar for the developing physician and continuing education dollar for the practitioner.

3. CLINICAL TRIALS

*3.1.*

*3.1.1. Type of study.* The development of cooperative group research is similar to the systematic approaches used for other clinical research programs in that treatment regimens are evolved from the basic science areas of pharmacology, biochemistry and physiology. Preclinical pharmacology is conducted in basic science laboratories and in animal laboratories. A variety of testing procedures are used to determine any neoplastic effect and toxicity. Once there is the suggestion of a possible usefulness for an agent, consideration is given to evaluation in humans. The initial step in humans is to go through dose and toxicity seeking procedures termed, 'Phase I' trials;

Phase I testing is rarely dealt with by cooperative groups as an initial evaluation process for a given treatment. Although, occasionally, an agent found to have problems with more advanced testing procedures may be reevaluated by a group using the Phase I technique. Patients enrolled in Phase I studies have exhausted all standard methods of treatment and either the drug being offered or no treatment at all are the only options for the patients.

When a reasonable dose level is established and dose limiting toxicity has been defined by Phase I testing, the agent is screened with every variety of cancer (Phase II). In the Gynecologic Oncology Group, Phase II testing of drugs is offered the patients with measurable lesions in whom standard therapy is no longer effective. The Gynecologic Oncology Group enrolls for each drug under evaluation a minimum of 25 patients and observes them for response and toxicity. Depending upon the disease and the performance of previously tested agents, efficacy of drugs ranges from minimal response to a response exceeding that previously observed for standard agents. Patients in the Gynecologic Oncology Group may be entered into a Phase II study by any member of the group. In contrast, the group has established a policy of carrying out studies of feasibility within single institutions. Like the Phase II tests, 25 patients constitute the limit but, in contrast, response of the tumor to the procedure or agent is not necessarily the objective of the test. This type of test is labeled the pilot study. At Phase III level of evaluation the determination is whether a new method, single or combined, drug, radiation, surgery, etc. is better than an established method. Once Phase II or pilot tests indicate promising leads the Gynecologic Oncology Group examines new approaches in a randomized comparison in which the patient is assigned to receive one or two or more therapeutic procedures. The design of such randomized clinical trials requires the determination of numbers of patients necessary to recognize a treatment difference of a desired magnitude with a predetermined minimal probability of error. The factors to be considered include: differences in patient and disease characteristics according to treatment difference, the condition of the patients and the target population, the appropriateness of the design for comparing the new regimen to the old, and the annual patient accrual rate. After consideration of all these factors, a decision has to be made as to whether the potential benefit of a study will exceed the risk. This determination has to be made within the group, long before participating institutions' individual human research committees make the same determination.

Because of the nature of referral patterns in gynecology and because of the Gynecologic Oncology Group's concentration on clinical trials, large numbers of patients have been available for Phase II testing. Ovarian cancer and cervical cancer are the most available for drug evaluation (Tables 4, 7).

Endometrial cancer runs a close third (Table 9). At the other extreme tubal carcinoma is so rarely encountered, that it is not worthwhile including it in a Phase II or Phase III study. Ovarian cancer's popularity is largely related to its high lethal quality and its potential to respond to most agents and yet not be cured.

In contrast to the Gynecologic Oncology Group, the multisystem groups conducting gynecologic investigations concentrated on Phase II screening procedures. The Gynecologic Oncology Group, when it was initiated in 1970, undertook studies which were essentially Phase III trials because of the need to confirm earlier results recorded by individual investigators who tended to use historical controls. Cooperative groups and particularly the Gynecologic Oncology Group have conducted studies using the natural history of disease instead of conducting only studies providing therapeutic information. The Gynecologic Oncology Group has been particularly interested in the study of patterns of tumor dissemination using operative procedures as a basis for surgical and pathologic investigation. Current surgical staging studies now include ovarian carcinoma, uterine sarcoma, endometrial carcinoma, and cervical carcinoma. Thorough examination of abdominal contents and biopsies of suspicious lesions have been required in staging studies. Peritoneal washings have been done as well as biopsies of the diaphragm, para-aortic and pelvic nodes. For the staging procedures, the dissection of nodes has not been of the same degree as that required for a radical hysterectomy. The term 'sampling' would be considered an appropriate descriptive word. An additional nontherapeutic approach used by groups has been the maintenance of a registry of all patients whether or not on protocols. When decisions are required on the practicality of undertaking studies, registry information may support the need for a study.

The Gynecologic Oncology Group has used registry surveys as a basis for establishing studies of relatively rare lesions. These include sarcomas and malignant germ cell tumors of the ovary. The Gynecologic Oncology Group recruits enough patients to conduct seven studies relating to these uncommon malignancies. The group has been able to accumulate enough patients with vulvar carcinoma to conduct two studies, one a staging procedure and another representing a contrast between pelvic node resection and pelvic radiation when there are positive groin nodes. In addition to the tubal carcinoma mentioned earlier, sex cord-stromal tumors of the ovary have been too rare for adequate accrual.

Multisystem groups have placed more emphasis on chemotherapy than on surgery and pathology. Radiation and immunotherapy also have had relatively less emphasis in the multisystem groups than in the Gynecologic Oncology Group. One group, the Radiation Therapy Oncology Group (RTOG) has through its membership stressed radiation therapy. The large patient volume available to the Gynecologic Oncology Group and the variety of diseases provide many opportunities to design and apply a spectrum of protocols that cover surgical treatment, pathology, immunotherapy, irradiation and chemotherapy. The Gynecologic Oncology Group is developing protocols combining an assessment of natural history with adjuvant treatment. In such situations, surgical and pathological staging acts as a form of quality control to properly assign patients to subsequent therapeutic procedures according to relative risk.

*3.1.2. Primary treatment.* Most of the studies of the Gynecologic Oncology Group could be classed as primary treatment, that is a study that is intended to provide the major attack upon the disease process, not to supplement some other therapeutic approach. Primary treatment of course is mostly utilized for newly diagnosed disease, but it could be considered as the approach when recurrence is treated. This has been particularly true for the Gynecologic Oncology Group sarcoma protocols when the disease is newly diagnosed in Stages III and IV. Primary treatment may be included in the ovarian protocols where little more than diagnostic surgery is carried out. The group has carefully provided in the study protocols, requirements that the patients must have not gone through similar previous therapy when they are about to be entered into a protocol. If chemotherapy is being evaluated, the patient must not have received previous chemotherapy. Thus, for a given modality or method, patients being entered particularly in Phase III studies would have primary treatment for that particular method regardless of whether the disease is new or recurrent.

*3.1.3. Adjuvant treatment.* Another area of investigation which is of importance to the clinical practitioner is the testing of agents which are added to the primary treatment, particularly when surgery is the primary treatment. This has been particularly observed in endometrial carcinoma where the cure of the disease particularly in Stages I and II basically depends upon surgery. Increased potential for cure is anticipated by the addition of chemicals, hormones, radiation, etc., which are intended to get rid of gross or microscopic residual disease after surgery. This approach is called adjuvant treatment. It requires an excellent knowledge of the usual results from the single procedure that is employed initially such as a hysterectomy for endometrial carcinoma. Tests are usually employed to establish the value of an adjuvant by contrasting the adjuvant with no adjuvant therapy before or after a surgical procedure.

*3.1.4. Treatment of advanced disease.* Advanced disease is usually the target of Phase II testing by groups. In Phase III testing, advanced disease has not been as responsive to treatment largely because of bulk. The GOG as well as other groups also exclude some advanced disease cases because they may not live long enough to evaluate therapeutic effects. In gynecology, especially in ovarian cancer, it appears that advanced bulky ovarian disease, when surgically debulked may respond to chemotherapy as if it had really been less extensive [3, 4]. The RTOG and the GOG are both looking at cervical cancer to see if for advanced disease there can be any way to potentiate the effect of radiation on massive advanced cancer.

*3.2. Protocol development*

In the Gynecologic Group the control of protocol development rests with

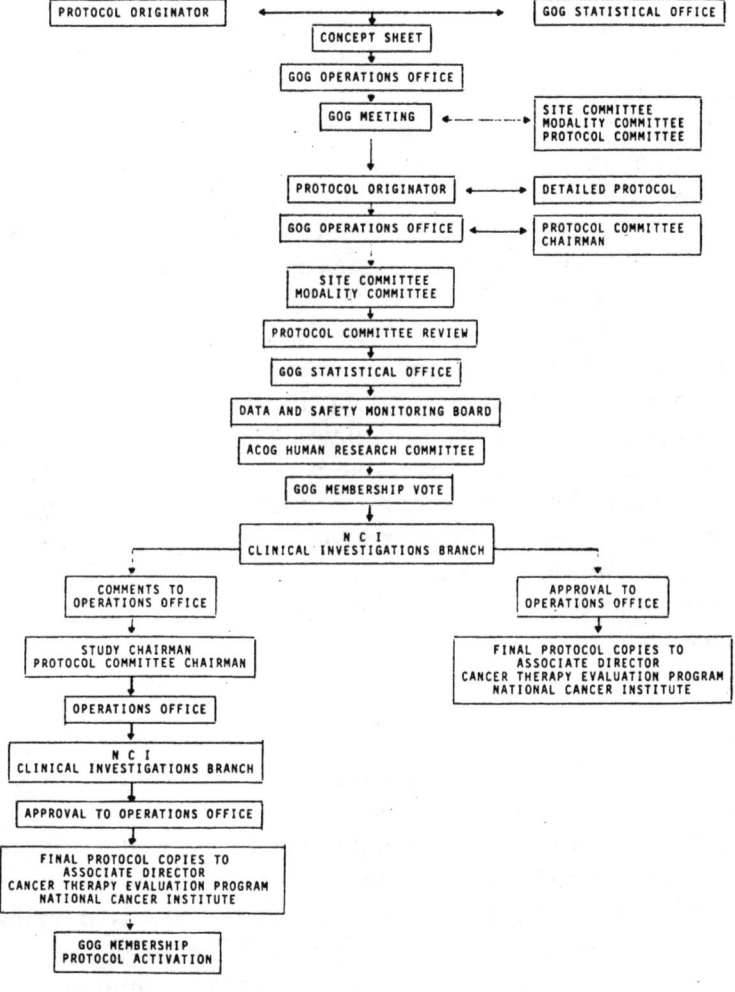

*Figure 1.* Protocol development.

the Protocol Committee, the biostatistician and the site and modality committees (Figure 1). Entirely new agents are introduced by the New Drug Liaison Committee through a master protocol which describes objectives, testing criteria and procedures for evaluation. In the Gynecologic Oncology Group the next step is to involve the site committees (a Cervix, Vulva, Vagina Committee, a Uterine Corpus Committee, an Ovarian Committee, and a Trophoblastic Disease Committee). They transcribe successful pilot and Phase II studies into new Phase III studies. The modality committees are consultants. They may suggest and plan new protocols, which they carry to the Protocol Committee for implementation. The modality committees also help with quality control reviews. The modality committees consists of Radiotherapy, Chemotherapy, Gynecologic Management, Immunology, Pathology and Nursing Committees. A site committee may initiate a study based on a suggestion of one of its members or a proposal from an institutional representative, particularly a Principal Investigator. Proposals may come from the Protocol Committee or possibly a site committee. The Protocol Committee may establish protocol chairmen, including modality representatives. The protocol chairmen compose a draft with the aid of headquarters. It is patterned after requirements defined in a group manual. Copies are distributed to the appropriate committee in advance of meetings. Suggestions are solicited and handled through the Operations Office. As the protocols are being developed, the Statistical Office carries out an audit to determine membership interest and the feasibility of the study based on the number of proposed entries. The Group Biostatistician makes basic decisions about opening and closing the studies. The various committees report to the Protocol Committee. After a vote is taken for approval, the protocol goes to the Human Research Committee of the American College of Obstetricians and Gynecologists. Once approval is received from this committee and the membership of the group have approved the study at a business meeting, the protocol is sent to the National Cancer Institute, Division of Cancer Treatment for review.

*3.3. Sequential study building*

Therapeutic trials may originate from a variety of sources. In the early phase of group development, established programs may be compared with each other on a prospective basis. The Gynecologic Oncology Group initially did this largely for ovarian and endometrial cancer (in its Protocols #2 and 3 for ovary, 17 and 18 for endometrium).

While getting started a group should also utilize Phase II and pilot testing to screen new procedures for promising leads. The GOG has particularly used pilot tests, that is up to 25 patients in a single institution, to check on the feasibility of giving combinations of drugs. Groups borrow successful pilot studies and Phase II studies from others and from promising but limited studies from nongroup sources. Initial encouraging results from preliminary testing programs may not be confirmed in larger group evaluations. In cooperative groups, 200 or more patients may demonstrate response rates from 1/2 to 3/4 of those reported in the original limited study. The difference may be related to the enthusiasm of the initial investigator, bias in patient selection, or factors that are never apparent, such as plain old statistical variation that is amplified by the small numbers. Pilot and Stage II studies are not controlled as critically as Phase III studies in that there is no randomization.

After the Gynecologic Oncology Group concluded its comparison of standard procedures and generally found no advantage of one over the other, particularly in #2 and 3 protocols, the next phase was to compare the most successful results from pilot or Phase II studies with the most successful standard procedure. That led, in ovarian carcinoma, to the development of Protocols #22, 25 and 47. The winning arm of a comparison establishes a new standard and the process is repeated. Successful cooperative groups are marked by having the process of building one study upon the results of another set up as a well-established cyclic event.

*3.4. Study conduct*

The National Cancer Institute, Division of Cancer Treatment, gets the protocols from the Group Chairman. There the staff acts on behalf of both the NCI and Food and Drug Administration. This is accomplished by carrying out a detailed review of the protocol by a staff representative representing different medical specialties and by one or more biostatisticians. Suggestions are then returned from this staff review to the Group Chairman. When these procedures are cleared, the protocol is activated by the Group, copies are filed with the National Cancer Institute and the Food and Drug Administration and copies are sent to member institutions. Attached to the protocols are standard sections of appendix which define toxicity grading, samples of informed consent, clinical staging, operative procedures, depending upon the nature of the protocol. Protocols are reviewed by each institution's human research committee. When the Operations Office is notified of the clearance, the Group accepts telephone entries of patients. At the time the participating institutions calls to enter patients, the reporting secretary or data clerk has on hand a form that has been filled out with the answers to a series of questions aimed at determining whether the patient is truly eligible. The staff person at the Operations Office has the same questionnaire termed, 'Fast Fact Sheet', except that it has listed on it what are considered to be the appropriate answers. After the patients minimal identifying criteria (relative to hospital record number, birth date, hospital, etc.) are provided, the GOG secretary at the Operations Office refers to the Fast Fact answers. If they are correct, the patient is accepted and the secretary checks a log book at the Operations Office to determine the therapy to be assigned. The Group Biostatistician provides a computer randomized listing to the Operations Office to assign therapy. A duplicate record, without randomization is provided to participating institutions to record the patient's registration number and arm of therapy selected when this is appropriate. Following entry of the patient, forms are submitted to the Operations Office as directed in each of the protocols. Multicopy forms are used. The Operations Office carries out further distribution of the form to the Group Biostatistician and protocol chairperson. Record submission is monitored by the Operations Office for timeliness and quality, with delinquencies and deficiencies reported to Principal Investigators.

Careful monitoring of complications is carried out on the basis of a standard classification. It is patterned after complications as defined by most of the multisystem groups, particularly that of the Eastern Cooperative Oncology Group.

It generally takes from six months to one year to get a study activated. It may take from one month to seven or eight months for an institution to clear a study through a human research committee. It may take anything from a few months for a Phase II study to six or seven years for a Phase III study involving rare tumors to be completed. Ovarian carcinomas of the recurrent or advanced type can be collected by a group like the Gynecologic Oncology Group at the rate of 200 to 300 patients per year. Endometrial cancer staging studies can be accomplished at the rate of 200 patients per year.

The number of open studies in the group varies from one or two pilot studies on group-wide protocols in gynecologic cancer to (for the GOG) 30 to 40 simultaneously operating gynecologic studies. Studies are termed 'open' when they are activated and 'closed' when they no longer accept patient entries. However, note that follow-up continues in such closed protocols. The protocol is 'terminated' when all data gathering is felt to be finished by the protocol chairperson and the group biostatistician. In a complex organization with concurrent studies in the same field there are priorities. In Phase II testing, priorities may be arranged by site of origin (Figure 2). Occasionally, when other sources report a particularly active drug in nongynecologic tumors, the priorities may be altered to permit earlier testing. The turnover of Phase II drugs for each disease causes a problem for the principal investigator as to the drug currently in use. As a result a month-by-month listing of drug priorities and disease is published by the Gynecologic Oncology Group. The selection process in Phase III studies is

1. FIRST TIME ON PROTOCOL 26

| | |
|---|---|
| OVARY - EPITHELIAL (See Reverse for List) | 26N (DHAD)    or    ***26O (AZQ) |
| UTERUS - ADENOCARCINOMA | 26G (ICRF-159) |
| CERVIX - SQUAMOUS | 26M (PALA) |
| CERVIX - ADENOCARCINOMA<br>ADENOSQUAMOUS CARCINOMA | 26E (DAG) |
| OVARY - GERM CELL TUMOR<br>UTERUS - SARCOMAS<br>REFRACTORY TROPHOBLASTIC DISEASE<br>VAGINA - ALL CELL TYPES | 26D (VP-16) |
| BARTHOLINS GLAND - ALL CELL TYPES<br>OVARY - OTHER THAN EPITHELIAL<br>PARAMETRIUM - ALL CELL TYPES<br>TUBE - ALL CELL TYPES<br>VULVA - ALL CELL TYPES<br>**UTERUS - SARCOMAS | 26C (CIS-PLATINUM) |

2. SECOND TIME ON PROTOCOL 26

CERVIX-SQUAMOUS AND OVARY-EPITHELIAL PATIENTS ARE NOT ELIGIBLE FOR MORE THAN ONE PROTOCOL 26 DRUG.

ALL OTHER CATEGORIES OF PATIENTS ARE ELIGIBLE FOR A MAXIMUM OF TWO PROTOCOL 26 DRUGS

***ONLY FOR PATIENTS WHO HAVE HAD ADRIAMYCIN, TOTAL DOSE OVER 400 MG/M2, OR PATIENTS WHO HAVE HISTORY OF CARDIAC DISEASE THAT WOULD MAKE THEM INELIGIBLE FOR PROTOCOL 26-N (DHAD)

**ONLY FOR PRIMARY CHEMOTHERAPY TREATMENT OF UTERINE SARCOMAS!!!

*Figure 2.* Sample priority list Phase II testing by site and drug for GOG.

guided for the investigator by an availability listing of protocols open to the investigator at a given time, plus schema to permit rapid perusal for determining patient suitability, and a detailed section in each protocol giving eligibility and ineligibility criteria. For a principal investigator the most difficult disease is ovary where stage, cell type, grade, surgical finding, and residual disease all may serve to define the eligibility of a patient for one or more of 10 to 12 protocols (Figure 3).

## 3.5. Quality control

Further illustration of the complexity of a group is the processing for quality as it affects eligibility and evaluability. At the Operations Office of the Gynecologic Oncology Group a small computer is used to monitor the

OVARY

| STAGE | PROTOCOL | | CHAIRMEN | DATE ACTIVATED |
|---|---|---|---|---|
| I | #46 | A RANDOMIZED COMPARISON OF MELPHALAN VS. INTRAPERITONEAL CHROMIC PHOSPHATE IN THE TREATMENT OF WOMEN WITH STAGE I (EXCLUSIVE OF STAGE IA(I) GI AND IB(I) GI) EPITHELIAL CARCINOMA OF THE OVARY (PHASE III) | DR. P.J. DISAIA<br>DR. C.P. MORROW<br>DR. J. ARSENEAU<br>DR. G. WEISBAUM | 2/5/79 |
| IA(I),<br>IB(I) | #7601 | OVARIAN CANCER STUDY GROUP PROTOCOL FOR SELECTED STAGE IA(I) - IB(I) OVARIAN CANCER WELL AND MODERATELY DIFFERENTIATED) | DR. L. WALTON<br>DR. T. JONES<br>DR. J. ARSENEAU<br>DR. A. MILLER | 9/18/78 |
| IC,<br>IIA,B,C,<br>IA(II),<br>IB(II) | #7602 | OVARIAN CANCER STUDY GROUP PROTOCOL FOR ALL STAGE IC AND IIA, B, AND C AND SELECTED STAGE IA(II) AND IB(II) (#7602-B PORTION OF STUDY IS CLOSED) | DR. L. WALTON<br>DR. T. JONES<br>DR. J. ARSENEAU<br>DR. A. MILLER | 9/18/78 |
| I,II,III | #41 | SURGICAL STAGING OF OVARIAN CARCINOMA | DR. H. BUCHSBAUM<br>DR. G. DELGADO<br>DR. A. MILLER | 2/5/79 |
| III OPT. | #52 | A PHASE III RANDOMIZED STUDY OF CYCLO-PHOSPHAMIDE PLUS ADRIAMYCIN PLUS PLATINOL (CAP) VS. CYCLOPHOSPHAMIDE PLUS PLATINOL (CP) IN PATIENTS WITH OPTIMAL STAGE III OVARIAN ADENOCARCINOMA | DR. G.A. OMURA<br>DR. H. BUCHSBAUM<br>DR. T. BONFIGLIO | 4/15/81 |
| SUBOPT. III,<br>IV | #60 | A PHASE III RANDOMIZED STUDY OF DOXORUBICIN + CYCLOPHOSPHAMIDE + CISPLATIN VS. DOXORUBICIN + CYCLOPHOSPHAMIDE + CISPLATIN + BCG IN PATIENTS WITH ADVANCED SUBOPTIMAL OVARIAN ADENOCARCINOMA, STAGE III AND IV. | DR. W.T. CREASMAN<br>DR. P.J. DISAIA<br>DR. J.T. THIGPEN<br>DR. G.A. OMURA | 2/9/82 |
| III | #61 | PHASE III RANDOMIZED STUDY OF CIS-PLATINUM + CYCLOPHOSPHAMIDE VS. HEXAMETHYLMELAMINE AFTER 2ND-LOOK SURGERY IN NON-MEASURABLE STAGE III OVARIAN ADENOCARCINOMA PARTIALLY RESPONSIVE TO PREVIOUS REGIMENTS CONTAINTING CIS-PLATINUM AND CYCLOPHOSPHAMIDE. (SEQUEL TO PROTOCOLS #47 AND #52) | DR. G.A. OMURA<br>DR. H. BUCHSBAUM<br>DR. S. WARD | 12/15/81 |

*Figure 3.* Typical listing of studies available at a given time for group clinical trials GOG.

flow of paperwork for timeliness and completeness. As an example, it will alert the Operations Office that a patient has been entered after a therapeutic procedure rather than before it as required by protocol. The computer provides a monthly print-out to each principal investigator indicating that records are delinquent and how long they are delinquent. The Operations Office of the GOG arranges for representatives of the modality committees to review pathology reports, tissue slides, cytologic preparations, gynecologic surgical records, forms outlining pretherapy work-up and radiation therapy records and films. The review of chemotherapy is carried out by the Statistical Office with the protocol chairmen. Preentry telephone screening clears 90% of patients; another 5 to 10% may prove ineligible as records are evaluated, slides are examined and X-rays are reviewed. The results of the reviews are transmitted to the group biostatistician, the study chairman and when there is a rejection of an entry, the principal investigator. The group biostatistician's office arranges a record check system before the onset of a study. The study chairman and the group biostatistician prepare a check-off and item completion type of form for evaluation called an EVL form, which is a vehicle allowing the study chairperson to review all abstracted data prior to each statistical analysis. Usually, the study chairman comes to the group biostatistician's office for a conference based on the findings. The Biostatistical Office analyzes and reports data twice yearly in a publication which is labeled, the 'Statistical Report'. Tables and life tables are presented, giving patient population characteristics, disease parameters, toxicity, and response to therapy. When it is appropriate, conclusions and future directions are provided in many reports.

The biostatistician and his staff constantly monitor the performance of the investigators. They note when there are deviations from the protocol prescribed therapy. Using the modality committee consultants and study chairmen, deviations from the protocol specifications are rated minor or major. Data is analyzed with and without the patients who have violations. Patients who have been found after entry to be ineligible or to have major protocol violations are considered exclusions. Patients not excluded are considered to be evaluable. Member institutions are required to have not less than an 85% evaluable rate. The Membership Committee of the Gynecology Oncology Group looks at ineligibility, and the evaluability and completeness of records in judging whether an institution shall continue as a member of the group. The same committee also considers contributions in terms of protocol development, participation in studies and publications.

Publications other than the biannual report are directed from the statistical office in collaboration with the study chairmen. Principal investigators and investigators whose institutions have contributed the largest numbers of patients are included as co-authors. Preliminary reports, particularly in the form of abstracts are used to report Phase II work. Phase III studies more often appear as full manuscripts. Broad exposure of the medical public to the information is sought by the Gynecologic Oncology Group as well as other groups with the major objective of promptly disseminating information derived from the clinical trials.

For a more detailed discussion of the entire concept of Clinical Trials and Cooperative Groups, the reader is referred to a publication entitled, 'Cancer Research – Impact of the Cooperative Groups', Barth Hoogstraten, M.D. (ed.), Mason Publishing, USA, New York, NY 1980 [1]. As a progress report for the Board of Scientific Counselors, Robert Hilgers, M.D., Joseph New, M.D., Robert Slayton, M.D. and George C. Lewis, M.D. formed a Gynecologic Oncology Task Force of the Cooperative Groups to prepare Chapter 11 of this book and provide a report for the Board of Scientific Counselors of Gynecologic Cancer. The publication reviewed the twenty-year period from 1958 to 1978. The material prepared by the Gynecologic

Task Force was extracted or revised for use in this chapter. The material is further expanded upon by reference to statistical reports made available by groups participating in gynecologic research for the years 1979–1981.

4. SPECIFIC STUDIES

*4.1. Ovarian cancer*

Though rare in comparison to other female genital cancer, ovarian malignancies gain importance through high mortality despite apparent sensitivity to a wide spectrum of therapeutic procedures. Investigation in this site category is hampered by the large number of variables that define 'ovarian cancer'. Patient populations have to be characterized and stratified. Other than Phase II and pilot-type projects of exploratory nature, studies require relatively large numbers for reliable conclusions. Even then, it pays to doublecheck results because of the potential undetermined extraneous influences. Quality control is essential, especially in terms of surgery, pathology and adjuvant therapy procedures. The multiple biologic variables have been important, well-recognized factors in the relatively slow progress for control of this category of cancers.

Prior to the development of chemotherapy, irradiation joined with surgical treatment in controlling ovarian carcinoma. When chemotherapy was introduced, the surgeon and radiation therapist was joined in the attack on ovarian cancer by internists, hematologists, pediatricians, and others. Practitioners generally not associated with cancer centers, and some who were, depended upon orally administered alkylating agents that had a reasonable latitude of safety for administration in patients who were ambulatory or lived some distance from the physician. Multisystem cooperative groups started out with single-agent Phase II testing (Table 4). More recently emphasis has shifted to multi-agent trials. Overwhelming attention was paid by investigators to advanced disease as contrasted to minimal cancer because patients with advanced lesions were more available. 'Early' disease was managed in every type of institution and did not tend to be referred to centers. With recurrence after operation, with or without adjuvant treatment, the patient was referred to more specialized centers. In the same manner, many advanced ovarian cancers had exploration with biopsy followed by referral to medical centers.

In the early 1970s, attention was being paid to ovarian cancer, but with limited emphasis on surgical staging. Surgery for the patient with early cancer was inconsistent and varied from surgeon to surgeon. Before 1975 inadequate surgical and pathological evaluation may have influenced the results appreciably. In GOG Protocol #1, IA and IB epithelial carcinomas were

Table 4. Ovary single agents in Phase II pilots.

| Agent | Group | Year activated | No. of evaluable patients | PR & CR % |
|---|---|---|---|---|
| Piperazinedoine | GOG | 1977 | 31 | 0 |
| Cis-platinum | GOG | 1977 | 35 | 28.6 |
| Galactitol | GOG | 1977 | 35 | 11.5 |
| VP-16 | GOG | 1977 | 24 | 0 |
| VP-16 | ECOG | 1977 | 11 | 0 |
| Baker's antifol | GOG | 1978 | 25 | 8 |
| ICRF | GOG | 1978 | 22 | 0 |
| Maytansine | GOG | 1978 | 29 | 0 |
| Yoshi | GOG | 1978 | 23 | too early |
| DepoProvera | ECOG | 1977 | 19 | 0 |
| MGBG | ECOG | 1977 | 10 | 10 |
| Phenestrim | ECOG | 1977 | 20 | 5 |
| MAMSA | SWOG | 1979 | 15 | 0 |

randomized postoperatively to no adjuvant therapy, pelvic irradiation therapy, or melphalan alone [5, 6, 7]. Thorough surgical staging as currently defined was not required. The study was one of the earliest efforts at prospective trials for Stage I disease. Problems in quality control resulted in reduced numbers of evaluable patients. Chemotherapy had fewer recurrences. Recognition of the deficiencies in that study led to the initiation of another study currently in progress (GOG #46), contrasting melphalan and radioactive chromic phosphate for stages IA and IB.

In GOG Protocols #2, 3, and 10-14, the major objectives were to check on nongroup claims as to the value of alkylating agents, radiation therapy, combinations of radiation therapy and alkylating agents and multidrug chemotherapy in the primary treatment of Stage III epithelial tumors, germ cell tumors, stromal tumors and sarcomas [3, 4, 8-13]. An important finding of the studies that were first undertaken by the GOG was that diagnosis and therapy differed from the protocol prescription. Radiation therapy was not always appropriately administered, borderline carcinoma was confused with invasive carcinoma and chemotherapy was applied with less error than surgery and radiation therapy. The studies did confirm the impressions of others that minimal residual disease after surgery was associated with a better prognosis than large postoperative residual tumor. In the GOG trial, no difference in survival or disease-free interval was found between melphalan, melphalan plus radiation or radiation alone [3, 4]. Melphalan appeared to be the least toxic treatment and it achieved results similar to results of various combinations (GOG #2, Table 5). In another study, mel-

Table 5. Ovary. Multiple agents – Randomized trials Phase II–Phase III.

| Agents and/or modality | Group protocol # | Year activated | No. of evaluable patients | CR & PR % |
|---|---|---|---|---|
| Vincristine/actinomycin/cytoxan Germ cell | GOG 10–11 44 | 1971 | 39 | 50–56% depending on cell type and stage |
| Actinomycin/5-fluoracil/cytoxan or irradiation (stromal) | GOG 14 | 1971 | 82 | registry only no contrast |
| Actinomycin/cytoxan vincristine/irradiation (mixed mullerian) | GOG 12 | 1971 | 28 | |
| Dactinomycin/methetrexate/chlorambucil (choriocarcinoma) | GOG 13 | 1971 | 5 | too few to analyze |
| Alkeran vs adriamycin cytoxan vs alkeran hexamethylemelamine | GOG 22 | 1976 | 369 | measurable 48–51% for combination 37% for single |
| Alkeran/C. parvum vs alkeran | GOG 25 | 1978 | 184 | still active |
| Vinblastine/bleomycin/platinum (Germ cell) | GOG 45 | 1978 | 21 | still active |
| Melphalan vs radioactive phospherous | GOG 46 | 1979 | 7 | still active |
| Adriamycin/cytoxan vs adriamycin/cytoxan/platinum | GOG 47 | 1979 | 190 | still active |
| No adjuvant vs melphalan Stage IA, IB | OCSG GOG 7601 | 1976 | 43 | still active |
| Melphalan vs radioactive phospherous or irradiation & melphalan Stage II and/or residual tumor | OCSG GOG 7602 | 1976 | 69 4 | still active |
| Actinomycin/5-fluorouracil/cytoxan vs methotrexate c.f. cytoxan vs vincristine, adriamycin vs methetrexate c.f. C. Parvum | OCSG 7603 | 1976 | | in progress |
| Levamisole/melphalan | GOG 7891 | 1978 | 23 | 35 |

Table 5. (continued).

| Agents and/or modality | Group protocol # | Year activated | No. of evaluable patients | CR & PR % |
|---|---|---|---|---|
| Cytoxan/adriamycin vs Melphalan | SECSG | 1975 | 36 | 33 vs 27 |
| Hexamethylmelamine cytoxan/ adriamycin platinum | SECSG NCOG | 1978 | 34 | 68 |
| BCNU/cyclophosphamide/adriamycin CCNU vs | SECSG | 1976 | 18 | 11 |
| MeCCNU | GOG 15 | 1972 | | |
| Low vs high dose platinum/hexamethylmelamine | ECOG | 1979 | 31 | 62.5% |
| Irradiation mid segment/ cytoxan/hexamethylmelamine/adriamycin/Cis-platinum | ECOG | 1978 | 43 | in progress |
| Cisplatinum/adriamycin Hexamethyl i.p. C. parvum | ECOG | 1979 | 8 | in progress |
| Melphalan vs 5-fluorouracil/ cytoxan/methotrexate | ECOG | 1975 | 114 vs 110 | 26 vs 41 |
| Alkeran vs thio-TEPA vs thio-TEPA (modified) methotrexate vs cytoxan, 5-fluorouracil, adriamycin, alternating with thio-TEPA, methotrexate | ECOG | 1975 | 346 | CAF and a CAF-TM most promising |
| Melphalan then hexamethylmelamine/adriamycin platinum/vs cytoxan, hexamethylmelamine, adriamycin platinum | ECOG | 1978 | 183 | 35% measurable |
| Cisplatinum cytoxan | ECOG | 1977 | 21 | 30 |
| Radiation vs radiation, melphalan vs melphalan | ECOG RTOG | 1977 | 47 | study abandoned not enough Stage II |
| Melphalan vs irradiation pelvic vs no therapy Stage 1 A, B | GOG 1 | 1971 | 87 | 6% vs 33% vs 17% |
| Melphalan vs chlorambucil | SWOG | 1970 | 24/23 | 12.5/22 |
| Melphalan vs melphalan 5-fluorouracil vs melphalan/ 5-fluorouracil/actinomycin | GOG 3 | 1971 | 94 69 74 | 25.4 26.0 28.4 |

Table 5. (continued).

| Agents and/or modality | Group protocol # | Year activated | No. of evaluable patients | CR & PR % |
|---|---|---|---|---|
| vs cytoxan/actinomycin/ 5-fluorouracil | | | 72 | 26.2 |
| Melphalan vs melphalan irradiation vs irradiation melphalan vs irradiation | GOG 2 | 1971 | 42 15 19 21 | no difference progression-free interval |
| Adriamycin/cytoxan vs adriamycin cytoxan, BcG | SWOG | 1976 | 65 56 | 43 57 |
| Adriamycin, cytoxan BcG vs adriamycin cytoxan, Cis-platinum vs adriamycin cytoxan platinum, BcG | SWOG | 1979 | 37 | in progress |
| Surgery/radiation/vinblastine/bleomycin/ Cis-platimum; actinomycin/cytoxan/adriamycin | CCG germ cell | 1978 | | in progress |
| Hexamethylmelamine/ Cis-Platinum/adriamycin/ cytoxan | ECOG Est PC 877 | 1977 | 12 | 70 |
| Hexamethylmelaimine/Cis-platinum vs hexamethyl-melamine/adriamycin/ Cis-platinum | ECOG EST PD877 | 1977 | 5 12 | 80 50 |
| Medoxyprogesterone vs VP-16 | ECOG | 1977 | 27 | 0 |
| Adriamycin/cyclophosphamide vs melphalan | NCOG | 2/78 | 45 | 69/32 |
| Adriamycin/cytoxan/ radiotherapy/surgery | NCOG | 1979 | 25 | 22 |
| Cytoxan Cis-platinum vs cytoxan | OCSG | 1977 | no data | |
| 5-fluorouracil/hexamethyl-melamine Cis-platinum vs adriamycin/ 5-fluorouracil/hexamethyle-melamine/Cis-platinum | SWOG | 1977 | 74 20 | 20 months survival approximately 25% 50% |

phalan was contrasted with the same agent plus antimetabolites or antibiotics or both. The toxicity of the combinations was excessive compared to the benefits gained from the single agent. It appeared that a single agent was certainly as effective as combinations, and certainly safer (GOG #3, Table 5) [8-10]. The GOG undertook a study of germ cell tumors employing a combination of vincristine, dactinomycin and cytoxan (GOG #10, Table 5) [8, 11, 12]. The efficacy of the combination has previously been considered in trials published by the M.D. Anderson Hospital [14]. In just over eight years, the group accumulated 39 patients and noted a 50-60% response rate depending on the pathologic type and stage of the lesion. These results confirmed earlier claims.

Cooperative groups are now progressing through a comparison of single agent with multiple agents (Table 5). Earlier data suggested there was no advantage to multiple drug programs as the GOG found in its Study #3. Recently, GOG Protocol #23 in measurable lesions indicated that combination therapy provides a more prolonged progression-free interval and a higher complete response rate [15, 16]. Currently, there is declining emphasis on radiation therapy and growing emphasis on chemotherapy in cooperative group research. The Eastern Cooperative Oncology Group has continued a pilot study for advanced ovarian cancer using cytoxan, hexamethylmelamine, adriamycin and Cis-platinum with intermittent radiotherapy. Three groups, ECOG, RTOG and GOG attempted a collaborative study for Stage II patients that contrasted abdominal and pelvic radiation with pelvic radiation plus chemotherapy *versus* chemotherapy alone. Because of the failure to accumulate enough patients and the competition of two studies for Stage I and II patients (OCSG 7601 and 7602) the protocol was closed after only 47 patients were entered. In uncontrolled studies, Cis-platinum employed as a single agent has been extremely active in ovarian carcinoma [17-20]. Groups have progressed to studies using this agent in combination. There remain questions as to whether any combination therapy using platinum will prove worthwhile, whether Cis-platinum by itself will be equivalent to other drugs and combinations, and whether long-term survival will be greatly influenced by any treatment method currently under evaluation, including Cis-platinum [21].

By the time the Gynecologic Oncology Group decided to take on surgical-pathologic staging studies, and by the time the Ovarian Cancer Study Group (an NCI Contract, 7601, 7602, 7603 – see Table 5) began to evaluate staging of early cancer, over 2,000 patients were entered into all the groups' protocols. Unfortunately the majority of studies by many groups have involved small numbers of patients even in Phase III studies so that not enough patients have been accumulated in any one study for appropriate evaluation. The largest early studies were conducted by the Eastern Cooperative

Oncology Group and the Southwest Oncology Group. More recent Phase III tests have been carried out on a larger scale by the Gynecologic Oncology Group enrolling hundreds of patients annually.

Immunotherapy has been evaluated by two groups. A Southwest Oncology Group Study [22] suggested that the addition of BcG, adriamycin and cytoxan for advanced ovarian carcinoma almost doubled the median survival time obtained by the two drugs alone. At the same time the Gynecologic Oncology Group evaluated *C parvum* plus melphalan *versus* melphalan alone (GOG #25), which to date has shown no advantage for the addition of *C parvum*.

Currently, certain generalizations can be made about ovarian cancer to the effect that: (1) the size of the largest residual mass appears to influence outcome; patients with less tumor bulk appear to have statistically significantly better survival than those with large tumor masses [4, 8]; (2) the philosophy of treatment of ovarian carcinomas has shifted away from radiation therapy and toward chemotherapy; (3) single agent therapy is less effective than multiple drug therapy; (4) advanced rare carcinomas of the ovary and very early epithelial carcinomas are difficult to accrue into studies; and (5) intergroup collaboration will be needed for studies of rare tumors. Nongynecologic groups appear quite suited for Phase I–II drug trials, pilot testing, and limited Phase III trials. Phase III programs are required to confirm the claims of pilot and Phase II tests and will continue to be the main contribution of the Gynecologic Oncology Group.

*4.2. Cervical cancer*

Cervical cancer has not received much attention from cooperative groups because successful primary therapy and predominance of early stage lesions have limited the available patients, and because few promising agents have been available. The optimistic prognosis for cervical as well as endometrial cancer prompted clinicians to deal with these malignancies in broad categories without the stratification that might have otherwise separated patients into relative risk categories. Stratification by other than clinical staging and grade has had limited research application since individual investigators have had only small numbers of patients available. Thus analytic reviews of treatment have tended to be indiscriminating until group investigation came into the picture and provided adequate numbers of patients for detailed studies of primary disease.

Cooperative group research has tried to better define some of the specific risk factors and their impact. The studies have spanned from surgical-pathological staging studies to the applications of single or combined therapeutic modalities. The Gynecologic Oncology Group in particular has looked at the entire spectrum of squamous cell cervical cancer of epithelial type from dysplastic changes through Stage IV disease. The GOG has just recently abandoned a pair of studies of the degree and extent of dysplasia in relation to a therapeutic program randomized between local excision, cryotherapy and conization. These are GOG Protocols #31 and 32. Too few patients were being accumulated to complete the studies in a reasonable period of time. Adequate long-term follow-up appeared to be impossible because of failure of the patients to return for evaluation.

In Protocol #5, the GOG looked at the diagnostic problems with microinvasive cancer [12, 13]. The group found that easily one-third of the entries were misdiagnosed according to erstwhile definition. In 111 cases there was positive correlation between depth and extent with morphologic features of invasion, that is, the wider and deeper the lesion, the more likely there was to be capillary permeation, confluence, dedifferentiation and lymphatic infiltration [23, 24].

Surgical staging studies with the disease beyond Stage IA for the Gynecologic Oncology Group were a natural extension of the analyses of microinvasive disease (see Table 6). The Gynecologic Oncology Group in Protocol #19, evaluated 292 patients and confirmed earlier observations about the lack of correlation between clinical and surgical staging [25]. From about 1/4 of Stage I to about 50% of Stage III patients had major discrepancies

Table 6. Surgical and pathologic staging in GOG studies for cervical cancer.

| Protocol number | Clinical stage of disease | Procedure |
|---|---|---|
| 5 | Microinvasive IA | Knife conization. Hysterectomy. |
| 19 | IB–IVA | For stage IB, radical hysterectomy pelvic and para-aortic node resection. For other stages pelvic and para-aortic node sampling, no hysterectomy. Biopsy of any gross tumor in abdomen. All transperitoneal. |
| 24 | II–IVA | Pelvic and para-aortic node sampling (trans or retroperitoneal) biopsy of any gross tumor. Peritoneal cytology. |
| 49 | IB | Radical hysterectomy pelvic and para-aortic node resection (transperitoneal). Peritoneal cytology, biopsy gross lesions. |
| 56–59 | IIB–IVB | Fine needle biopsy suspicious nodes from noninvasive studies. For negative studies trans or retroperitoneal para-aortic node sampling, peritoneal exploration, peritoneal cytology. For positive para-aortic nodes, scalene node biopsy. |

between clinical and surgical findings. Six % of Stage IB, 18% of Stage IIA, 32% of Stage IIB, and 32% of Stage IIIB had involvement of para-aortic nodes. Over 25% of the patients had modification of their therapy as a result of the surgical findings. Survival for these patients has not been analyzed. For surgical treatment alone and the combination of radiation and surgery no excessive morbidity was encountered. The findings from Protocol #19 led to the use of surgical staging prior to entry in later protocols (GOG #24, 49, 56, 59). This was true for Protocol #24 applying a standard program of radiation therapy after surgical staging [26]. Patients were stratified according to positive and negative nodes in addition to the standard stratification for stage. Patients so stratified and given radiation were randomized between no additional therapy or immunotherapy with *C parvum*. Surgical staging was intended to avoid maldistribution of positive nodes

*Table 7.* Cervical cancer Phase II pilot single-agent/single-modality type studies.

| Agent/modality | Group | Year activated | No. of evaluable patients | CR & PR % |
|---|---|---|---|---|
| Porfiromycin | SWOG | 1966 | 34 | 27 |
| Adriamycin | SWOG | 1970 | 6 | 33.3 |
| CCNU | SWOG | 1971 | 7 | 28.5 |
| Bleomycin | SWOG | 1971 | 9 | 22.2 |
| Bleomycin (pelvic infusion) | GOG | 1971 | 16 | 12.5 |
| Bleomycin | SWOG | 1972 | 26 | 7.6 |
| CCNU | GOG | 1972 | 58 | 3 |
| Methyl CCNU | GOG | 1972 | 62 | 5 |
| Methyl CCNU | SWOG | 1972 | 31 | 13 |
| 5-Azacytadine | SWOG | 1972 | 4 | 0 |
| Adriamycin | GOG | 1974 | 61 | 19.7 |
| Adriamycin | WCSG |  | 9 | 55 |
| Cis-platinum | SWOG | 1974 | 7 | 0 |
| Cis-platinum | GOG | 1977 | 34/22 | 29.4/50.0[a] |
| Piperazinedione | GOG | 1977 | 33 | 6 |
| VP-16 | GOG | 1977 | 30 | 0 |
| Galactitol | GOG | 1977 | 32 | 21.9 |
| Cis-platinum | GOG | 1978 | 226 | in progress |
| Baker's antifol | GOG | 1978 | 32 | 15.6 |
| ICRF | GOG | 1978 | 28 | 17.8 |
| Maytansine | GOG | 1978 | 29 | 3.4 |
| M-AMSA | GOG | 1979 | suspended 1980 – toxicity | |
| M-AMSA | SWOG | 1979 | 4 | in progress |
| YOSHI | GOG | 1979 | 3 | in progress |
| Hexamethylmelamine | WCSG |  | 34 | 24 |

[a] No prior chemotherapy.

since such an inbalance could outweigh the effects of therapy. This is still in the follow-up phase and results are not available.

For an earlier study, GOG #4 [27-29], the Gynecologic Oncology Group evaluated hydroxyurea, a radiosensitizer against a placebo without stratification by nodal status. Stages IIB-IVA were treated with conventional radiation therapy. Ninety patients were studied. With hydroxyurea the complete response rate was 68% and the progression-free interval 13.6 months. Estimated median survival time was 19.5 months. A complete response rate of 49%, a progression-free interval of 7.6 months and an estimated median survival time of 10.7 months was reported in the group of patients assigned to the placebo arm. Hematologic toxicity was more common and more severe in patients receiving the hydroxyurea.

High-LET radiation therapy is being investigated by two national clinical trial groups (RTOG and NCOG). A four-arm prospective randomized study utilizing photons, neutrons, and mixtures of both was designed to study patients with Stage III-IVA carcinoma of the cervix. The NCOG studied heavy charged particles in the form of helium ions in a contrast against conventional radiotherapy to the pelvic and para-aortic lymph nodes. Only a limited number of patients have been entered into these studies, and it is too early to report results.

Studies employing chemotherapy alone outweigh other types of studies. Most numerous have been single agent Phase II studies (Table 7) [30-46]. Relatively few combinations have been evaluated [15, 16, 47-50]. Studies have been limited, not exceeding 60-65 patients. Responses were poor, though, one study under the Southwest Oncology Group for mitomycin, vincristine and bleomycin twice weekly had 60% response in 50 evaluable patients [49] (Table 8). The numerous single-drug studies still indicate that with one exception there is only minimal activity. Cis-platinum in a Phase II study of the GOG, achieved a 29.4% response rate in 34 previously treated patients [37, 38]. In 22 patients treated primarily there was a 50% response rate. The GOG is pursuing this investigation further in a dose-seeking investigation (GOG #43) using $50 \text{ mm/M}^2$ vs $100 \text{ mm/M}^2$ vs $20 \text{ mgm/M}^2$ daily times five days. This study has just been closed and results are not available. Among other agents tested by the GOG, galacticol, Baker's antifol, and ICRF 159 are the only agents showing any promise (Table 7). Various combinations of Cis-platinum with other drugs are being screened in Phase I-II and pilot testing. The GOG has prepared a series of studies of cervical carcinoma from Stage I through Stage IV looking at potential surgery, radiation therapy and chemotherapy combinations. In Protocol #49, patients in Stage IB with one to three unilateral positive nodes are randomized between radiation and no radiation as adjuvant therapy. In Protocol #56, patients in Stage II-IV are given radiation therapy

*Table 8.* Cervical cancer Phase II/III multi-agent/multi-modality type studies.

| Agent/modality | Group | Year activated | No. of evaluable patients | CR & PR % |
|---|---|---|---|---|
| Adriamycin/bleomycin | WCSG | | 11 | 0 |
| Adriamycin/bleomycin vs CCNU/bleomycin | COG | 1971 | 6<br>9 | 14<br>22 |
| Adriamycin/vincristine | GOG 23 | 1974 | 54 | 18.5 |
| Adriamycin/cytoxan | GOG 23 | 1974 | 39 | 15.4 |
| Mitomycin/vincristine/ bleomycin once weekly | SWOG | 1974 | 27 | 19 |
| Mitomycin/vincristine bleomycin 2× weekly | SWOG | 1974 | 54 | 56 |
| Adriamycin/5-fluorouracil vincristine vs cytoxan | SECSG | 1975 | 60 | no different |
| Mitomycin/vincristine bleomycin infusion | SWOG | 1976 | 49 | 32 |
| Adriamycin/Cis-platinum mitomycin/bleomycin | GOG P 14 | 1976 | 19 | 32 |
| Vincristine/Cis-platinum | SWOG | 1978 | 13 | 31 |
| Mitomycin/bleomycin | SWOG | 1978 | | 18 |
| Mitomycin/vincristine bleomycin/Cis-platinum vs Cis-platinum/ Mitomycin vs Cis-platinum | SWOG | 1979 | 3 | too early |
| Dianhydrogalactitol/ Cis-platinum | ECOG | 1979 | 3 | in progress |
| Cytoxan/Cis-platinum | GOG 7992 | 1979 | 16 | in progress |
| Adriamycin/Cis-platinum | GOG 7993 | 1979 | 7 | in progress |
| Bleomycin/Mitomycin C sequential | NCOG | 6/78 | 18 | 0% 22% |
| Mitomycin/vincristine/ bleomycin/Cis-platinum | SWOG | 1978 | 13 | 38 |
| Cis-platinum/bleomycin methotrexate/leukovoria | ECOG | 1981 | 2 | too early |

and randomized between receiving hydroxyurea or misonidazole during radiation. In Protocol #59, the patients with positive para-aortic nodes are given extended field radiation plus hydroxyurea followed by randomization between no subsequent therapy or the addition of Cis-platinum. It is likely that with continued application of early screening techniques, the lead taken by the Gynecologic Oncology Group in studying early disease will be more profitable in the future.

## 4.3. Endometrial cancer

Because of the reluctance of many investigators to depart from their own standard approaches for endometrial cancer which for them have been most successful, it is difficult for the Gynecologic Oncology Group to initiate randomized trials for Stage I and early Stage II endometrial cancer. In order to achieve more information the group initiated a study to evaluate disease risk factors using surgical-pathological evaluations of tissues and fluids in GOG Protocol #33 [51]. Patients entered into this study must have clinical Stage I or occult Stage II disease and, as a preentry requirement, must not have any preoperative radiation. A total abdominal hysterectomy and bilateral salpingo-oophorectomy with peritoneal fluid aspiration (or washing) and node dissection are required in order to evaluate cervical involvement, myometrial penetration, grade, involvement of the adnexa and status of peritoneal cytology. After 200 patients with Stage I, Grade 1 disease were operated upon, the incidence of positive nodes, adnexa or peritoneal fluid was so low, that the patients at that stage and grade were thereafter excluded from the study as being very low risk. At the same time, the GOG decided that the patients with more than half the myometrium penetrated, with positive nodes, occult cervical involvement or adnexal involvement were suitable for adjuvant treatment employing pelvic radiation and randomization between adriamycin and no adriamycin. Based on preliminary findings of Pilot #1 of the GOG [52], which is very similar to GOG Protocol #33, patients with positive peritoneal cytology were placed in a high risk category for which it was felt there should be adjuvant chemotherapy. Therefore, patients with positive peritoneal cytology are placed onto GOG Protocol #48 which provides CT Provera 50 mg tid p.o. until there is evidence of progressing disease; then the patients are randomized between adriamycin alone and adriamycin plus cytoxan. For the staging study GOG Protocol #33, there is an intermediate group, neither Stage IA, Grade 1 nor any of the positive findings suggested above. Currently the intermediate group is being considered for management under protocols yet to be developed.

At the other end of the scale of endometrial cancer investigation is the treatment of recurrent or advanced endometrial cancer, unsuitable for treatment by standard radiation or surgical treatment, or both. Advanced or recurrent disease is the most common target of most groups. There have been no programs completed for the prospective evaluation of preoperative and/or postoperative radiation in endometrial cancer. In 1980, the RTOG initiated a study of intracavitary radiation *vs* external radiation *vs* a combination of intracavitary and external therapy for Stage I, Grade 2 and 3 endometrial carcinoma. There are still too few patients entered. In groups, there is a reluctance to abandon traditional methods of therapy in favor of developing studies for early or moderately early disease. One factor is that in patients who are surgically staged and found to have disease limited to the uterus, the anticipate survival rate is so high that it is virtually impossible to get a large enough group in a reasonable period of time to determine if there may be significant differences between variations in therapy. In the surgical endometrial adjuvant study with over 500 patients, the four-year survival for hysterectomy alone or radium plus hysterectomy was 86.5% [2]. To demonstrate that any modification of treatment would improve upon this survival would prove impractical in terms of the number of patients that would have to be accumulated. The alternative elected by the GOG is to separate by risk the patients under the general category 'Stage I' and then seek to improve at least the poor risk patients, that is patients with more than half the myometrium penetrated, occult cervical involvement, positive nodes, positive adnexa, positive peritoneal cytology.

Single-agent new drug screening in Phase II trials has been carried out predominantly through the Gynecologic Oncology Group [40, 53, 54]. Other groups have participated more in combination programs with particular emphasis on adriamycin as one of the agents employed [55] (see Tables 9 and 10). Adriamycin seems to be the most active agent but the combina-

*Table 9.* Endometrial single agent – phase II.

| Agent | Group | Year activated | No. of evaluable patients | CR & PR % |
|---|---|---|---|---|
| Adriamycin | GOG | 1975 | 49 | 39 |
| Piperazinedione | GOG | 1977 | 20 | 5 |
| Cis-platinum | GOG | 1977 | 21 | 0 |
| VP-16 | GOG | 1977 | 38 | 0 |
| Galactitol | GOG | 1977 | 17 | 6 |
| High-dose methotrexate with rescue/radiation | SWOG | 1977 | No specification by site | |
| Intracavitary External Irradiation combined with intracavitary external | RTOG | 1980 | 4 | too early |
| Baker's antifol | GOG | 1978 | 1 | 0 |
| ICRF | GOG | 1978 | 0 | – |
| Maytansine | GOG | 1978 | 0 | – |
| Tamoxifen | GOG | 1980 | 22 | too early |

Table 10. Endometrial multiple agent – Phase II and III.

| Agent | Group | Year activated | No. of evaluable patients | CR & PR % |
|---|---|---|---|---|
| Megace Adriamycin cytoxan vs Alkeran 5-fluorouracil megace | GOG | 1977 | 31 | 38% both arms |
| Irradiation alone vs irradiation & adriamycin | GOG | 1977 | 78 | too early |
| Provera then adriamycin vs adriamycin cytoxan | GOG | 1979 | 62 provera 21 randomized | too early |
| DepoProvera vs placebo – adjuvant | SEAG | 1963 | 540 | no benefit documented |
| Megace cytoxan adriamycin vs same plus 5-fluorouracil | ECOG | 1976 | 149 | MCA = 27% MCAF = 16% MLF = 17% |
| Adriamycin cytoxan vs adriamycin cytoxan BcG | SWOG | 1975 | 24/22 | 45/38 |
| Cis-platinum adriamycin cyclophosphomide | NCOG | 1979 | | 56% |
| Adriamycin vs cytoxan | ECOG | 1974 | 40 | 20% vs 0% |
| CCNU vs Methyl/CCNU | GOG | 1972 | 6 | 1/1 2/5 |
| AMSA | SWOG | 1979 | | in progress |

tions containing adriamycin do not have significantly higher response rates than adriamycin alone.

In the future investigation and treatment may be tied to progesterone receptors. One study is underway in the Gynecologic Oncology Group after an earlier pilot study indicated a correlation between grade of tumor and level of cytoplasmic progesterone receptors [56–58]. In the future such determinations may serve as a guide for selection of hormone and other anticancer therapy.

### 4.4. Vulvar cancer

Very few studies of vulvar carcinoma exist. Eastern Cooperative Group, ECOG has a pilot (PE 879) for Cis-platinum, bleomycin and radiation therapy. Only three patients have been entered to date. GOG has had two studies. One, GOG #37, has been a surgical pathologic study of patients with Stages I–IV squamous cell carcinoma of the vulva. It compares the clinical factors of FIGO stage and histopathologic findings with the patterns of tumor spread to determine prognostic significance. In this study, the surgical procedure consists of radical vulvectomy, bilateral inguinal and femoral lymphandectomy. Patients with positive groin nodes are randomized between deep pelvic lymph node dissection or external pelvic and inguinal radiation. One hundred fifty-five patients have been staged and sixteen patients randomized. Not enough information has accumulated for analysis. Vulvar carcinoma occasionally is included in various Phase II studies but insufficient patients are included in any study to draw conclusions. One other group, the Eastern Cooperative Oncology Group, initiated a pilot study in June, 1980 to evaluate Cis-platinum and bleomycin with radiation therapy in advanced carcinoma of the vulva and vagina.

*4.5. Sarcoma*

The Gynecologic Oncology Group evaluated adriamycin compared to no adjuvant treatment in postoperative patients with Stage I and Stage II uterine sarcomas. To date, about 152 evaluable patients have been accumulated. All the histological variants were equally divided between the two arms. Recurrences are still similar in both groups. Significant cardiac toxicity has not been encountered. Follow-up continues but because of the relatively large number of mixed mesodermal tumors with no benefit from adjuvant therapy, further entry of these patients into the GOG Protocol #20 has been discontinued.

In a second GOG study, GOG #21, there was an evaluation of adriamycin *vs* adriamycin and DTIC for Stages III–IV sarcomas [59]. This study has been closed after entering 326 evaluable patients. The combination chemotherapy seemed to have a greater response rate but the difference was not significant. Toxicity was greater in the combination arm. Leiomyosarcoma appeared to be more responsive than heterologous or homologous mixed mesodermal tumors. There was no difference in progression-free interval or survival of patients with nonmeasurable disease for either regimen.

In GOG Pilot #P-2, the distribution of metastatic disease in Stage I and Stage II uterine sarcomas (limited to the uterus) was studied [60]. The work involved patients with heterologous and homologous mixed mesodermal tumors and showed 35.7% positive pelvic lymph nodes and 14% positive para-aortic nodes. A total of 28 patients were evaluated. This was followed by a group-wide study of surgical-pathologic type. This was GOG Protocol #40 and was opened in 1979 and to date 55 evaluable patients have been entered. In 1979, the GOG opened another study for advanced or recurrent uterine sarcoma (GOG #42). In this study patients were randomized between adriamycin alone and adriamycin plus cytoxan. Ninety-three evaluable patients were entered. This study was just closed because indications were the results would be the same or worse than the previous study (GOG

Protocol #21). The GOG decided that because their Phase II studies suggested Cis-platinum might be as good or better than adriamycin, patients with advanced or recurrent sarcoma are being placed on Cis-platinum 50 mg/M$^2$ every three weeks.

REFERENCES

1. Hoogstraten B (ed): Cancer Research: Impact of the Cooperative Groups. New York: Mason Publishing, USA Inc, 1980.
2. Lewis GC, Jr, Slack NH, Mortel R, Bross ID: Adjuvant progestogen therapy in the primary definitive treatment of endometrial cancer. Gyn Oncol 2:368-376, 1978.
3. Brady L, Blessing J, Homesley H, Lewis GC Jr: Radiotherapy (RT), chemotherapy (CT) and combined therapy in Stage III epithelial ovarian cancer. (For the Gynecologic Oncology Group.) Proc Am Assoc Cancer Res 20:218, 1979.
4. Brady LW, Blessing JA, Slayton RE, Homesley HD, Lewis GC Jr: Radiotherapy (RT), chemotherapy (CT), and combined therapy in Stage III epithelial ovarian cancer. (For the gynecologic Oncology Group.) Cancer Clinical Trials 2:111-120, 1979.
5. Hreshchyshyn MM, Norris HJ: Postoperative treatment of women with resectable ovarian cancer with radiotherapy, melphalan, or no further treatment. (For the Gynecologic Oncology Group.) Proc Am Assoc Cancer Res 18:195, 1977.
6. Hreshchyshyn MM, Norris HH, Park R, Lagasse LD, Blessing J: Postoperative treatment of women with resectable malignant and possibly malignant epithelial ovarian tumors with radiotherapy, melphalan, or no further treatment. Proc UA Int Contra Ca, Buenos Aires, 1978.
7. Hreshchyshyn MM, Park RC, Blessing JA, Norris JH, Levy D, Lagasse LD, Creasman WT: The role of adjuvant therapy in Stage I ovarian cancer. (From the Gynecologic Oncology Group.) American Journal of Obstetrics & Gynecology 138:139-145, 1980.
8. Lewis GC Jr, Blessing JA: Ovarian cancer. Use of multiple modality programs involving surgery, radiation therapy and chemotherapy. Cancer 40:588-594, 1977.
9. Blom J, Park R, Blessing J: Treatment of women with disseminated and recurrent ovarian carcinoma with single and multichemotherapeutic agents. (For the Gynecologic Oncology Group.) Proc Am Soc Clin Oncol 19:338, 1978.
10. Park RC, Blom J, DiSaia JP, Lagasse LD, Blessing JA: Treatment of women with disseminated or recurrent advanced ovarian cancer with melphalan alone in combination with 5-fluorouracil and dactinomycin or with the combination of cytoxan, 5-fluorouracil and dactinomycin. (From the Gynecologic Oncology Group.) Cancer 45:25-29-2542, 1980.
11. Slayton R, Hreshchyshyn M, Silverberg S, Blessing J: Response of malignant ovarian germ cell tumors to vincristine (V), dactinomycin (A) and cyclophosphamide (C). (For the Gynecologic Oncology Group.) Proc Am Soc Clin Oncol 18:311, 1977.
12. Slayton RE, Hreshchyshyn MM, Silverberg SG, Shingleton HM, Park RC, DiSaia PJ, Blessing JA: Treatment of malignant ovarian germ cell tumors: Response to vincristine, dactinomycin and cyclophosphamide. (Preliminary Report.) Cancer, 42:390-309, 1978.
13. Slayton RE, Johnson G, Brady L, Blessing J: Radiotherapy (RT) and chemotherapy (CT) in malignant tumors of the ovarian stroma (MTOS) (For the Gynecologic Oncology Group.) Proc Am Soc Clin Oncol 21:430, 1980.
14. Smith JP, Rutledge F: Advances on chemotherapy for gynecologic cancer. Cancer 36: 669-674, 1975.
15. Wallace HJ Jr, Hreshchyshyn MM, Blessing JA: Comparison of the therapeutic effects of

adriamycin *versus* adriamycin and vincristine *versus* adriamycin and cyclophosphamide in the treatment of advanced carcinoma of the cervix. Proc Am Assoc Cancer Res 18:131, 1977.
16. Wallace HJ Jr, Hreshchyshyn MM, Wilbanks GD, Boronow RC, Fowler WC Jr, Blessing JA: Comparison of the therapeutic effects of adriamycin alone *versus* adriamycin plus vincristine *versus* adriamycin plus cyclosphosphamide in the treatment of advanced carcinoma of the cervix. Cancer Treatment Reports, 62:1435–1441, 1978.
17. Rossof AH, Drukker BH, Talley RW *et al.*: Randomized evaluation of chlorambucil and melphalan in advanced ovarian cancer. Proc Am Assoc Cancer Res 17:300, 1976.
18. Thigpen T, Lagasse L, Bundy B: Phase II Trial of Cis-platinum in Treatment of Advanced Ovarian Adenocarcinoma (For the Gynecology Oncology Group.) Proc Am Assoc Cancer Res 20:84, 1979.
19. Thigpen T, Shingleton H, Homesley H, Lagasse L, Blessing JA: Cis-dichlorodiammineplatinum (II) in the treatment of gynecologic malignancies: Phase II trials by the Gynecologic Oncology Group. Presented 9/21/78 at the National Cancer Institute. Cancer Treatment Reports, 63:1549–1555, 1979.
20. Thigpen JT, Lagasse L, Homesley H, Blessing JA: Cis-platinum in the treatment of advanced or recurrent adenocarcinoma of the ovary: A Phase II study of the gynecologic Oncology Group (submitted to Am J Clin Oncol).
21. Briscoe K, Posmantier M, Brown J, Kennedy BJ: Cis-diamminedichloroplatinum (II) and adriamycin in the treatment of advanced ovarian carcinoma. Proc Am Soc Clin Oncol 19:378, 1978.
22. Alberts DS, Moon TE, Stephans RA, Wilson H, Oishi N, Hilgers RD, O'Toole R, Thigpen JT: Randomized study of chemo-immunotherapy for advanced ovarian carcinoma: A preliminary report of a Southwest Oncology Group study. Cancer Treatment Reports, 63: 325–332, 1979.
23. Sedlis A, Sall S: Micro-invasive carcinoma of uterine cervix clinical-pathological study (For the Gynecologic Oncology Group.) Proc Am Soc Clin Oncol 18:306, 1977.
24. Sedlis A, Sall S, Tsukada Y, Park R, Mangan C, Shingleton H, Blessing JA: Micro-invasive carcinoma of uterine cervix: A clinical-pathological study. (For the Gynecologic Oncology Group.) American Journal of Obstetrics and Gynecology 133:64–74, 1979.
25. Lagasse LD, Creasman WT, Shingleton HM, Ford HJ, Blessing JA: Results and complications of operative staging in cervical cancer. (Experience of the gynecologic Oncology Group.) Gynecologic Oncology, 9:90–98, 1980.
26. DiSaia PJ, Levy D, Bundy B: A preliminary report on the treatment of women with cervical cancer, Stages IIB, IIIB, and IVA confined to the pelvis and/or para-aortic nodes with radiotherapy alone *versus* radiotherapy plus immunotherapy (intravenous *C-parvum*), Phase III. Presented at the 2nd International Meeting of Immunotherapy of Cancer at the NCI, 4/28-30/80. To be published in Proceedings of Immunotherapy Meeting. Terry W, Rosenberg S (eds). New York: Elsevier/North-Holland Biomedical Publishing Co.
27. Hreshchyshyn MM: (Report 1) Description of the GOG, its structure and functions. (Report 2) Treatment of women with cervical cancer Stage IIIB and IV confined to the pelvis with hydroxyurea or placebo both in combination with radiation therapy. (For the Gynecologic Oncology Group.) Gynecologic Oncology 3:251–257, 1975.
28. Hreshchyshyn MM, Aron BS, Boronow RC, Franklin EW III, Shingleton HM, Blessing JA: Hydroxyurea or placebo combined with radiation to treat Stage IIIB and IV cervical cancer confined to the pelvis. International Journal of Radiation Oncology, Biology and Physics 5:317–322, 1979.
29. Keys H, Blessing JA *et al.*: Hydroxy urea and radiation for Stage IIIB and IV cervix cancer: Analysis of recurrence patterns and radiation factors. International Journal of Radiation Oncology, Biology and Physics 6:1429, 1980.

30. Quagliana JM, O'Bryan RM, Baker L, Gottlieb J, Morrison FS, Eyre HJ, Tucker WG, Costanzi J: Phase II study of 5-azacytidine in solid tumors. Cancer Treatment Reports 61:51–54, 1977.
31. Omura GA, Shingleton HM, Creasman WT, Blessing JA, Boronow RC: Chemotherapy of gynecologic cancer with nitrosoureas: A randomized trial of CCNU and methyl-CCNU in cancers of the cervix, corpus, vagina and vulva. Cancer Treatment Reports 62:833–835, 1978.
32. Haas CD, Coltman CA, Gottlieb JA, Haut A, Luce JK, Talley RW, Samal B, Wilson HE, Hoogstraten B: Phase II evaluation of bleomycin. A Southwest Oncology Group Study. Cancer 38:8–12, 1976.
33. Tranum BL, Haut A, Rivkin S, Weber E, Quagliana JM, Shaw M, Tucker WG, Smith FE, Samson M, Gottlieb J: A Phase II study of methyl CCNU in the treatment of solid tumors. Cancer 35:1148–1153, 1975.
34. Thigpen JT, Homesley H, Prem K, Mladineo J: Phase II trial of piperazinedione in treatment of advanced squamous cell carcinoma of the cervix. Proc Am Assoc Cancer Res 19:162, 1978.
35. Stolinsky DC, Bateman JR: Further experience with hexamethylmelamine in the treatment of carcinoma of the cervix. Cancer Treatment Reports 60:907–911, 1976.
36. Thigpen T, Shingleton H: Phase II trial of Cis-platinum in treatment of advanced squamous cell carcinoma of the cervix. Proc Am Soc Clin Oncol 19:332, 1978.
37. Thigpen T, Shingleton H: Phase II trial of Cis-platinum in treatment of advanced squamous cell carcinoma of the cervix. (For the Gynecologic Oncology Group.) Proc Am Soc Clin Oncol 19:332, 1978.
38. Thigpen T, Shingleton H, Homesley H: Phase II trial of Cis-platinum as first or second line treatment for advanced squamous cell carcinoma of the cervix. (For the Gynecologic Oncology Group.) Proc Am Soc Clin Oncol 20:388, 1979.
39. Thigpen T, Shingleton H, Homesley H, Lagasse L, Blessing J: Cis-platinum in treatment of advanced or recurrent squamous cell carcinoma of the cervix: A Phase II study of the Gynecologic Oncology Group. Cancer 48:899–903, 1981.
40. Thigpen T, Shingleton H, Homesley H, DiSaia P, Lagasse L, Blessing J: Cis-diamminedichloroplatinum (II) in the treatment of advanced or recurrent cervix and uterine cancer: Phase II trials of the Gynecologic Oncology Group. Presented at Symposium on Cis--platinum, Atlanta 9/27–28/79. In: Cisplatin: Current Status and New Developments. Prestayko W, Crooke T, Carter K (eds). New York: Academic Press, 1980.
41. Slayton R, Creasman W, Bundy B: Phase II trial of VP-16 in treatment of advanced squamous cell carcinoma of the cervix. (For the Gynecologic Oncology Group.) Proc Am Soc Clin Oncol 20:365, 1979.
42. Slayton RE, Creasman WT, Petty W, Bundy B, Blessing J: A Phase II trial of VP-16 in the treatment of advanced squamous cell carcinoma of the cervix and adenocarcinoma of the ovary. (A Gynecologic Oncology Group Study.) Cancer Treatment Reports 63:2089–2092, 1979.
43. Arseneau JC, Bundy B, Dolan T, Homesley H, DiSaia P: Phase II trial of Baker's antifol (NSC 139, 105) in advanced cervical carcinoma. (For the Gynecologic Oncology Group.) Proc Am Soc Clin Oncol 21:424, 1980.
44. Arseneau JC, Bundy B, Dolan T, Homesley H, DiSaia P: Phase II study of Baker's antifol (Triazinate, TZT, NSC-139, 105) in advanced squamous cell carcinoma of the cervix. (For the Gynecologic Oncology Group.) Am J Clin Oncol (CCT) 5:61–64, 1982.
45. Thigpen T, Ehrlich C, Blessing J: Phase II study of maytansine in treatment of advanced or recurrent squamous cell carcinoma of the cervix: A Gynecologic Oncology Group Study. Proc Am Soc Clin Oncol 21:424, 1980.

46. Thigpen, JT, Ehrlich CE, Conroy J, Blessing JA: Phase II Study of maytansine in the treatment of advanced or recurrent squamous cell carcinoma of the cervix: A Gynecologic Oncology Group Study (submitted to Am J Clin Oncol).
47. Hoogstraten B, Hass CD, Haut A, Talley RW, Rivkin S, Isaacs BL: CCNU and bleomycin in the treatment of cancer. A Southwest Oncology Group Study. Medical and Pediatric Oncology 1:95–106, 1975.
48. Greenberg BR, Kardinal CG, Pajak TF, Bateman JR: Adriamycin *vs* adriamycin and bleomycin in advanced epidermoid carcinoma of the cervix. Cancer Treatment Reports 61:1383–1384, 1977.
49. Baker LH, Opipari MI, Wilson H, Bottomley R, Coltman CA: Mitomycin C, Vincristine and bleomycin therapy for advanced cervical cancer. Obstet Gynecol 52:146–150, 1978.
50. Slayton RE, Mladineo JP: Adriamycin (A) and Cis-diamminedichloroplatinum (DDP) in recurrent and mestastatic squamous cell carcinoma of the cervix. Proc Am Soc Clin Oncol 19:335, 1978.
51. Lewis GC Jr, Bundy B: Surgery for endometrial cancer. Presented at the American Cancer National Conference - Gynecologic Cancer, Los Angeles. Cancer 48:568–574, 1981.
52. Creasman WT, Boronow R, Morrow CP, DiSaia PJ, Blessing JA: Adenocarcinoma of the endometrium: Its metastatic lymph node potential. A Preliminary Report. (Gynecologic Oncology Group - George Lewis MD, Chairman). Gynecologic Oncology 3:239–243, 1976.
53. Thigpen T, Torres J, Buchsbaum H: Phase II trial of adriamycin in the treatment of advanced endometrial adenocarcinoma. (For the Gynecologic Oncology Group.) Proc Am Soc Clin Oncol 18:352, 1977.
54. Thigpen T, Buchsbaum H, Mangan C, Blessing JA: Phase II trial of adriamycin in the treatment of advanced or recurrent endometrial carcinoma: A Gynecologic Oncology Group Study. Cancer Treatment Reports 63:21–27, 1979.
55. Horton J, Begg CB, Arseneau J, Bruckner H, Creech R, Hahn RG: Comparison of adriamycin with cyclophosphamide in patients with advanced endometrial cancer. Cancer Treatment Reports 62:159–161, 1978.
56. Ehrlich CE, Cleary RE, Young PCM: The use of progesterone receptors in the treatment of recurrent endometrial cancer. In: Endometrial Cancer. Brush MG, King RJB, Taylor RW (eds). London: Bailliere-Teindall, 1978, pp 258–264.
57. Young PCM, Ehrlich CE: Progesterone receptors in human endometrial cancer. In: Steroid Receptors and the Management of Cancer. Cleveland, Ohio: CRC Press. (In press).
58. Ehrlich MD, Young PCM, Cleary RE: Progesterone receptors – A New approach to recurrent endometrial cancer. Proc Am Assoc Cancer Res 18:7, 1977.
59. Omura GA, Blessing JA: Chemotherapy of Stage III, IV and recurrent uterine sarcomas: A randomized trial of adriamycin (AD) *versis* AD-dimethyl triazeno imadazole carboxamide (DTIC). (For the Gynecologic Oncology Group.) Proc Am Assoc Cancer Res 19:26, 1978.
60. DiSaia PJ, Morrow CP, Boronow R, Creasman W, Mittelstaedt L: Endometrial sarcoma – Lymphatic spread pattern. American Journal of Obstetrics and Gynecology 130(1):104–105, 1978.

# Subject Index

Abdominal irradiation, 284, 286, 287
Active immunotherapy, 209–10
Adenocarcinoma of the Fallopian Tube, 252
Adjuvant therapy in Ovarian cancer, 285–6
Adnexa, 377
Alpha Fetoproteins (AFP), 69, 104, 145–7, 197
Agar, 327–334
Androgen receptors, 84
Androgenic moles, 156
Angiogenesis, 237
Animal models, 19, 196, 201–2, 214, 313–41
Antibodies, 33, 188, 198
Antibody-directed therapy, 74
Anticoagulation, 238
Antigen identification, 324–6
Antigen shed, 194
Antigenic modulation, 188
Antigens, 195–202
    as biological markers, 63
    in ovarian cancer, 238
    tumor-specific, 187
Anti-lymphatic serum, 319
Ascites, 194, 205–6, 283
Ataxia telangiectasia, 197

BCG, 210
Benign cystic teratoma, 124–5
Bias, in clinical studies, 265
Blood vessels, 238
Bragg's Peak, in irradiation, 301
Brain metastases, 163

Cancer screening, by HSV, 44
Carcinoembyronic antigen (CEA), 64–66, 196–7
    as monitor of neoplastic recurrence, 197
    in ovarian cancer, 64, 196
    plasma concentration, 64
Carcinoid teratoma, 127
CEA – see Carcinoembryonic antigen

Cell cycle,
    in radiotherapy, 300, 304
    in release of antigens, 188
Cell survival curve, 303
Central nervous system metastases, in trophoblastic cancer, 181
Cervical cancer, 1–62
    CEA levels, 65
    chemotherapy, 356
    clinical studies, 372
    etiology, 3
    history, 228
    Herpesvirus Hypothesis, 3
    immune response, 27
    metastases, 239, 245–8
    precursor lesions, 19
    radiotherapy, 232
    sexual transmission, 40
    staging, 373
Cervical Cancer Antigen (TA-4), biological marker, 72
Chemical radiosensitizers, in radiotherapy, 300, 304
Chemotherapy (*see also under* specific disease)
    compared to radiotherapy, 293, 371
    group research organization, 357
    with immunotherapy, 211
    immunosuppressive side effects, 204
Chlorambucil, 280, 288
Choriocarcinoma, 134–35, 155, 160–61, 198
    chemotherapy, 157
Chromosomal alterations, in radiotherapy, 304
Chromosomal analysis, 327
Chromosome breakage, in radiotherapy, 304
CIS-platinum, 178, 371–81
Clinical trials, 343–84
    history, 343
    phases of study, 264, 355
    structure and organization, 355–6
Clonogenic Stem-cell Assay, 327–34
Combination therapy, 145, 211, 246, 279

Common pathway hypothesis, lymphatic
    metastases, 234–5
Corynebacterium parvum (C. Parvum),
    210, 211, 216, 264, 326, 372
    in cervical cancer, 374
CSF (Cerebro-spinal fluid),
    concentration of HCG, 163, 166–7
Cure rates, 265–66
    difficulty of measurement, 264
Curative therapy and palliation, 264
Curettage, 158, 160
Cyclophosphamide, 292
Cyst rupture, 283
Cystadenocarcinoma,
    mucinous, 65
    serous, 65
Cytoxan, 372, 377
Cytotoxic drugs, 156

Diaphragm, 237
Diethylstilbestrol, 84
Differentiation antigens, 195, 198–202
DNA, 13, 15, 25, 81
    radiation effects, 300–1
Drug-resistance, 177
Dynamic state, theory of viral
    persistence, 7
Dysgerminoma, 106
Dysplasia, 19

Electric charge, 305
Electrons, 300
Embryonal carcinomas, 128–34, 198
Endocrinological status of patient, 87
Endodermal sinus tumors, 110–6, 198
End-points, in clinical research, 263–5
Endometrial cancer, 81–102
    CEA levels, 65
    clinical trials, 377–79
    drug evaluations, 357
    hormonal receptors, 81–102
    metastases, 249–52
Endometrium, steroid receptors, 82–3
Enzymes, 81–2
Epidemiology, 2, 35
Epithelial ovarian carcinoma, 193–5
Estrogenic control of virus replicative
    cycle, 11
Estrogens, 81–3, 159
Evacuation of the Uterus, 158

Fallopian tubes, adenocarcinoma of, 252
Fever, 7
Fibrin, 238

Freund's adjuvant, 210
Funding, of clinical research, 352

Gamma rays, 299, 300, 304, 305
Gene expression, 14
Gene mapping, 12
Genetic studies, 326–7
Genetic template, 4
Germ cell tumors of the ovary, 103–154
    clinical appearance, 106
    histogenesis, 106
    pathogenesis, 103
    pathology, 107
    staging, 104
    therapy, 108
Glycoproteins, 196–8
Gonadoblastoma, 140–3
Gynecologic Oncology Group, 349

Hazards model, proportional, 271
HCG – see Human chorionic gonadotropin
Heavy ions, 310–11
HeLa cell line, 314
Helium ion beam radiotherapy, 310
Herpesvirus hypothesis, 12
Herpes Simplex Virus, 4–9
    asymptomatic presence in host, 10
    in cervical cancer, 1–63
    oncogenic potential, 12
Herpetic infections, 7–11
Heteroantisera, 198, 209, 213
Heterografts, 313–341
Heterotransplantation, 334–5
High-LET radiation – see Linear Energy
    Transfer, high
Histocompatibility antigens, 195
History, of gynecologic cancer research,
    347
Hormonal therapy, in endometrial
    cancer, 94
Hormones, 81
Host defense, 188
Host/virus relationship, 8
Host immune response, 238–42
Human chorionic gonadotropin, (HCG),
    145–7
    as biological marker, 66, 104
    cancer screening, 158
    trophoblastic cancer, 156
Human subjects in research, 350
Hybridomas, 326
Hydroxyurea, 376
Hyperbaric oxygen, 300
Hyperthermia, 300

Hypoxic tumor cells, 299–304
Hysterectomy, 156–8
Hysterotomy, 158

Immune response, 34
Immune surveillance, 236–8
Immunity, exogenous, 209
Immunocompetence, 203–9
Immunoglobulins, 194
Immunological destruction of Tumor cells, 190–1
Immunologically privileged sites, 318–9
Immunostimulants, 210
Immunosuppression, 204
Immunotherapy, 209–17
    active/passive, 209
    clinical trials, 371
    in trophoblastic cancer, 183
Immunotherapy, active, 209
Immunotherapy, passive, 209
Incubation period, in viral cancer, 2
Infections, asymptomatic, in Koch Postulates, 1
Interpretation of treatment results, 263
Inflight pions, 300
Informed consent, 350
Ionizing radiation, 300, 304
Irradiation of the upper abdomen, 288

Karyotypic analysis, 326–7
Koch Postulates, 1–2

Laparotomy, second-look, 266
Latency, of viral infection, 7
Leiomyosarcoma, 380
Leukocyte migration enhancement, 208
Linear energy transfer, high, 300–5, 375
Linear energy transfer, low, 305
Liver metastases, 168
Liver shielding, in post-operative irradiation, 287
Log-rank test, statistical technique, 271–3
Lung metastases, 165
Lymph node metastases, 227–56
Lymphadenectomy, 240

Macrophage-mediated cytotoxicity, 190
Malignant mixed germ-cell tumors, 136
Markers, 63–81
    biochemical, 161
    experimental work, 324
    treatment monitoring, 146

Markers (Cont'd)
    tumor-specific, 63
Melphalan, 372
Menstruation, 7
Metastases, 227–262
    anatomic hypothesis, 231
    choriocarcinoma, 160
    direction of, 246
    distant, 232
    in ovarian cancer, 194
    in trophoblastic cancer, 155, 157, 165, 172
Mice, athymic nude, 313, 320
Mice, LASAT, 324
Mitosis, 81
Mucinous tumors, 197
Mixed germ cell-sex cord stromal tumors, 143–4
Moles, in trophoblastic cancer, 155–60
    androgenic moles, 156
    invasive, 155
    transformation to malignancy, 160
Multivariate analysis, 273–8
Murine ovarian cancer, 214
Mutations, in radiotherapy, 304

National Cancer Institute, 353
Natural killing cells (NK cells), 190, 237
Neutron therapy, 306–7
Nutrition of cells in culture, 315

Oncofetal antigens, 195–8
Oncogenic potential of Herpes virus, 12–30
Oncogenic transformation, 17
Oral contraceptives, 159
Ovarian cancer, 81–102, 187–226, 263–98
    antigenic markers, 195–202
    chemotherapy, 275, 287–92, 367
    clinical trials, 282, 366–72
    drug evaluations, 356
    hormonal effects, 81–102
    immunobiology, 187–226
    immunotherapy, 210
    metastases, 194–224
    prognosis, 269–82
    radiotherapy, 263–98
    staging, 267
    surgery, 285
    therapy, 275
Ovarian cancer antigen (OCA), 71
Ovarian cystadenocarcinoma antigen

(OCAA), 70
Ovarian teratomas, 116
Oxygen enhancement, 304

Palliation, 265–66
   index of, 266
Particulate radiation, 306–11
Passive immunotherapy, 213–4
Patient profile, in clinical trials, 350
Patient registries, 158
Pelvic arteriography, 164
Pelvic irradiation, 284–5
Peritoneal metastases, 195
Photons, 305
Pilot studies, 356
Pions, 307–10
   inflight pions, 300
   stopping pions, 300
Placenta, 156
Polyembryoma, 139
Postoperative irradiation, 292
Postoperative therapy, 278
   statistical analysis, 282–5
Precursor lesions, 19
Progesterone, 82, 92, 159
Progesterone receptors, 379
Prognostic variables, interdependence, 269
Promiscuity, 40
Promotion/maintainance genes, 15
Prostatic fluid, 10
Protocols, 345–6
Protons, 300

Radiation, 299–312
   damage to normal tissue, 310
   deposit of radiation, 301
   dose localization, 304
   electromagnetic, 305
   finite depth of penetration, 302
   focused distribution at depth, 303
   shape of radiation, 302
Radiobiological interaction, 301
Radioactive isotopes, 305
Radiography, of lungs in trophoblastic cancer, 165
Radioimmunoassay, 280
Radiolabelling, 66, 74, 169
Radioresistance, 304
Radiosensitivity, 108
Radiotherapy, 263–98, 299–312
   compared to chemotherapy, 287, 293, 371
   complications, 299

Radiotherapy (Cont'd)
   doses, 299
   heavy particle, 299–311
   multifractionated, 304
   murine ovarian cancer, 214
   ovarian cancer, 263–298
   side effects, 264, 290
   trophoblastic cancer, 181
Rare lesions, 351
Reactivated virus, 2
Receptors, 84
Recurrence, 265
Reduced intercellular adhesiveness, 235
Regional node dissection, 242
Relative biological effectiveness (RBE), 304
Research, 343–84
   Cooperative Group Research, 343–84
   costs, 354
   funding, 346
   critical analysis, 263–67
Residuum, of tumor, 269, 289
Response rates, 266
Retroperitoneal lymphatics, 194
Risk, 169–70
   groupings of patients by risk, 172–6, 279

Sarcoma, 357, 380–1
Sequencing of clinical studies, 359–61
Seroconversion, 2
Serous histology, 197
Serum, 324
Sex rates, in herpesvirus, 10
Sexual transmission, of herpesvirus, 10
Shed, of virus, 10
Specific immune response, in ovarian cancer, 207
Staging
   Cervical cancer, 373
   classifications, 267
   germ cell cancer, 104
   limitations, 267
   ovarian, 275–8
   standardization, 268
Static state, theory of viral persistence, 7
Statistical analysis, 263–98
   in protocol design, 361
Steroid receptors, 82
Stopping pions, 300
Stopping region, 302
Stress, emotional, 8
Strumal carcinoid, 128
Subrenal capsule assay, 335

Suppression, of lymphocytes, 240
Surgery, in trophoblastic cancer, 180
Survival curve, 264
   in treatment evaluation, 265
   interpretation, 266
   shape of curve, 265
Syncytial endometritis, 156
Systemic circulation, of tumor cells, 236
Systemic immunosuppression, 319

T and B cells, 188–9, 240
T cell mediated cytotoxicity, 170
Teratoma, 116
   mature cystic teratoma, 123–4
   monodermal teratomas, 125
   mature teratomas, 116
   immature teratomas, 116
Thymectomy, in animal models, 319
Thymus, 189
Time factors,
   in cervical cancer, 39
   in mole transformation to choriocarcinoma, 160
Tissue culture techniques, 313–8
Toxicity of therapy, 264–8
Transformation, mechanism of neoplasia, 12, 17
Treatment modality selection, statistical analysis, 273
Transplantation resistance antigens, in tumors, 196
Trophoblastic pseudotumors, 156
Trophoblastic tumors, 155–86
   chemotherapy, 157
   chlinical features, 159–61
   diagnosis, 161–9
   HCG values, 156
   hormonal influence, 159
   prevention, 158–9
   prognosis, 169
   risk, 169
   treatment, 155–80

Tumor cell composition, 328–9
Tubal carcinoma, 357
Tumor differentiation, 197, 272–82
Tumor immunology, 187–95
Tumor kinetics,
   adherence, 283
   arrest, 237
   dormancy, 236–8
   expansion, 235
   growth, 240
   recurrence, 299
Tumor markers, biological, 63–80
   germ cell tumors, 104, 144–47
Tumor metastases, 235–8
Tumor registries, 357
Tumor-specific antigens, 198, 326
Tumor-associated antigens, 70–72, 187
Tumor staging, 284
Tumor vaccine studies, 325–6
Tumors, chemically induced, 196
Tumors, virally induced, 196

Ultrasound, 164
Uterine sarcoma, 357, 380

Vaccination, against tumor, 210
Vaccum extraction, of uterus, 158
Variable fractionation patterns, 300
Vincristine, 371, 375
Viral carcinogenesis, 14
Viral etiology, in cervical cancer, 1–62
Viral proteins, 22–27
Virus expression, 27
Vulvar cancer, 242–5
   clinical trials, 379–80
   diagnosis, 242
   prognosis, 242

X-rays, 299, 304, 305

Yolk sac tumor, 110–116

CPSIA information can be obtained
at www.ICGtesting.com
Printed in the USA
LVHW051927170623
750084LV00005B/292

9 780898 385557